Immunology of ENT Disorders

IMMUNOLOGY AND MEDICINE SERIES

IMMUNOLOGY

SERIES · SERIES · SERIES · SERIES AND SERIES · SERIES · SERIES · SERIES

MEDICINE

Volume 23

Immunology of ENT Disorders

Edited by

G. K. Scadding

Consultant Rhinologist
Royal National Throat, Nose & Ear Hospital
Gray's Inn Road,
London, UK

Series Editor: K. Whaley

KLUWER ACADEMIC PUBLISHERS
DORDRECHT/BOSTON/LONDON

Distributors

---

for the United States and Canada: Kluwer Academic Publishers, PO Box 358, Accord Station, Hingham, MA 02018-0358, USA
for all other countries: Kluwer Academic Publishers, Distribution Center, PO Box 322, 3300 AH Dordrecht, The Netherlands

A catalogue record for this book is available from British Library.

ISBN 0-7923-8914-X

Library of Congress Cataloging-in-Publication Data

Immunology of ENT disorders / edited by G.K. Scadding.
p. cm.—(Immunology and medicine series ; v. 23)
Includes bibliographical references and index.
ISBN 0-7923-8914-X (casebound)
1. Ear—Diseases—Immunological aspects. 2. Nose—Diseases—Immunological aspects. 3. Throat—Diseases—Immunological aspects.
I. Scadding, G.K. II. Series.
[DNLM: 1. Otorhinolaryngologic Diseases—immunology.
2. Otorhinolaryngologic Diseases—therapy. W1 IM53BI v. 24 1994 / WV 150 133 1994]
RF46.5.I464 1994
617.5′1079—dc20
DNLM/DLC
for Library of Congress 94-20882
CIP

Published in the United Kingdom by Kluwer Academic Publishers, PO Box 55, Lancaster, UK.

Kluwer Academic Publishers BV incorporates the publishing programmes of D. Reidel, Martinus Nijhoff, Dr W. Junk and MTP Press.

Typeset by Lasertext Ltd, Stretford, Manchester, U.K.
Printed and bound in Great Britain by Hartnolls Ltd., Bodmin, Cornwall

Contents

Series Editor's Note vii

Preface viii

List of Contributors ix

1 Basic immunology 1
P. Fitzharris

2 The ENT presentation of HIV infection and the acquired immunodeficiency syndrome 31
J. M. Parkin

3 The immunology of the tonsil 45
G. K. Scadding

4 Fungal infections 57
R. J. Hay

5 Immunocytochemistry in the diagnosis of pathological conditions of the ear, nose and throat 73
L. Michaels

6 Allergic rhinitis 93
G. K. Scadding

7 Food and allergic rhinitis 117
L. J. Hawk

8 Wegener's disease 123
V. J. Lund

9 Sarcoidosis 135
V. J. Lund

10	Nasal polyps *A. B. Drake-Lee*	151
11	Inner ear disorders *G. B. Brookes*	169
12	Middle ear disorders *G. B. Brookes*	199
13	Future prospects for immunological involvement in ENT disorders *G. K. Scadding*	217
	Index	225

Series Editor's Note

The interface between clinical immunology and other branches of medical practice is frequently blurred and the general physician is often faced with clinical problems with an immunological basis and is expected to diagnose and manage such patients. The rapid expansion of basic and clinical immunology over the past two decades has resulted in the appearance of increasing numbers of immunology journals and it is impossible for a non-specialist to keep apace with this information overload. The *Immunology and Medicine* series is designed to present individual topics of immunology in a condensed package of information which can be readily assimilated by the busy clinician or pathologist.

K. Whaley, Leicester
August 1994

Preface

Until recently, the contribution of immunological knowledge to the understanding and management of ENT disorders was slight, being largely confined to the appreciation that many rhinitic patients were allergic. Happily, this situation is rapidly changing: the immunological basis of many disorders of the ears, nose and throat is becoming recognized and the mechanisms of the reactions involved are being elucidated. From this, rational therapy should evolve.

This book aims to highlight some of the areas in which immunological mechanisms are involved in otorhinolaryngology. It is written by experts in their respective fields of immunology and allergy, otology, rhinology and pathology. It opens with an overview of the pathways of the immune response and the cells and molecules involved, leading to an appreciation of the normal defence mechanisms of the upper respiratory tract and possible areas of failure. There is then a chapter on HIV infection and how this may present to otorhinolaryngologists. The normal function of the tonsil and the immunological effects of tonsillectomy are then considered. The varying roles of fungi in ENT disorders ranging from commensal through allergen to invasive organisms is assessed by Professor R. J. Hay.

Perhaps the most obvious immunological contribution to management thus far lies in the immunocytochemical diagnosis of pathological conditions of the ears, nose and throat and this is covered in a chapter by Professor Leslie Michaels.

Diseases in which immune mechanisms appear to be harmful or destructive rather than protective are then considered. These include Wegener's granulomatosis and sarcoidosis. An update on the rapidly changing information on allergic rhinitis, on the effects of food and on nasal polyposis are given in three further chapters. The final chapter deals with future prospects for immunological involvement in ENT disorders.

This volume should provide interesting insights, with possible novel therapeutic approaches, not only to otorhinolaryngologists, but also to audiologists, allergists and respiratory physicians. It should also provide an up-to-date background for any immunological researcher in this field.

List of Contributors

G. B. Brookes
Consultant ENT and Neuro-Otological Surgeon
The Royal National Throat, Nose and Ear Hospital
Gray's Inn Road;
National Hospital for Neurology and Neurosurgery
Queen Square;
Honorary Senior Lecturer
Institute of Laryngology and Otology and Institute of Neurology
University of London;
London
UK

A. B. Drake-Lee
Consultant ENT Surgeon
Queen Elizabeth Hospital
Birmingham
B15 2TH
UK

P. Fitzharris
Consultant Allergist
Department of Medicine
Wellington School of Medicine
Mein St, Newtown, Wellington
PO Box 7343, Wellington South
New Zealand

L. J. Hawk
Princess Christian's Hospital
12 Clarence Road
Windsor
Berkshire
UK

R. J. Hay
St John's Institute of Dermatology
Guy's Hospital, UMDS
London Bridge
London
SE1 9RT
UK

V. J. Lund
Reader in Rhinology
Professorial Unit
Institute of Laryngology and Otology
University College London;
Honorary Consultant in Otorinolaryngology
The Royal National Throat, Nose and Ear Hospital
Gray's Inn Road;
and Moorfields Eye Hospital
London
UK

L. Michaels
Department of Pathology
The Royal National Throat, Nose and Ear Hospital
Gray's Inn Road
London
WC1X 8DA
UK

J. M. Parkin
Department of Immunology
St Bartholomew's Hospital
38 Little Britain
London
EC1A 7BE
UK

G. K. Scadding
Consultant Rhinologist
The Royal National Throat, Nose and Ear Hospital
Gray's Inn Road
London
WC1X 8DA
UK

1
Basic Immunology

P. FITZHARRIS

Survival of the individual depends on protection from pathogenic organisms, including protozoa, bacteria, viruses and fungi. This protection of the integrity of the individual is the major function of the immune system. Failure of components within the system results in a wide variety of immunodeficiency-associated diseases, frequently recurrent infections. The problems associated with immunodeficiency are explored further in the following chapter.

With increased complexity and sophistication of the immune defences, these mechanisms have themselves become a potential source of damage to the host in circumstances where normal control mechanisms are lost. When this occurs, normal or modified host tissues may become targets for immune attack – autoimmune disease. Tissues may also become involved in damage mechanisms as innocent bystanders. This occurs in certain hypersensitivity reactions. Furthermore, an inappropriate response may be mounted to an inert or harmless foreign substance: much allergic disease is caused in this way.

The balance between pathogenicity, damage and immune protection is delicate.

IMMUNITY TO INFECTION

Protective immune mechanisms are usually classified into two categories:

1. Non-specific innate or natural immunity,
2. Specific acquired or adaptive immunity.

These mechanisms do not function in isolation from each other, but interact in ways which result in their increased efficiency. Both non-specific and specific mechanisms utilize soluble factors and effector cells.

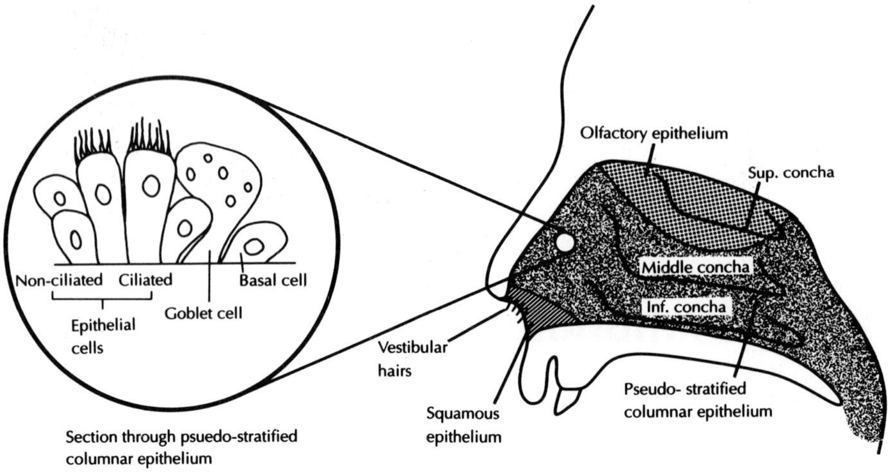

Figure 1 Lateral view of the nasal cavity showing the distribution of the pseudostratified columnar epithelium. The inset shows the epithelial cells in more detail

NON-SPECIFIC IMMUNITY

Mechanical factors

Physical barrier function is provided by skin and mucous membranes. Skin bearing hairs lines the nasal vestibule. The hairs provide a barrier function, albeit to relatively large objects, e.g. insects attempting entry! Other than the specialized olfactory region, the remainder of the nasal mucosa and paranasal sinuses is lined with a pseudostratified respiratory epithelium of approximately $120\,cm^2$. The epithelium comprises four cell types: ciliated and non-ciliated epithelial cells, goblet cells (unicellular mucous glands) and basal cells from which the columnar and goblet cells develop on a basement membrane (see Figure 1).

Secretions cover the respiratory epithelium in both upper and lower respiratory tracts. Mucociliary clearance is a major defence mechanism comparable to gastrointestinal motility in reducing colonization by micro-organisms and enhancing their expulsion. Nasal fluids contain the secretions of goblet cells, seromucous glands and lachrymal glands together with substances transported across the specialized epithelial cells, condensed water from humidified expired air and micro-organisms or deposited materials.

The lower layer of mucus is a serous fluid, the sol layer over which the viscid gel layer moves transported by the cilia[1]. The cilia beat in the sol layer at 12–15 Hz with a rapid 'stiff-armed' effect or stroke during which claw like projections from the tips of the cilia propel the viscid gel layer towards the nasopharynx[2]. The cilia subsequently bend in a plane at right angles to the effector beat to return during the slower recovery phase (Figure 2).

Ciliated cells bear 50–100 cilia per cell. Nasal cilia are 5–6 μm in length and 0.33 μm in diameter. A surface membrane encloses an organized structure of a ring of 9 paired outer microtubules surrounding 2 central microtubules

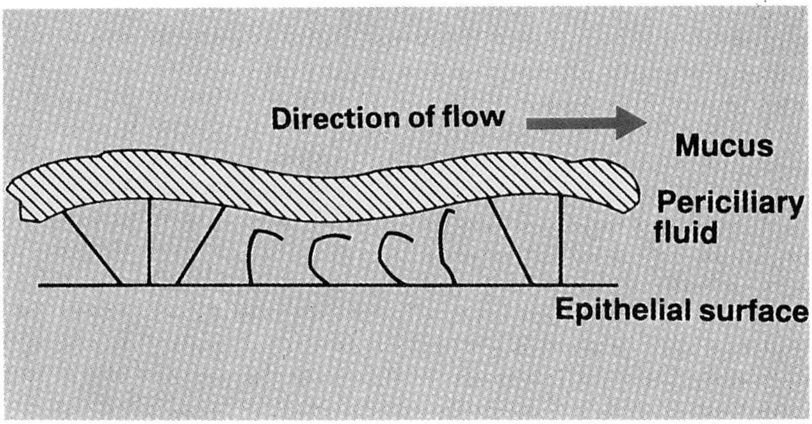

Figure 2 Ciliary action. Ciliary beating occurs with a rapid stiff-armed forward stroke during which the gel layer of mucus is moved forward by the tiny hooks at the tips of the cilia. There is then a slower recovery phase during which the cilia bend down into the sol phase before returning for another effector beat. Ciliary beat frequency can be tested in vitro by the measurement of the interruption of a light beam[4,5]

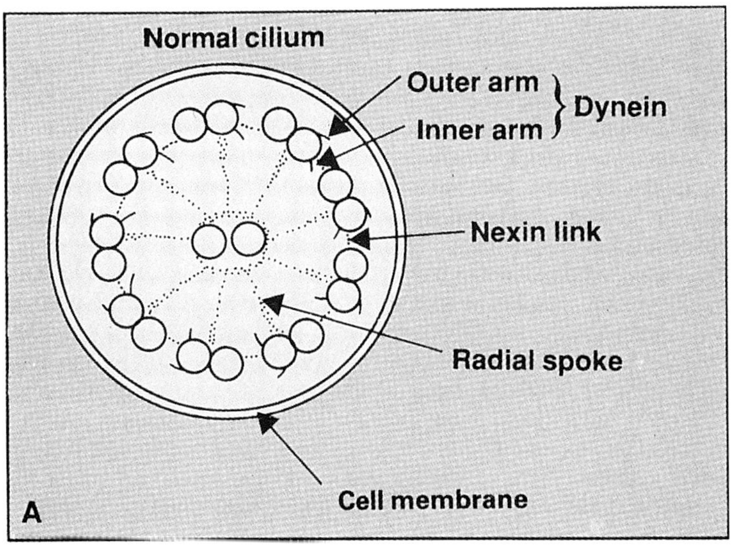

Figure 3 Transverse section of a cilium showing the ring of nine paired outer microtubules surrounding two central microtubules to which they are linked by central spokes. The outer doublet microtubules have inner and outer dynein 'arms', which are absent in various forms of ciliary dyskinesia

(Figure 3). Nexin links join the outer tubules together while central spokes link them to the inner microtubules. The enzyme, dynein, breaks down adenosine triphosphate (ATP) to adenosine diphosphate (ADP) in a magnesium-dependent reaction providing the energy for ciliary movement. Inner

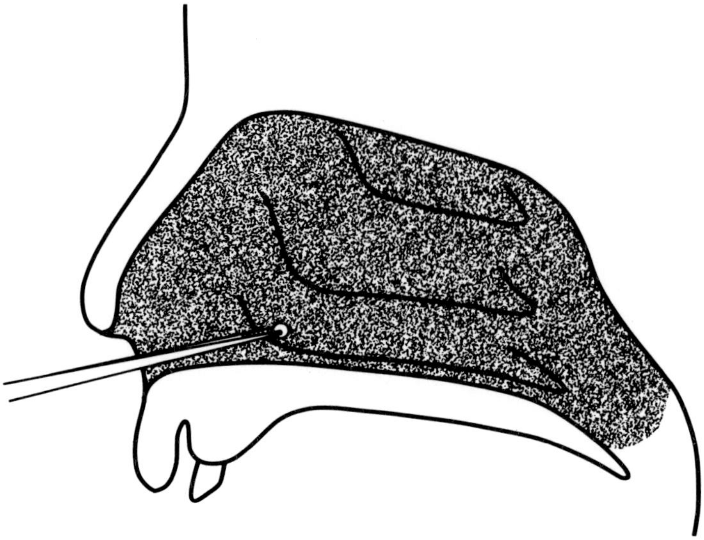

Figure 4 A test for nasal mucociliary clearance – the saccharin test. A simple test of mucociliary activity can be undertaken by placing a fragment of saccharin on the inferior turbinate and noting the length of time taken for the patient to experience a sweet taste. The subject should be unaware of the nature of the substance and must not eat, drink, blow the nose or sneeze during the test. Normally, it takes between 5 and 20 minutes for the taste to appear

and outer dynein 'arms' are found associated with the 9 outer doublet microtubules and it is these which are absent in Kartagener's syndrome of sinusitis, bronchiectasis and situs inversus. In Kartagener's syndrome, the microtubules become the basal body, the outer pairs become triplets and the inner pair disappear.

Both ciliated and non-ciliated epithelial cells bear 200–400 microvilli, approximately one third the size of cilia and with a central core of actin filaments. These microvilli are non-motile and probably play a role in the regulation of ion and fluid transport between cells and in the periciliary cells[3]. Mucus flows from the front to the back of the nose at approximately 6 mm/min. Although there is considerable variation, the time taken for the transport of mucus from the anterior part of the nose to the nasopharynx is usually 5–20 min. This is easily tested by the saccharin test (Figure 4). Mucus from the sinuses drains through ostia and joins the mucus on the lateral wall of the nose. After passing around the Eustachian orifice, it is swallowed. Ciliary activity, which can be measured in vitro on a nasal brushing by photometric methods[4,5], is reduced by drying, cigarette smoke and upper respiratory tract infection. Recent evidence suggests ciliary beat frequency may be reduced in the acute allergic response[6]. Apposition of two mucosal surfaces in structural abnormalities prevents ciliary activity as do certain topical applications, e.g. adrenaline and cocaine, and extremes of pH. Corticosteroids have been shown to reduce the rate of saccharine clearance following one week's therapy[7]. Sneeze and cough reflexes provide additional protection for the mucosa.

Cells

Multipotential stem cells in the bone marrow give rise to more specialized offspring in a highly regulated and controlled process (Figure 5). The cellular components of the first line of host defence are: macrophages and monocytes, neutrophils, eosinophils, basophils, platelets, natural killer (NK) cells and endothelial cells. These produce or interact with the soluble or molecular factors including cytokines, complement, acute phase proteins and arachidonic acid metabolites. Cell-surface receptors and adhesion proteins are of particular importance in the interactions of these components. Invasion of a tissue site by microbial pathogens creates an acute inflammatory focus with rapid increase in vascular permeability, changes in blood flow and the mobilization, accumulation and activation of leukocytes, mainly neutrophils and monocytes. There has been a considerable amount of recent work in these areas.

Polymorphonuclear granulocytes

Granulocytes are shortlived cells produced in the bone marrow at a rate of approximately 80 million/minute. They are released as mature cells and make up approximately two thirds of the total intravascular leukocyte pool. Mature forms contain a multilobed nucleus and numerous granules containing proteolytic and hydrolytic enzymes. They are classified according to their staining reactions into neutrophils, eosinophils and basophils. Their effects are non-specific although specificity may be contributed by the involvement of specific antibodies, and interaction with antibodies and complement is important in their protective role. Neutrophils make up over 90% of these circulating granulocytes and are 12–16 μm in diameter. They have an important role in phagocytosis. At sites of inflammation, neutrophils migrate out of the capillaries and into the surrounding tissue. Once in the tissue, they migrate towards the site of inflammation by a process known as chemotaxis.

Granulocytes (both neutrophils and eosinophils) have been implicated in the pathogenesis of a variety of inflammatory and allergic diseases. They have the capacity to release a large number of agents which may not only injure tissues but also degrade matrix proteins into chemotactic fragments which have the potential to amplify the inflammatory response. In many situations, however, it is assumed that the beneficial protective effects of neutrophils outweigh the tissue damaging effects. The functional state of the neutrophil can be modulated with its secretory state, in particular, being profoundly influenced by environmental factors.

Neutrophil-mediated injury/matrix degradation occurs in a highly specialized micro-environment created by the adhesive cell; mononuclear cells influence neutrophil emigration by the generation of neutrophil chemotactic factors. Neutrophil fate is not necessarily by disintegration – a recent mechanism for the removal of intact senescent neutrophils has been demonstrated.

Neutrophils show a low level of constitutive protein synthesis producing

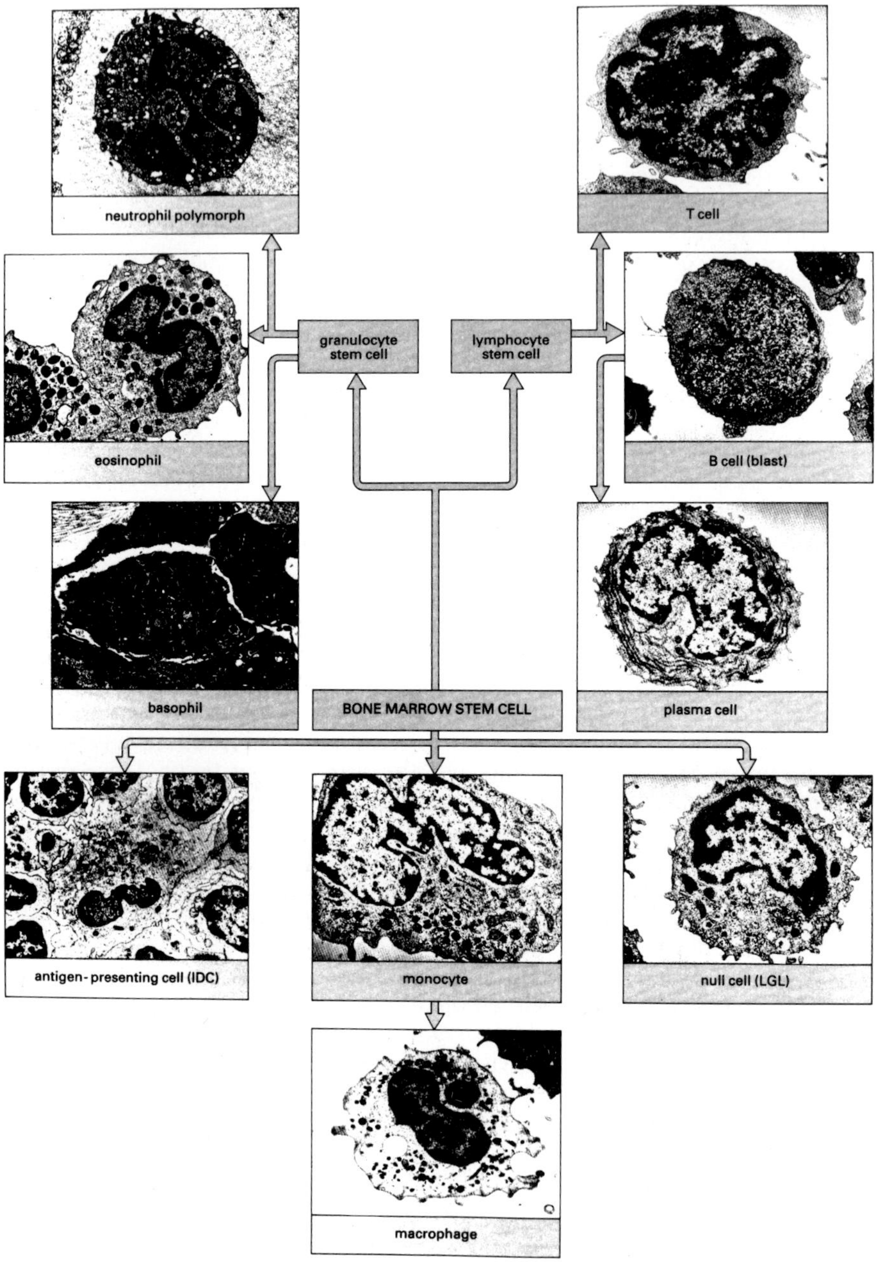
neutrophil polymorph
T cell
eosinophil
granulocyte stem cell
lymphocyte stem cell
B cell (blast)
basophil
BONE MARROW STEM CELL
plasma cell
antigen-presenting cell (IDC)
monocyte
null cell (LGL)
macrophage

the complement receptor (CR) 1, Fc receptor (FcR), major histocompatibility complex (MHC) Class I and CR3 α chain proteins. Recently, they have also been shown to produce heat shock proteins[8] in response to environmental changes. Rapid priming of neutrophil function, not requiring protein synthesis, can result from exposure to traces of bacterial lipopolysaccharide (LPS), tumour necrosis factor (TNF) or platelet activating factor (PAF). These agents, which themselves cause little secretion, prime the neutrophils such that subsequent exposure to secretagogues such as C5a, immune complexes or formyl-methionyl-leucyl-phenylalanine (fMLP) now causes marked neutrophil secretion. Experimental studies confirming these results demonstrate damage to microvasculature in vivo[9] and endothelial cells in vitro[10] by the combination of LPS and C5a, but not by either agent alone.

The molecular mechanisms involved in cellular priming and activation are a subject of great interest. The chemotactic factor, fMLP, triggers a rapid rise in intracellular cytosolic calcium and increased cellular permeability, resulting in uptake of extracellular calcium. Intracellular calcium mobilization appears associated with the metabolism of phosphatidyl inositol 4,5-bisphosphate (PIP2) 2,1,5-triphosphate (1,4,5-IP3). Whether different patterns of inositol lipid metabolism are involved in distinguishing the migration response from the respiratory burst pathway, or between the mechanisms involved in priming and in activation, is not yet clear.

Neutrophil adhesion to endothelial cells is the first step in neutrophil migration and is also the site of early injury in many diseases. The leukocyte-function-associated molecule (LFA1) plays a key role in cell adhesion among leukocytes and between leukocytes and other cell types. The LFA1 family of adhesion receptors consists of three structurally related glycoproteins, LFA1, CR3 and p150,95, which make up the CD11–CD18 group of adhesion molecules. They have similar architecture and are composed of two non-covalently linked polypeptides; a unique α subunit (CD11a–c) and a common β subunit (CD18). The LFA1 group belongs to the integrin family of adhesion receptors but, unlike other integrins, is found only on leukocytes. Antibodies to the CD11–CD18 complex of adhesive molecules on the neutrophil surface inhibit the adherence of neutrophils to endothelial cells under stimulated conditions in vitro and prevent neutrophil migration into inflamed skin in vivo[11]. These antibodies, however, have little effect on 'background' adhesion of unstimulated neutrophils. Endothelial cells after treatment with cytokines, e.g. IL1 and TNF, show a protein-synthesis-dependent increase in expression of surface-adhesive molecules, for example endothelial leukocyte adhesive

Figure 5 Cells of the immune system. Bone marrow stem cells can mature either to form cells of the granulocyte lineage or the lymphoid cell lineage. T and B cells are both derived from lymphocytic stem cells following differentiation in the primary lymphoid organs. They both have large nuclei and a thin cytoplasmic rim. After activation, lymphocytes become blast cells with an expanded cytoplasm with more endoplasmic reticulum and Golgi apparatus. B lymphocytes may develop into antibody-synthesizing plasma cells. Null cells (otherwise known as large granular lymphocytes) look like lymphocytes but develop along a separate pathway. Other cells derived by this path are the monocytes, which can leave the blood and become tissue macrophages, and other antigen-presenting cells. The granulocyte stem cell can become a neutrophil, an eosinophil or a basophil. The first two are actively phagocytic whereas the basophil is not, but shares many of the characteristics of the tissue mast cell

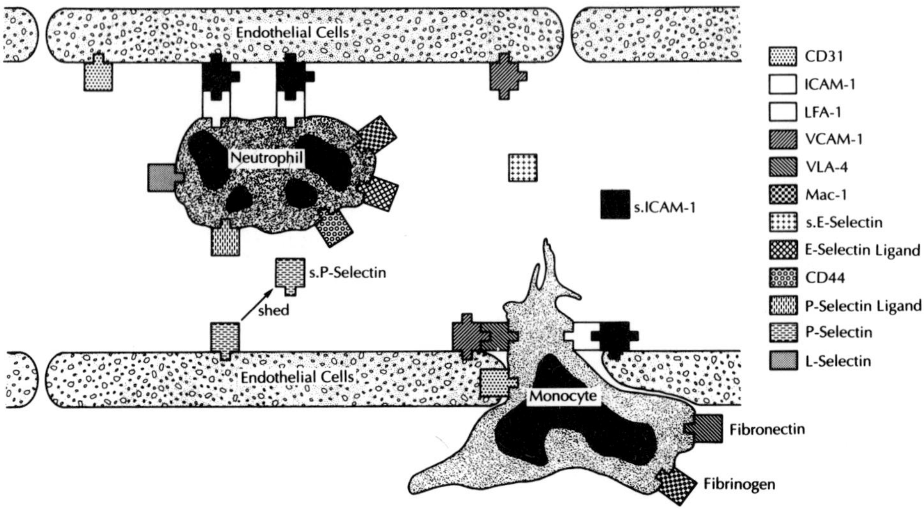

Figure 6 Adhesion molecules and diapedesis. Cells circulating in the blood can become attached to the endothelium via specific adhesion molecules which are increased in inflammation. The cells then undergo diapedesis through the endothelial wall, are attracted by chemo-attractants to the site of inflammation where they may be able to phagocytose foreign material

molecule (ELAM)-1. Intercellular adhesive molecule (ICAM)-1 and ICAM-2 appear to be the ligands for neutrophil CD11a–CD18 (Figure 6).

Numerous substances, termed chemotaxins, are capable of inducing directed cellular migration. The movement of cells (both leukocytes and monocytes) from intravascular compartment to extravascular space (tissue) involves a series of events including ligand-induced cellular activation, deformity and polarization of the cells, adherence to the endothelium and diapedesis or movement through the endothelium via a gradient-dependent process. These events result in sequestration of the phagocytes in target tissue sites. The biological consequences of chemotaxis may be beneficial, as in traumatic injury and infection, or detrimental, as in a variety of autoimmune and arthritic diseases.

Well-known chemotactic factors include the complement-derived molecule, C5a, the bioactive lipid leukotriene (LT) B4 and the bacterial peptide fMLP. Although these classic chemotactic factors have defined receptors on the leukocyte surface, many other chemotaxins have not been shown to have unique cellular receptors, suggesting that many factors may act on common receptors or induce chemotaxis by an indirect effect, such as causing the release of chemotactic factors from the stimulated cell. LPS from Gram-negative bacteria, for example, may promote neutrophil accumulation by the induction of production of TNF, IL-1α and IL-1β or a monocyte-derived neutrophil chemotactic factor (e.g. IL-8) from macrophages. Cytokines may influence the density and/or affinities of chemotactic receptors or other surface receptors, e.g. adhesive proteins on neutrophils. Conflicting reports from different groups regarding the effects of certain lymphokines including

TNFα and -β may result from the use of different methods of assessment of locomotion and possibly from dose effects. Similarly, there are conflicting reports on the relationships between the respiratory burst and chemotaxis in neutrophils and monocytes.

Knowledge of the control of neutrophil migration and fate in inflammation are important in understanding the determinants of tissue neutrophil load and of the persistence or resolution of inflammation. Ageing neutrophils undergo 'apoptosis' (programmed cell death), a process associated with endonuclease activation and leading to macrophage recognition and ingestion of the intact senescent cell. This prevents the disgorgement of large amounts of toxic substances by the neutrophil. Interestingly, inflammatory mediators, such as LPS, appear to inhibit apoptosis, thus prolonging tissue neutrophil life.

Eosinophils and basophils

These are dealt with in Chapter 4 on allergic rhinitis.

Mononuclear phagocytes

Bone marrow stem cells give rise to the cells of the mononuclear phagocyte system. These cells are widely distributed throughout the body and additionally are recruited to the sites of injury, infection and immune stimulation. Their properties vary a great deal depending on their functional state and on local interactions with cells and extracellular molecules. Monocytes enter the bloodstream in an immature form during fetal and adult life. Once in the tissues, they differentiate further into resident macrophages which may have characteristic morphology and often become associated with epithelia, e.g. Langerhans cells in the skin. Their life span is of weeks or months. An inflammatory stimulus will recruit additional monocytes from the blood to the local site; these newly recruited cells may have different properties from the resident macrophages. The main functions of the mononuclear phagocyte system are two-fold: (1) removal of particulate antigens and (2) antigen presentation to specific lymphocytes. Mononuclear phagocytes and neutrophils are often referred to as 'professional phagocytes' to distinguish them from other less-effective phagocytic cells. The phagocytic tissue macrophages form a network – the reticuloendothelial system which is found in many organs. Adherence and ingestion by monocytes is enhanced when the cells bind the micro-organisms by specialized receptors. The term 'opsonization' describes the preparation for phagocytosis of micro-organisms which are otherwise not recognized or which have developed strategies for preventing their engulfment. Opsonization is primarily carried out by antibodies and by complement. Mannosyl-fucosyl receptors (MFR) on human monocytes can bind to non-encapsulated organisms carrying these surface sugars. Receptors for fibronectin are also expressed. Monocytes also bear receptors for the Fc portion of IgG. The Fcγ RI has high, the Fcγ RII medium and the Fcγ RIII (CD16) low affinity. Other surface receptors enhancing effective function include CR1 (C3b receptor, CD35) and CR3 (CD11b) which are present particularly on activated macrophages and important in adherence, CR3 binds C3bi. LFAI (CD11a) and p150,95 (CD11c) are also expressed by macrophages. Opsonization is to the benefit of the host when phagocytosed infectious agents succumb to intracellular killing. Pathogens which can resist intracellular killing can, however, abuse these receptors by entering professional phagocytes. The mobility of phagocytes permits dissemination of such micro-organisms. Class II MHC antigens are present on some of the monocyte/macrophage series and are important in the presentation of antigen to T cells. The low-affinity IgE receptor (CD23) is also found on monocytes.

Phagocytosis usually involves pseudopodia moving roughly symmetrically around the organism and fusing on the distal side. A variant, 'coiling phagocytosis', has also been described for particular intracellular parasites. Complement receptors, including both CR1 which recognizes C3b and CR3 which recognizes C3bi, mediate a major role in phagocytosis. In the absence of serum, phagocytosis in general is much diminished and the identity of the ligand recognized by CR3 not definitely defined. Monocytes can generate complement components. Recently, it has been suggested that β-glucan binds to the lectin-like domain of the CR3 receptor. Interestingly, ligation of CR1 and CR3 receptors with particles coated in C3b or C3bi does not consequently stimulate the release of oxygen metabolites or the release of arachidonic acid metabolites. In contrast, stimulation of CR3 with β-glucan particles stimulates a strong oxidative burst. Other receptors which may play a role in phagocytosis include the mannosyl-fucosyl receptor, LFA1 and p150,95 receptors, fibronectin receptors and Fc receptors.

Microbicidal mechanisms

Once the organism has been internalized, the phagosome fuses with lysosomes to form a phago-lysosome and killing mechanisms are usually activated. These include enzymes and other antibacterial proteins in association with reactive oxygen intermediates (ROIs). The importance of these systems depends on the organism involved.

Oxygen-independent killing mechanisms

After an initial rise, the pH within the phago-lysosome falls within ten to fifteen minutes. Cysteine-arginine-rich cationic peptides, which include bactericidal permeability increasing protein which may act by damaging membranes, and defensins are most active during the initial rise in pH. These proteins are azurophil granule constituents. At more acidic pH, lysosome enzyme function becomes optimal. In addition, acidity itself may damage or kill some organisms. Lysozyme kills some Gram-positive organisms with readily accessible peptidoglycan. Cathepsin G shows a broad spectrum of antimicrobial activities. Lactoferrin remains effective in binding iron and making it unavailable to bacteria even at low pH.

Oxygen-dependent killing mechanisms

Stimulated phagocytic cells generate superoxide (O_2^-) through activation of a latent reduced NADPH oxidase system, the active enzyme being localized in the neutrophil plasma membrane, most likely consisting of a flavoprotein and a unique low-potential cytochrome b559. The superoxide is converted into toxic oxygen derivatives – hydroxyl radicals ($OH^{\cdot}$), singlet oxygen (O^-) and hydrogen peroxide (H_2O_2). These may act alone, following internalization of the phagosome. If lysosomal fusion occurs, the presence of peroxidase plus halides may produce additional toxic oxidants, e.g. hypohalite. Oxygen radicals can catalyse lipid peroxidation, DNA damage and protein damage and degradation.

Secretory products of phagocytes

Lysozyme is the main secretory product of macrophages; following phagocytosis other lysosomal hydrolases are released. Neutral proteases are important in the extracellular environment. These include collagenase, elastase, plasminogen activator and a cytotoxic proteinase; their secretion varies according to the level of cellular activation. Activated macrophages also secrete complement components, keeping up the levels at sites of inflammation where continual consumption is occurring.

Soluble mediators

The complement system

More than 30 glycoproteins are now recognized to be associated with this pathway which was first described almost one hundred years ago as a heat-labile activity in serum which led to lysis of bacteria coated with antibody.

Complement is a major defence system which can be activated directly if a foreign particle or organism offers a suitable binding site for self-activation of the early complement components. Bound C3 acts as an opsonin and a nidus for deposition of the lytic membrane attack complex (MAC). Complement can also be activated via immunoglobulins once the particle has bound immunoglobulin molecules. The physiological consequences of complement activation include opsonization, cellular activation and cell lysis (Figure 7).

The immunoglobulin-triggered pathway (the classical pathway) is composed of eleven distinct plasma proteins defined as 'components', each with a number and a prefix 'C'. The C1–C9 are components of the classical pathway and the membrane attack complex (MAC). The MAC is composed of activated C5 together with components of C6–C9. All of these components are distinct plasma proteins apart from C1 which is a complex of three glycoproteins, C1q, C1r and C1s.

The 'alternative pathway', an activation pathway not necessarily involving antibody, involves two proteins known as 'factors', factor B and factor D, with a third protein known as properdin (P). Two of the control proteins are also known as factors (I and H) while other control proteins are referred

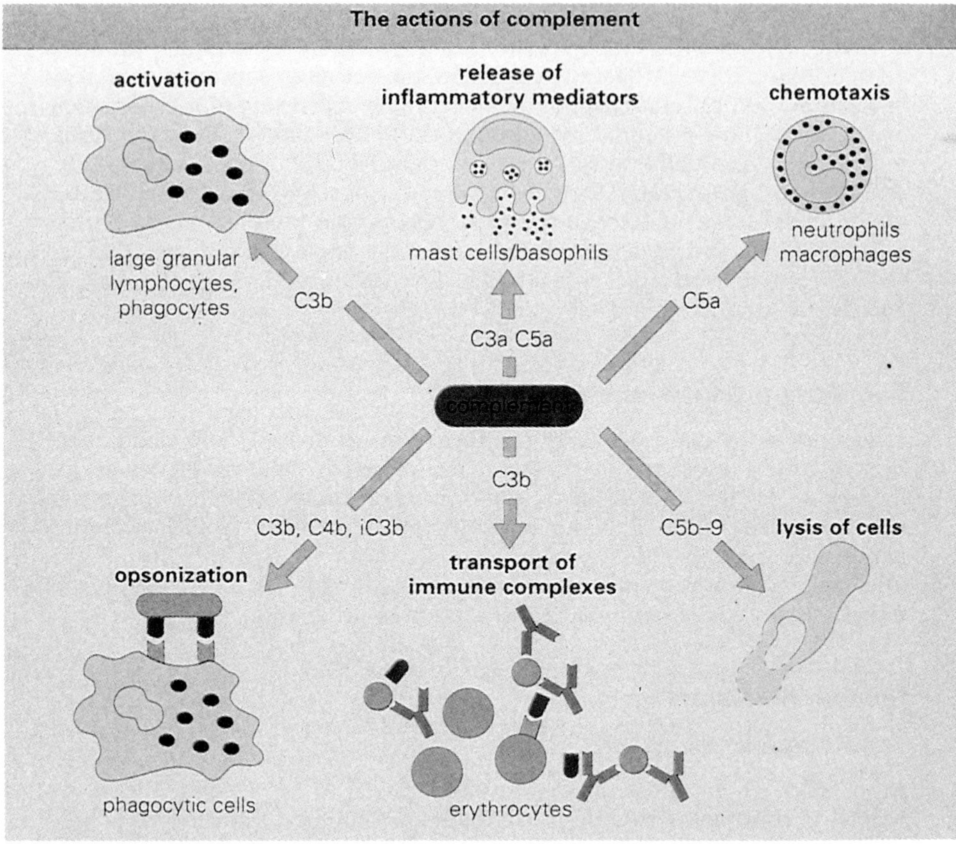

Figure 7 The functions of complement (Reproduced from Brostoff J, Scadding GK, Male D, Roitt IM. Clinical Immunology. London: Gower Medical Publishing; 1991 by kind permission)

to by their substrate, e.g. C1-inhibitor (C1-Inh). Six enzymes, serine proteases, are involved in the activation of this pathway. Enzymatically active forms of components generally have a bar over the symbol, e.g. $\overline{\text{C1r}}$, $\overline{\text{C1s}}$. The complex which contains an active site is also designated with a bar, e.g. $\overline{\text{C3b}}$, $\overline{\text{Bb}}$. Proteolytic fragments are indicated by suffixed letters, e.g. C4a and C4b are the activation fragments of C4. The smaller fragment is usually designated a, the larger b. Figure 8 shows the two pathways of complement activation. These pathways merge at the C3 activation step, thus components C5–C9 are common to both pathways and responsible, as the MAC, for target cell damage and lysis. The major constituent of the system is C3, present in the plasma at approximately 1 g/L. Activation of C3 by spontaneous hydrolysis or proteolytic cleavage by a C3 convertase enzyme is the central step in complement activation.

Activation of the classical pathway in vivo is primarily by the interaction of the C1q component of C1 with IgG or IgM. C1q has a complex structure

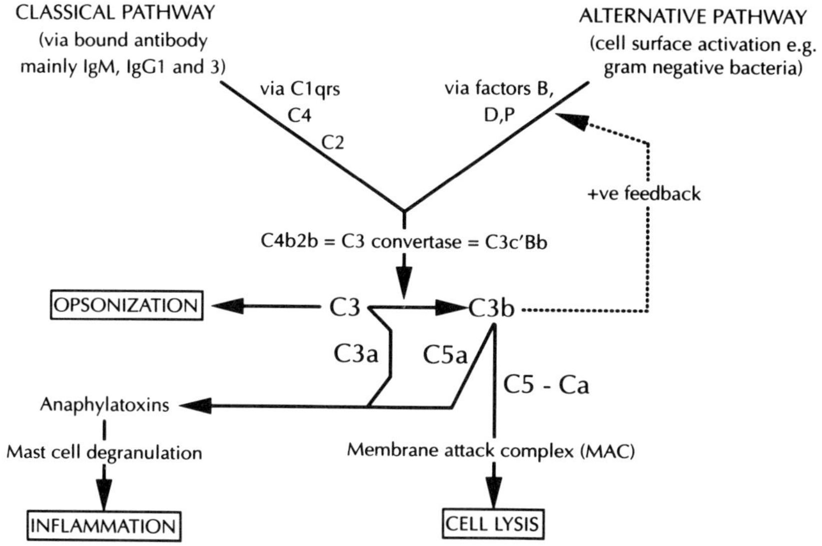

Figure 8 The complement pathways

of eighteen polypeptide chains which form six triple helices aligned in parallel for half their length then diverging towards their globular head regions. The structure has been likened to a 'bunch of tulips'. The enzymic activity of C1 is derived by activation of the two molecules of pro-enzyme C1r with two molecules of pro-enzyme C1s. Binding to monomeric IgG is weak but much increased in IgG immune complexes and in antigen-bound IgM. In man, IgG1 and IgG3 are the major C1q binding subclasses – IgG2 binds weakly and IgG4 is inactive. Interaction of two or more heads of C1q with an appropriate activator appears to induce a conformational change which releases the inhibitory effect of C1-Inh. Activation of C1r then C1s, then effects splitting of the C4 molecule, yielding C4a anaphylotoxin (molecular weight (MW) 9000) and the larger unstable C4b fragment. C4b can interact with the CR1 receptor, and can also bind C2. With C1s the C2 is split yielding C2a (MW 30 000) and C2b (MW 70 000): originally C2a was the larger fragment, C2b the smaller, a change has been suggested to further rationalize the nomenclature. C4b2b is the classical pathway C3 convertase enzyme, cleaving C3 into C3a and C3b. C3a is an anaphylotoxin of 77 amino acids and the exposed thioester in C3b is subjected to nucleophilic attack by water or the hydroxyl or amino groups of other molecules. C3b may thus become covalently bound to cell surface molecules. The range of activated C3b is limited by hydrolysis and deposition is thus largely restricted to binding to the activating surface rather than to host cells which do not activate complement.

Native C3 in plasma undergoes continuous low-grade hydrolysis of the internal thioester bond without the loss of the C3 fragment, yielding C3i which acts as a binding site for factor B. Factor B is structurally and functionally homologous to C2. The bound factor B is converted to Ba and Bb by factor D with the resulting complex C3iBb being a C3 convertase, cleaving C3 and producing C3b which may bind to cell surfaces and provide a binding site for more factor B, initiating a positive feedback amplification loop. The C3bBb enzyme dissociates fairly rapidly unless stabilized by the binding of properdin. Fluid phase regulatory proteins include factors H and I. Perhaps more critical is the regulation of cell-bound C3b. Surface-membrane molecules, CR1, membrane co-factor protein and decay-activating factor, function to limit the formation of C3 convertase enzymes on host cell surfaces. Deposition of C3b on non-cell surfaces, however, is followed by the production of a relatively stable C3bBbp C3 convertase which will focus more C3 deposition in the vicinity. Immune complexes also represent 'protected sites' for C3b.

The final phase of the complement cascade is the formation of the MAC. C5 is activated by C4b2b3b from the classical pathway and by C3bBb3b from the alternative pathway with the production of a small fragment C5a, a potent anaphylotoxin and major inflammatory mediator, and C5b. The subsequent formation of the MAC is non-enzymatic and follows the successive binding of C6, C7 and C5b to form a C5b67 complex. A hydrophilic–hydrophobic transition results in insertion into lipid bilayers. The subsequent binding of C8 and C9, which polymerizes, results in the formation of the typical cylindrical 'lytic plugs'.

The major site of production of plasma complement proteins is the liver, but local production, for example by tissue macrophages, also occurs and may be important at sites of inflammation. Increased catabolism occurs in many inflammatory diseases but is usually compensated for by increased synthesis. Modulators of complement levels include various hormones, lymphokines and endotoxins of bacterial origin, as well as at least one activation product of complement itself, C5a.

The study of complement deficiencies has provided valuable information on complement function. In deficiencies of C5 and subsequent components, there is, in general, no impairment of handling of immune complexes. People having a homozygous deficiency in any of the early classical pathway components, i.e. C1q, C1r, C1s, C4, C2 and C3, however, show a high incidence of immune complex disease, consistent with the importance of the classical pathway in preventing the function and deposition of large immune complexes during the early stages of antibody–antigen interaction. The alternative pathway is important in solubilizing preformed precipitates of immune complexes. Deficiency of C3 or of its inactivator C3bi is very rare and is associated with recurrent severe bacterial infections.

Complement and inflammation

Activation of the complement system is a potent trigger for the initiation and amplification of inflammation. Three anaphylotoxins of similar structure and activity, i.e. C4a, C3a and C5a, are released from their parent molecules. C5a is the most potent, C4a the least. They stimulate chemotaxis of leukocytes and degranulation of mast cells and basophils. In addition to chemotaxis, ligation of complement receptors on neutrophils and monocytes may also stimulate exocytosis of granule contents and free radical production via respiratory burst. The anaphylotoxins induce vasodilatation, increase vascular permeability and induce smooth muscle contraction. A large part of these effects is probably indirect via the release of histamine, arachidonic acid metabolites and other mediators from mast cells and basophils. C5a induces the production from monocytes of IL1 with its potent pro-inflammatory properties. C5a also appears to mobilize to the cell surface a pool of complement and adherence receptors, including CR1, CR3 and p150,95 thus enhancing adherence and phagocytosis.

Complement and phagocytosis

The major phagocytic receptors are the Fc receptors which recognize the Fc portion of antibody and CR1 and CR3 whose ligands are C3b and iC3b respectively. Although a high level of antibody on target organisms may be sufficient to initiate phagocytosis, a low level of antibody may not effectively bind and stimulate phagocytosis. It may, however, be sufficient to activate complement with the deposition of C4 and C3 fragments, thus amplifying the opsonization signal and much enhancing the efficiency of phagocytic binding. Ligand-receptor signalling mechanisms are incompletely understood, but result in involvement of the actin network in the cytoskeleton since drugs which disrupt actin filaments inhibit the ingestion phase of phagocytosis although the adherence to opsonized targets of phagocytes remains unimpaired. After ingestion, the resultant internalized vesicles, phagosomes, fuse with lysosomes where lysosome enzymes degrade the opsonized target.

Complement and defence against infection

Activated complement components can bind to a wide variety of surfaces via hydroxyl or amino groups. Complement has an important role in the destruction and clearance of Gram-negative and Gram-positive bacteria, parasites and viruses. The specificity of the reaction is an attribute of the specific antibody involved. Resistance to complement-mediated destruction is an important determinant of pathogenicity of many bacterial strains and a variety of mechanisms is used. Most Gram-negative bacteria can activate complement by both the classical and alternative pathways. Intact Gram-positive bacteria, however, do not usually activate the classical pathway in the absence of antibody. Probably the difference is caused by the different cell wall composition of these two classes of bacteria. Gram-negative bacteria display typical MAC lytic lesions while Gram-positive bacteria are resistant to lysis but are readily opsonized for phagocytosis. There is no definite evidence that complement plays a major role in the recovery from viral infection, but it does appear to be involved in the mechanisms of antiviral immunity. Certain viruses can activate classical and alternative pathways. The Epstein–Barr virus uses the CR2 to gain intracellular access. Other viruses may gain access to cells indirectly via immunoglobulin and C3 fixed to the virus.

Complement and the induction of specific immune responses

Complement plays a role in the induction of specific antibody responses by enhancement of localization of antigen and localization of antigen–antibody complexes. Antigen-presenting cells bear complement receptors, for example follicular dendritic cells bear all three receptors, CR1, CR2 and CR3. The role of complement appears to be accessory rather than vital, however. Human C3-deficient patients do have recurrent severe infections, but these appear to be primarily a result of deficiencies in opsonization, bactericidal activity, immune adherence and chemotaxis. They do not show overt evidence of impaired antibody production. C2-, C4- or C3-deficient guinea pigs, however, show a depressed primary antibody response to low immunizing doses of T cell-dependent antigens.

Lactoferrin

Lactoferrin is produced by glandular epithelium and is present in nasal secretions, saliva and milk. It binds iron in a similar way to transferrin and inhibits the growth of certain bacteria, particularly *Staphylococcus* and *Pseudomonas* spp., by the removal of iron.

Lysozymes

These are produced by serous glands, including those in the nose, and are also present in tears, as well as being produced by macrophages. Lysozyme is an enzyme which splits the mucopeptides of the bacterial cell wall by cleaving *N*-acetylmuramic acid from *N*-acetylglucosamine. Lysozyme is particularly toxic to non-encapsulated Gram-positive bacteria, but can also kill damaged Gram-negative organisms.

SPECIFIC IMMUNITY

Unlike innate immunity, specific immunity involves immunological memory with increased resistance to second or subsequent infections with the same organism. This ability to recognize and remember a diverse range of antigenic structures resides with the lymphocytes.

Lymphocytes

Lymphocytes of two main types are produced from stem cells in the bone marrow: B lymphocytes develops in the bone marrow or fetal liver, differentiating into antibody-forming cells, while T lymphocytes differentiate in the thymus and have several functions, including helping B cells make antibody, killing virally infected cells, regulating the immune response and stimulating microbicidal and cytotoxic activity of other immune effector cells. Lymphocytes migrate via the blood to secondary lymphoid organs,

MHC: major histocompatibility complex

including the spleen, lymph nodes and the mucosa-associated lymphoid tissue, e.g. tonsils and Peyers patches. An adult human has approximately 10^{12} lymphoid cells which make up about 20% of circulating blood cells. Lymphocytes may live as memory cells for several years. Communication between cells is both by cell–cell contact and by soluble factors. In the primary lymphoid organs, the lymphocytes develop their repertoire of specific antigen receptors and develop 'self-tolerance'. Both B and T cells recognize antigens. Each lymphocyte carries one type of receptor and therefore can recognize one type of antigen, but the receptors on different lymphocytes have different specificities. The enormous diversity of receptors is generated during lymphocyte development, before the cells encounter antigen, by the processes of somatic mutation and recombination, from a relatively small number of germline genes.

B lymphocytes recognize antigens in their native conformation, either free in solution, on membranes or on the surface of cells using surface immunoglobulin (Ig) as their surface receptor. This is a cell surface form of the antibody which the cell will secrete. The T cell receptor (TCR) is structurally different from antibody. It is encoded by a different set of genes and usually recognizes antigen which has been processed or degraded and is physically associated with molecules encoded by the MHC. These MHC molecules thus act as a guidance system for T cells in their recognition of antigens. Antigen is presented to lymphocytes by a group of antigen-presenting cells, including many cells of the phagocytic series. MHC molecules are also extremely polymorphic, again presumably related to the need to be able to present many different antigens. Unlike antigen receptors, however, the polymorphism of the MHC molecules is maintained in the germline MHC genes. Different MHC haplotypes vary in their ability to bind and present different antigens. Thus MHC genes control immune responses at the level of T cell antigen recognition and ultimately determine the individual's capacity to respond to pathogens and his susceptibility to autoimmune diseases.

When an antigen first enters the immune system, there may be relatively few lymphocytes which recognize it via specific surface receptors. Interaction with antigen induces a response in those cells usually manifested by proliferation and further differentiation resulting in expansion of the clone of cells which has the capacity to recognize the particular antigen. If the antigen is re-encountered there will be a larger clone of specific cells and these may be further differentiated. Secondary responses are thus faster and usually more effective than primary ones. Antigen-stimulated lymphocytes may either differentiate fully into immune effector cells or may become memory cells which will respond to further challenge with the same antigen.

B lymphocytes

B cells produce antibody and are classically defined by the presence of endogenously produced Ig. The surface Ig acts as an antigen-specific surface receptor. B cells develop initially in the fetal liver and subsequently in the bone marrow and make up 5–15% of circulating lymphoid cells. Fluorochrome-labelled anti-immunoglobulins can be used to quantitate B cells bearing different Ig classes. The majority of these circulating cells bear IgM while cells bearing other Ig classes are predominantly found in specialized tissues, e.g. IgA-bearing cells are predominantly found in mucosa-associated lymphoid tissue. Other surface molecules found on B cells include MHC Class II, important in co-operation with T cells. Complement receptors CR1 (CD35) and CR2 (CD21) are associated with activation and may play a role in homing responses. CR2 is also the receptor for the Epstein–Barr virus. Fc receptors for IgG (FcRII, CDw32) are present. A subpopulation of B cells possibly involved in autoantibody production bears CD5. Although most antigens cannot induce B cell antibody production without T cell help (T cell-dependent antigens), a number of antigens (T cell-independent antigens) can induce a B cell response in the absence of T cell help.

T lymphocytes

These cells differentiate in the thymus before entering the peripheral lymphoid tissues. The TCR is expressed on the surface of T cells associated with a glycoprotein CD3 which appears involved in signal transmission after interaction of antigen with TCR. Two types of TCR have been defined. Both are heterodimers of two disulphide-linked polypeptides, either α and β chains, or γ and δ. While the great majority of circulating blood lymphocytes bear the $\alpha\beta$ TCR, $\gamma\delta$ TCR-bearing cells have been shown to occur primarily at epithelial sites, particularly gut and skin. There is great current interest in the function of this T cell population. T cells have been separated into two main functional subpopulations. Regulatory helper T (TH) cells recognize antigen in association with MHC Class II determinants and bear the CD4 antigen. Effector cytotoxic (TC) T cells usually use MHC Class I as a restriction element and bear CD8. A second regulatory subset, suppressor cells, have proved much more difficult to define. TH cells have been subsetted in different ways. 'Naive' and 'memory' subpopulations can be separated by their expression of CD45 and CD45R. In the mouse, subpopulations TH1 and TH2 producing different lymphokines have been defined. This differentiation is less clear in the human.

All T cells express the receptor for sheep erythrocytes (CD2) – this was the basis of the original separation method for T cells. CD5 is also expressed on T cells.

'Null' cells

A third population of lymphocytes, morphologically large granular lymphocytes (LGLs), make up 10–20% of blood lymphocytes and bear neither TCR nor surface Ig. They possess electron-dense granules and share a number of surface markers with both T cells and cells of the myelomonocytic series. CD16 (FcγIII) is expressed by these cells and commonly used as an identifying marker, although it is also expressed on granulocytes and some macrophages. These cells have the ability to kill certain tumour cells, virus-infected cells and targets coated with IgG. These lytic activities are known as natural killer (NK) activity and antibody-dependent cellular cytotoxicity (ADCC) respectively.

T cells, B cells and null cells also share other common leukocyte antigens, including LFAI important in cell adhesion and intercellular communication.

Lymphocyte activation

Antigen-induced lymphocyte proliferation usually occurs in the secondary lymphoid tissues rather than in the blood. In vitro, mitogenic lectins which bind and cross-link specific cell-surface carbohydrate residues will polyclonally stimulate lymphocytes. Monoclonal antibodies to cell-surface molecules CD3, TCR and (for some antibodies) CD2 are also mitogenic. These reagents are used extensively for in vitro studies of T and B cell activation, although T and B cells are activated by different mitogens. Activation of the T cell surface receptor induces lymphokine secretion, the expression of IL2 receptors and the cells are driven into the cell cycle. Activated T cells bear IL2 receptors (IL2R) made up of a low-affinity receptor (CD25) and a larger medium-affinity molecule of 70 kDa. These together make up a high-affinity IL2R. Class 2 MHC, transferrin receptors and CD38 are also expressed on activated T cells. Activated B cells also bear high-affinity IL2R, transferrin receptors and elevated levels of MHC Class 2. CD23 (low-affinity IgE receptor) is also present on activated B cells and is involved in their activation. Particular markers of differentiated B cells include CD38 and PCA1.

Structure of immunoglobulins

The immunoglobulins are a group of glycoproteins present in plasma and tissue fluids of all mammals. They are produced by terminally differentiated plasma cells which develop from precursor B cells which carry membrane-bound immunoglobulin as their antigen receptors. Circulating antibodies are structurally identical to membrane-bound antibody apart from the lack of the transmembrane and intracytoplasmic portions.

The basic immunoglobulin structure is of four polypeptide chains, two identical heavy (H) and two identical light (L) chains, linked by disulphide bonds (Figure 9). This basic structure was proposed in 1962 by Rodney Porter. Enzymatic cleavage with papain cleaves the molecule in the hinge region into three fragments – two identical Fab fragments and one Fc fragment. The Fab fragments bind antigen, although they do not precipitate it because they are univalent. The Fc fragment mediates effector functions, such as complement fixation, binding to effector cells and placental transmission. Digestion with the enzyme pepsin yields two major fragments – the F(ab′)2 fragment encompassing the two Fab fragments joined by the hinged region and fragments of the Fc region.

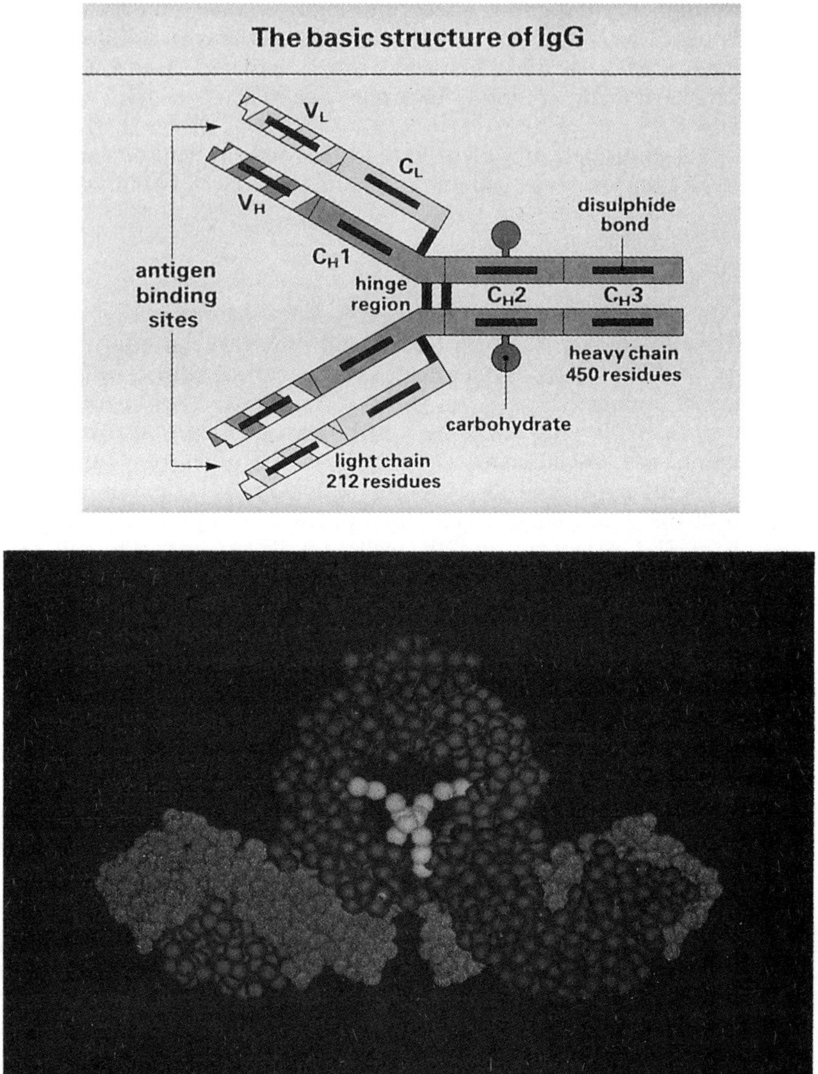

Figure 9 Basic structure of antibody (top) and a three dimensional picture (bottom). The antibody has two light and two heavy chains. The variable regions make up the antigen-combining site or F(ab)2 portion. The tail or Fc portion is responsible for many of the functional properties of antibody (see Table 1) (Reproduced from Brostoff J, Male D, Roitt IM. Immunology, 2nd edn. London: Gower Medical Publishing; 1993, by kind permission)

The smaller (light) chain has a molecular weight of approximately 22 000 while the larger (heavy) chain has a molecular weight of 50 000 to 77 000 and is structurally different for each class/subclass. Light chains consist of variable (V_L) and constant (C_L) domains, each of approximately 100 and 110 amino acid residues. Heavy chains consists of one V_H and a number of C_H

domains which vary with the class of antibody. For IgG, IgA and IgD, there are three VH domains; for IgM and IgE there are four, the additional domain being on the carboxy terminal side of CH1. The V and C domains themselves have little sequence homology, whereas CH1 and CL and CH2 and CH3 domains show homology. Each domain contains 90 to 100 amino acids with a centrally placed disulphide loop. X-ray crystallography shows domains to be oval or cylindrical.

Antibody classes

IgG

The four IgG subclasses are determined by their heavy chains: γ_1, γ_2, γ_3 and γ_4 respectively. Differences in amino acid composition between the heavy chains of subclasses are less than those between the different classes of heavy chains. There are differences in number and distribution of interchain disulphide bonds. The approximate proportions of IgG made up by these subclasses are 66%, 23%, 7% and 4% respectively. The immune response to a particular antigen may lie largely within one subclass; hence, a subclass deficiency can lead to failure of immunoprotection. Antibodies to organisms with carbohydrate on their surface, e.g. *Streptococcus pneumoniae* and *Haemophilus influenzae*, are mainly IgG_2. About 5% of patients with chronic infective lower respiratory tract problems are IgG_2 deficient. IgG is the major immunoglobulin in normal human serum. It has a molecular weight of 146 000, a sedimentation coefficient of 7S and makes up 70–75% of the total immunoglobulin pool. It is present in both intra- and extravascular pools and is the major antibody in secondary immune responses.

IgM (Figure 10a)

This has a pentameric structure, the whole molecule having a molecular weight of 970 000. IgM makes up 10% of the immunoglobulin pool and is largely intravascular. IgM is important in primary antibody responses. Subunits are each made up of two new heavy chains and two light chains. The subunits are held together by disulphide bonds between adjacent $C\mu3$ and $C\mu4$ domains of adjacent units. Flexion appears to occur between $C\mu2$ and $C\mu3$ domains. There are multiple oligosaccharide side chains associated with the μ chain and a peptide, J (joining) chain, is thought to be involved in polymerization prior to secretion by the antibody-producing cell. One J chain (137 amino acids) is bound by disulphide bridges between the $C\mu4$ regions of two adjacent subunits. There are few IgM-secreting plasma cells in the nasal mucosa and only traces of IgM in nasal fluid. IgM is the most effective complement-fixing immunoglobulin.

IgA (Figure 10b)

IgA is the second most abundant immunoglobulin in the blood making up 15–20% of human serum immunoglobulin where it is found mainly as the

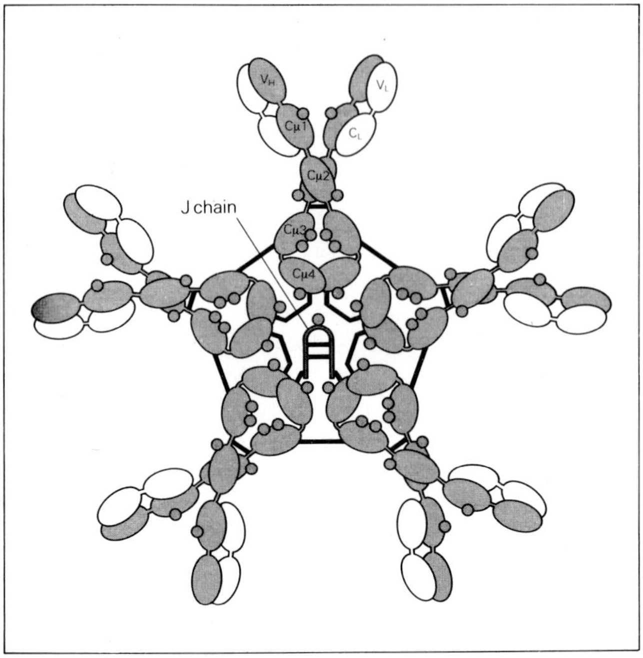

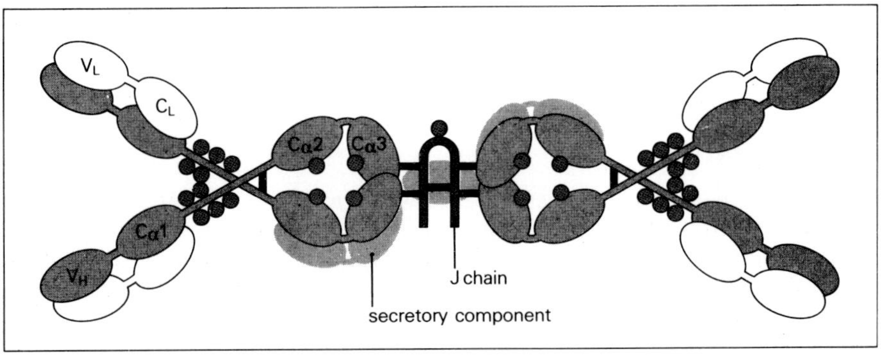

Figure 10 Structure of (a) IgM and (b) IgA. IgM is the most primitive antibody and is formed first during an immune response. It is extremely effective at fixing complement. sIgA is the predominant secretory antibody and is protected from enzymatic digestion by secretory piece

monomer, although 15–20% is found as dimers and trimers. The subclasses are IgA_1 and IgA_2. IgA_1 predominates in the blood while both are found in secretions. IgA is the predominant immunoglobulin in sero-mucus secretions, not only those of the upper respiratory tract but also saliva, colostrum, milk and those of the genito-urinary tract. The IgA in secretions (sIgA) is predominantly dimeric with a molecular weight of 385 000. The complete molecule is made up of two 4-chain units of IgA, one J chain (MW 15 000) and one secretory component (SC, MW 70 000). The J chain is synthesized by plasma cells and the dimer assembled within the plasma cells, the J chain holding the two subunits together. SC is synthesized by epithelial cells and acts as a receptor for dimeric IgA. It is present within the epithelial cell membrane on the basolateral surface of some mucosal epithelial cells. The IgA–SC complex is internalized by adsorptive endocytosis, transported in vesicles through the cell and released at the luminal surface. In the nose, mainly the serous type of nasal acinar and duct cells are involved in this process. The binding of SC also appears to protect IgA from proteolytic attack. Many micro-organisms present in the respiratory tract, including *Haemophilus influenzae* and *Streptococcus pneumoniae*, produce proteases which cleave the IgA_1 subclass at a Pro–Thr bond within the hinge region, perhaps contributing to the altered subclass ratio in secretions. There are additional differences in the proportion of IgA_2-bearing plasma cells in the respiratory lamina propria compared with bone marrow, tonsil and peripheral nodes. Additionally, SC has been shown to stabilize a form of IgA_2 which is otherwise liable to dissociation of the light and heavy chains. The ratio of IgA- to IgG-bearing cells is higher in the upper airways, including trachea and main bronchi, than in the more peripheral lung. Although the functions of IgA in the secretions remain only partly understood, its main actions appear to be neutralization of viruses and toxins, inhibition of the adherence and growth of micro-organisms on epithelial and other cell surfaces and 'antigenic exclusion' – the prevention of access of antigen to the systemic immune system. It has also been suggested that binding of antigen to IgA may interfere with the opsonic role of specific IgG antibodies by blocking the binding of antigen to IgG. IgA is not thought to play a major role as an opsonin although a capacity to enhance macrophage phagocytosis has been demonstrated. IgA does not activate complement.

IgD

Although present on the membrane of many circulating B cells, IgD makes up less than 1% of circulating immunoglobulin. It appears to play a role in B lymphocyte differentiation.

IgE

Present in the serum in only small amounts, IgE binds to high-affinity receptors on the surface of basophils and mast cells and to a lower-affinity receptor present on the surface of several other cell types, including monocytes, platelets and B lymphocytes. The ε heavy chain has a molecular weight of 72 500 and is heavily glycosylated. Cross-linking of the high-affinity receptors on mast cells and basophils results in cell activation with production of both granule-derived mediators, including histamine and proteases, and of newly formed arachidonic acid metabolites, including prostaglandins, leukotrienes and platelet activating factor (PAF). IgE plays an important role in the tissue responses to metazoan parasites and in allergic disorders (see Chapter 6).

Table 1 Functions of antibody

Fab combination with antigen	
	Neutralization, e.g. toxins
	Prevention of attachment, e.g. IgA in secretions
Fc binding	
	Neutrophil attachment and phagocytosis (IgG)
	K cell killing (antibody-dependent cellular cytotoxicity) (IgG)
	Complement activation (classical pathway) (IgM and IgG)
	T and B lymphocyte binding (immune regulation) (IgA, M, G and E)
	Mast cells → degranulation (IgE)
	Epithelial cell → transfer to mucosal secretions (IgA)

Antibody effector functions (Table 1)

Essentially each immunoglobulin molecule is bi-functional with the Fab portion of the molecule concerned with binding to antigen and the Fc region with binding to host tissues, including lymphoid cells and phagocytes, and to the first component of the classical complement system. These effector functions are determined by the structure of the Fc region. Activation of the complement system is most effective with IgM, IgG_1 and IgG_3. IgG_2 is less effective while IgG_4, IgA, IgD and IgE are ineffective.

In man, IgG molecules of all subclasses cross the placental syncytiotrophoblast to provide the newborn with passive immunity. Antibody binding to a variety of effector cells is via the Fc receptors.

Generation of antibody diversity

Antibodies show great diversity with more types of antibody than the number of genes in the human genome. How is this diversity generated? The immunoglobulin genes comprise three separate loci which encode the H chain (on chromosome 14q32), the kappa chain (chromosome 2p12) and lambda chain (chromosome 2q11). Each cluster contains genes coding for the variable and constant regions (Figure 11). Within both light and heavy chain variable regions variations between different antibodies are concentrated in three 'hypervariable regions' in each chain. These hypervariable regions make contact with antigen and thus largely determine the antigen-binding capacity of the antibody.

Light chain genes

Initial work on the lambda light chains showed that two separate areas of DNA coded for constant and variable regions and that these gene segments were brought closer together in antibody-forming cells. Between the V and C regions is a short joining (J) segment. The exact numbers of V, J and C genes are not known in the human. The kappa chain genes are similar although there appears to be a greater number of V kappa genes as well as five J kappa genes.

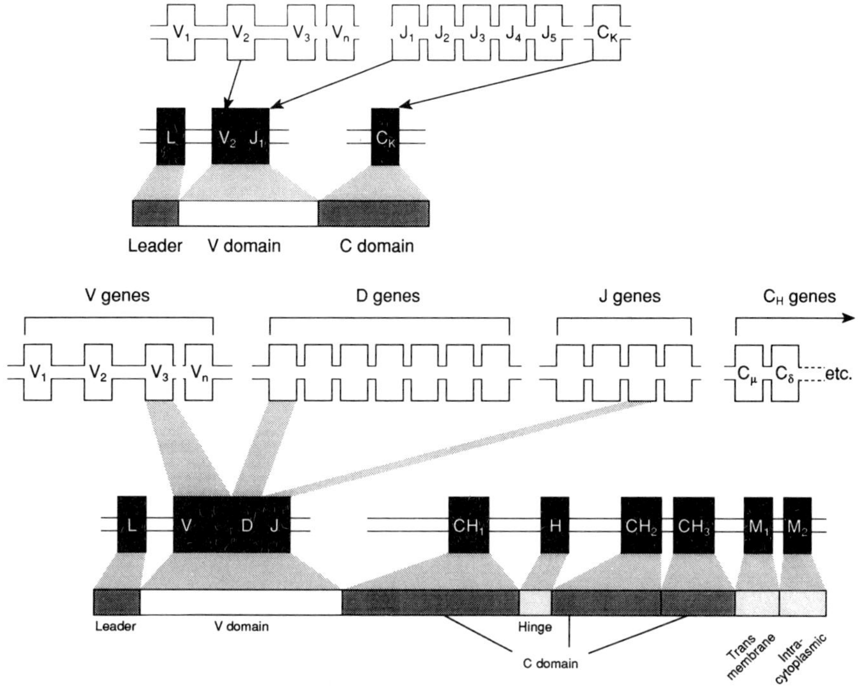

Figure 11 The genetics of antibody formation. DNA recombination takes place during B cell development and maturation in two stages. First there is the recombination of one of many germline V genes with one of a few J genes (light chain) or with one of several D genes and then a J gene (heavy chain). This occurs during the transition from lymphoid stem cell to B cell. Later, in the differentiated B cell, irreversible class switching may occur (vide infra).

The light chain gene comprises 3 exons: a leader (L) exon, which is necessary for polypeptide translation across the endoplasmic reticulum, an exon formed from the combination of a V and a J gene which encodes the variable region, and a C exon encoding the constant domain.

The heavy chain gene is similar with a leader (L), a variable domain formed from the recombination of three separate gene segments, V, D and J, and separate exons for each constant domain, with a hinge exon (H) between CH_1 and CH_2. For a membrane antibody, there are also two exons, M1 and M2, coding for the transmembrane and intracytoplasmic portions.

The segments encoding V domains are several kilobases upstream of the C region genes and a V gene may link with any one of the C genes. Thus, a B cell may initially produce IgM using an IgM C gene but can later switch to a different C gene isotype (e.g. IgG), thus changing antibody class while retaining specificity for antigen

Heavy chain variable region genes

The H chain variable region is encoded by three separate DNA segments: variable (V), diversity (D) and joining (J) gene segments together encoding a V region of 100–130 amino acids. A functional IgH or L chain gene is generated during B cell development by a series of rearrangements which generate a V region coding block from the constituent gene segments. A 'productive' VDJ rearrangement within the H chain locus triggers L chain rearrangement.

Heavy chain constant region genes

All classes of immunoglobulin use the same set of variable region genes. The constant region of the heavy chain is switched when antibody class is changed. Lymphocytes may bear both IgM and IgD on their surface. These antibodies have the same specificity indicating usage of identical VH genes but associated with different constant region genes. All the constant region genes are downstream from the J segment genes. In man, the order of the genes is μ, δ, γ_3, γ_1, ε_2, α_1, γ_2, γ_4, ε_1, α_2.

Just upstream to the μ gene is a switch sequence, repeated upstream of the other constant-region genes (except δ) which is a recombination site allowing class switching to other constant region genes and thus other antibody classes.

Diversity is thus generated by a variety of genetic mechanisms:

1. The presence of multiple V region genes in the germ line (both VH and VL).
2. Recombination between the different elements forming a V gene 'block'.
3. The association of particular VH with a particular VL, although combinations may in practice be limited.
4. Junctional diversity – 'looseness' in the precision of VDJ joining.
5. Somatic mutation – this operates in late B cell development with base changes in VH or VL segments and is probably involved in increasing antibody affinity during an immune response.

Antibody–antigen interactions

Epitopes recognized by antibodies are usually a number of amino acid residues brought together by the conformation of the antigen, but may also be linear polypeptides. Most proteins appear to have 'immunodominant' regions although these may differ between different species or strains. Areas of protein involved in loops and turns with high mobility are often associated with antigenicity.

Antigen recognition is determined by HLA constitution acting at the level of the T cell receptor, thus the repertoire of antibodies formed to a particular protein will vary between individuals. Some of these antibodies will bind to the antigen better than others and will provide a more effective immune response. Certain individuals have 'gaps' in their immune repertoire, rendering them unable to mount an effective response against a particular pathogen.

IMMUNE DEFICIENCY IN ENT DISORDERS

Susceptibility to infection is increased by several factors (Table 2). Immune deficiencies can underlie chronic ear, nose and throat infections. Secondary immune deficiencies (Table 3) are commoner than primary ones and can usually be diagnosed by a careful history and relevant blood tests (Table 4). Approximately one or two patients a year are found to have such a deficiency at the Royal National Throat, Nose and Ear Hospital Special Rhinology

Table 2 Causes of increased susceptibility to infections

Immunodeficiency	– primary
	– secondary
Circulatory disorders	
Obstructive defects	
Integument defects	
Unusual microbiological factors	
Foreign bodies	

Table 3 Secondary immunodeficiency

Iatrogenic
Malnutrition
Prematurity
Lymphoma
Splenectomy
Uraemia
Infections
Protein-losing enteropathy

Clinic.

Primary immune deficiency is rarer, with hypo-γ-globulinaemia occurring in approximately 1 in 50000 of the population. Minor forms of immunoglobulin deficiency are more common; that of IgA occurring in between 1 in 500 and 1 in 700 of the population. Since the effects of immunoglobulin deficiency are frequently apparent initially in the upper respiratory tract, early diagnosis is possible if ENT surgeons are aware of this and send clotted blood samples from patients with repeated infections for immunoglobulin analysis. Early diagnosis and prompt immunoglobulin replacement therapy not only prevents or delays lower respiratory tract problems, but is also more effective in the treatment of upper respiratory tract problems.

References

1. Lucas AM, Douglas LC. Principles underlying ciliary activity is the respiratory tract. Arch Otolaryngol. 1934;20:518–41.
2. Jeffery PK, Reid L. Electron microscopy of rat airway. J Anat. 1975;120:295–320.
3. Petruson B, Hansson HA, Karlsson G. Structural and functional aspects of cells in the nasal mucociliary system. Arch Otolaryngol. 1984;110:576–81.
4. Rutland J, Cole PJ. Non-invasive sampling of nasal cilia for measurement of beat frequency and study of architecture. Lancet. 1980;2:564–5.
5. Greenstone M, Logan-Sinclair R, Cole PJ. An automated method of recording nasal ciliary beat frequency. IRCS Med Sci. 1984;12:715–6.
6. Holmstrom M, Lund VJ, Scadding GK. Nasal ciliary beat frequency following nasal allergen challenge. Am J Rhinol. 1992;6:101–5.
7. Holmberg K, Pipkorn U. Mucociliary transport in the human nose. Effect of topical glucocorticoid treatment. Rhinology. 1985;23:181–5.
8. Eid NS, Kravath RE, Lanks KW. Heat shock protein synthesis by human polymorphonuclear cells. J Exp Med. 1987;165:1148–52.
9. Worthen GS. Lipid mediators, neutrophils and endothelial injury. Am Rev Resp Dis. 1987;136:455–8.

Table 4 Immunodeficiency causing ENT disorders

Innate immune system	
Ciliary dysfunction	– primary – Kartagener syndrome – secondary to – infection – pollution – allergy
Mucus abnormalities	– cystic fibrosis Young syndrome
Neutrophil abnormalities	– ?lazy leukocyte syndrome
Complement defects	– absence of C3 or its inactivator causes severe infections – absence of C9 results in increased susceptibility to *Neisseria* spp.
Acquired immunity	
Humoral (antibody-mediated)	– IgA deficiency ← may – IgG deficiency $\pm$ other Ig classes occur – IgG subclass deficiency ← together
Cellular	– usually results in severe infections, notably with fungi, mycobacteria and viruses, and in an increase in neoplasia

The major known immunological defects leading to ENT problems are shown. Situs inversus occurs in approximately half of those patients with Kartagener syndrome. Affected individuals are sterile as are those with Young syndrome, a genetic disorder involving abnormal mucus of unknown aetiopathology. IgA deficiency is relatively common, occurring once in 500–700 individuals, but only half of these suffer an increase in infections (see Chapter 12). Hypo-γ-globulinaemia is rarer, although probably underdiagnosed. In any individual with recurrent ENT infections, a sample of clotted blood should be sent for serum immunoglobulin determination. Affected individuals can benefit from immunoglobulin replacement therapy (which can now take place at home). Early diagnosis and treatment confer a better prognosis, probably because chronic infection leads to secondary irreversible changes in the upper respiratory tract mucosa. IgG_3 subclass abnormalities have been described in chronic rhinosinusitis – the significance of these observations remains to be elucidated. Primary cellular immune defects are very rare, although secondary deficiencies due to the HIV virus are becoming more common. (See Chapter 2.)

10. Smedly LA, Tonnesen MG, Sandhaus RA, et al. Neutrophil-mediated injury to endothelial cells. Enhancement by endotoxin and essential role of neutrophil elastase. J Clin Invest. 1986;77:1233–43.
11. Nourshargh S, Rampart M, Hellewell PG, et al. Accumulation of 111In-neutrophils in rabbit skin in allergic and non-allergic inflammatory reactions in vitro with a monoclonal antibody recognising the CD18 antigen. J Immunol. 1989;142:3193–8.
12. Scadding GK, Lund VJ, Navas-Romero J, Darby YC, Seymour N, Turner MW. IgG3 subclass deficiency in chronic rhinosinusitis. Rhinology. 1994; 32: 15–19.
13. Tonegawa S. Somatic generation of antibody diversity. Nature. 1983;302:575.
14. Yancopoulos GD, Alt FW. Regulation of the assembly and expression of variable region genes. Annu Rev Immunol. 1986;4:339.
15. Alt FW, Blackwell TK, Depinho RA, et al. Regulation of genome rearrangement events during lymphocyte differentiation. Immunol Rev. 1987;89:5.
16. Allison JP, Lanier LL. The structure, function and serology of the T-cell antigen receptor complex. Annu Rev Immunol. 1987;5:503.
17. Ashwell JD, Klausner RD. Genetic and mutational analysis of the T cell antigen receptor. Annu Rev Immunol. 1990;8:139.
18. Matis L. The molecular basis of T cell specificity. Annu Rev Immunol. 1990;8:65.
19. Clevers H, Alarcon B, Wileman T, et al. The T cell receptor/CD3 complex: a dynamic protein ensemble. Annu Rev Immunol. 1988;6:629.
20. Ahmed A, Smith AH. Surface markers, antigens and receptors on murine T and B cells.

CRC Crit Rev Immunol. 1983;4:19.
21. Muller-Eberhard HJ. The membrane attack complex of complement. Annu Rev Immunol. 1986;4:503.
22. Porter RR, Reid KBM. Activation of the complement system by antigen-antibody complexes: the classical pathway. Adv Protein Chem. 1979;33:1.
23. Fearon DT. Activation of the alternative complement pathway. CRC Crit Rev Immunol. 1979;1:1.

Further reading

Roitt I. Essential immunology, 7th edn. Oxford: Blackwell Scientific Publications; 1991.
Brostoff J, Scadding GK, Male D, Roitt IM, eds. Clinical immunology. London: Gower; 1991.
Brostoff J, Male D, Roitt IM, eds. Immunology, 3rd edn. London: Gower; 1993.
Male D, Champion B, Cooke A. Advanced Immunology, 2nd edn. London: Gower; 1992.

2
The ENT Presentation of HIV Infection and the Acquired Immunodeficiency Syndrome

J. M. PARKIN

THE VIROLOGY AND IMMUNOPATHOGENESIS OF HIV – AN OVERVIEW

The human immunodeficiency viruses (HIV)

Two types of HIV have been recognized to date. HIV-1, the first to be isolated, is the most common, found in individuals from Europe, the USA, Australasia and Central Africa. This retrovirus ('retro', as it translates its RNA to DNA, the reverse of cellular transcription mechanisms) is the cause of a range of clinical disorders varying from an asymptomatic 'carrier' state to the severe immunodeficiency of the acquired immunodeficiency syndrome (AIDS). The more recently discovered HIV-2 is found most frequently in those from Western African countries, but also occasionally in other groups. Initial natural history studies suggest that although HIV-2 causes the same spectrum of disease as HIV-1, it may be less pathogenic, with more individuals remaining asymptomatic. Dual infection with HIV-1 and HIV-2 occurs. However, as most published work relates to HIV-1, most of the discussion in the following pages relates to the effects of this virus.

Viral replication

HIV consists of core (p24) and matrix proteins wrapped in an icosahedral envelope, consisting of multiple units of the transmembranous protein (gp41) and its external projection (gp120) (see Figure 1). The latter bears the binding site for the host cell-surface protein CD4, found mainly on 'helper' T lymphocytes, but also on monocytes, macrophages and some cells of the

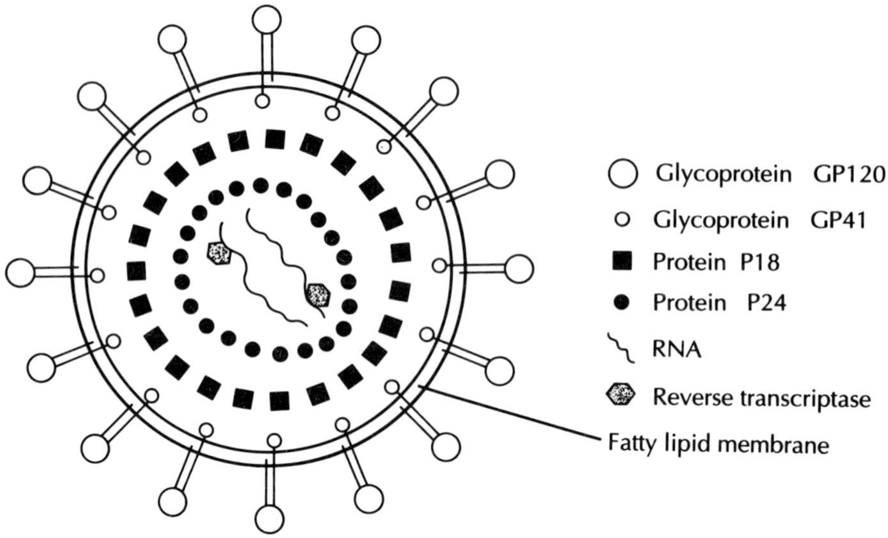

Figure 1 Structure of human immunodeficiency virus. The external projection gp120 of the transmembrane protein bears the binding site for the host cell surface protein CD4. Recently another cell surface protein CD 28 (?) has been shown to be involved in the binding and uptake of HIV particles

nervous system. The presence of the CD4 molecule appears to determine the site of damage of HIV, which is mainly confined to the immunological and neurological systems. Although HIV-1 has been shown to infect CD4-negative cells, such as the epithelium of the gastrointestinal tract, the infection is many-fold less productive, and the significance uncertain.

After binding to CD4 via gp120, the viral and host cell membrane fuse and the uncoated viral particle enters the cell. Using the 'reverse transcriptase' enzyme that is carried with the virion, HIV is transcribed into a DNA copy that is inserted into the host genome. It is this integration that leads to a life-long infection of the cell. During cell activation, viral transcription is also switched on (and amplified by virally coded control proteins). A productive infection results and new viral particles are formed which bud through the host cell membrane and are released to infect other cells (Figure 2).

Immunopathogenesis of HIV infection

Despite extensive investigation into the immunological defects induced both *in vivo* and *in vitro* in the course of HIV infection, the exact mechanism of the immunodeficiency observed in patients remains uncertain. HIV has well-described direct cytopathic effects leading to syncytia formation and cell lysis, and this could account completely for the CD4+ lymphocyte depletion which is a hallmark of AIDS[1]. Indirect effects may also lead to CD4+ cell loss, for example by: 'bystander' killing of non-infected cells that have passively bound soluble gp120 to their surface CD4, and are therefore

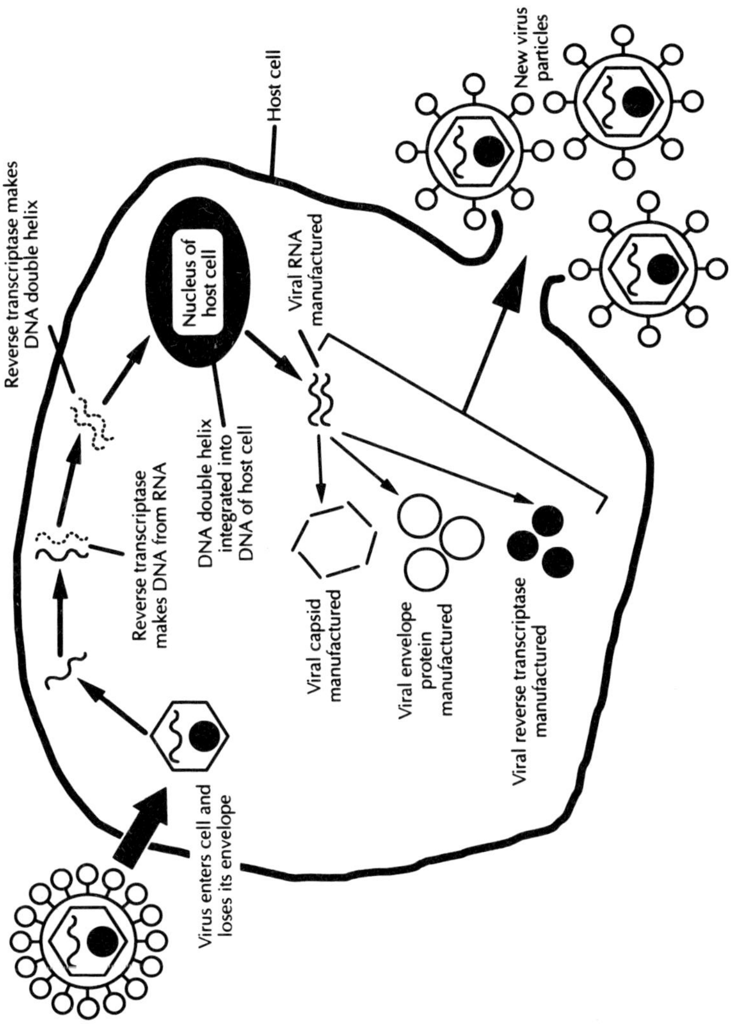

Figure 2 Cellular events in HIV replication. A DNA copy of the virus RNA is inserted into the host cell genome, leading to life-long infection of that cell

recognized by HIV-specific cytotoxic lymphocytes; or induction of autoimmune antilymphocyte responses, as there is homology between gp120 and the human MHC proteins.

However, there is evidence of immunological defects even at the early stages of HIV infection, before CD4 depletion has occurred and when only a small number of cells appear to be infected[2]. This may be due to immunosuppressive effects of viral proteins released from infected cells. Cells other than CD4+ lymphocytes are also abnormal: B cells show signs of activation and immature phenotype[3,4]; monocytes, macrophages and Langerhans cells have defective phagocytic and antigen presentation function; and cytokine production is dysregulated. Whether these effects are a direct result of HIV infection, due to the HIV-induced loss of a regulating cell population, or to the effects of intercurrent infections complicating the immune deficiency, cannot as yet be unravelled. An area of intense research is the role of co-factors in enhancing the development of immunodeficiency (suggested candidates being cytomegalovirus, human herpes virus type 6, HTLV-1 and mycoplasma). It seems most likely that the pathogenesis is multifactorial.

CLINICAL CONSEQUENCES OF HIV INFECTION

Whatever the mechanism of the immunodeficiency, the outcome is clear – a defect in the cell-mediated response leading to susceptibility to opportunist infections and tumours. It is these which will most often bring the patient to the physician or surgeon.

Types of infections and tumours frequently observed

The infections observed are with organisms normally controlled by the T cell and macrophage arm of the cellular immune system. These are predominantly intracellular organisms, in particular viruses (cytomegalovirus, herpes simplex, varicella zoster and polyomavirus), fungi (*Candida*, *Cryptococcus*, *Histoplasma*) and protozoa (*Pneumocystis carinii*, *Toxoplasma* and *Cryptosporidium*). Facultative intracellular bacteria, such as *Salmonella* and *Mycobacteria* spp., also cause disease. These infections and the tumours, Kaposi's sarcoma and non-Hodgkins lymphoma, are the major causes of death. Control of most bacterial infections is under the antibody, complement and phagocyte systems (the eradication of extracellular organisms not requiring the elaborate antigen-processing and presentation/recognition systems of the cellular immune components). However, as the antibody response is under the regulation of CD4+ lymphocytes, this is also partly defective, patients having a 'functional dysgammaglobulinaemia' being able to produce antibodies to previously encountered antigens, but not to neo-antigens. This is most apparent in paediatric HIV disease (as infants infected *in utero* have not yet developed an antibody repertoire), where disseminated bacterial infection is a common cause of mortality. In adults, there is also an increased susceptibility to bacterial infections, this leading to morbidity rather than mortality[5].

Effect of past exposure to infectious agents on disease presentation

As the majority of opportunist infections are due to reactivation of previously acquired infection, rather than *de novo* disease, the lifetime history of a patient's residence and travel will give valuable clues to the likelihood of various infections occurring. For example, African patients with HIV infection are most likely to present with tuberculosis as this infection is ubiquitous and individuals are very commonly infected at some stage in their lives. The organism is not eradicated and infection will re-emerge as the immune deficiency develops. Cryptococcal meningitis is also frequent in this group. Conversely, *Pneumocystis carinii* infections are extremely rare as this does not appear to be a common environmental organism in Africa. This contrasts with the situation in the Western world, where *Pneumocystis carinii* pneumonia is the most common presenting infection in patients with AIDS (unless prophylaxis is used). Likewise, patients visiting regions endemic for *Histoplasma* or *Leishmania* may have contracted these infections asymptomatically, but will be at risk of reactivation.

Infections due to non-HIV-related immunosuppression

A more recent factor in the host defence defect in HIV-positive patients is the use of bone marrow suppressive drugs such as the anti-HIV agent, azidothymidine, the cytomegalovirus-suppressive, ganciclovir, and chemotherapeutic agents for Kaposi's sarcoma and lymphoma. These induce neutropenia, lowering another arm of the immune system and exposing the patient to an additional range of infections, such as Gram-negative sepsis with *Pseudomonas*, *Escherichia coli* and *Klebsiella* spp., and disseminated fungal infections, in particular with *Aspergillus* spp.

Changing pattern of disease in HIV infection

As effective drugs become available for the control of HIV infection (in particular the nucleoside analogue inhibitors of reverse transcriptase, azidothymidine and dideoxyinosine) and regimens for the primary and secondary prophylaxis of *Pneumocystis carinii*, *Cryptococcus*, *Toxoplasma* and mycobacterial infections are developed, the pattern of disease observed in HIV-infected individuals has changed[6]. Patients are surviving longer due to the decreased incidence of some of the opportunist infections (mainly *Pneumocystis carinii* pneumonia, PCP) and the slowed progression of HIV damage to the immune and neurological systems by the use of anti-retroviral drugs. However, the improved treatments have brought new problems. An example is the use of nebulized pentamidine as prophylaxis for PCP. Patients on this topical treatment are at risk of extrapulmonary pneumocystosis[7]. Also, as patients live longer, the complications of HIV infection that are less amenable to treatment are gaining prominence in morbidity and mortality, tumours now accounting for a much higher proportion of deaths. More aggressive chemotherapy regimens, and possible prophylactic approaches, will be the next stage in improving the quality and quantity of life for the patient with AIDS.

MANIFESTATIONS OF HIV INFECTION IN THE EAR, NOSE AND THROAT

The most frequent presentation of HIV-related ENT disease is in the mouth, and therefore this will be considered first.

Oropharynx

The most common abnormalities to be observed in the mouth are candidiasis and hairy oral leukoplakia. These are of particular importance as, although not AIDS-defining events in their own right, they carry a prognostic risk for the ultimate development of AIDS.

Candidiasis

The typical white plaques of pseudomembranous candidiasis are seen on the mucous membrane of the tongue, palate (especially under dental plates), fauces, and on the gums and buccal mucosa. The hypertrophic and atropic forms are less frequent. Angular stomatitis is also seen. The lesions can be asymptomatic, but can cause considerable discomfort and eating difficulties. If accompanied by burning dysphagia, this is strongly suggestive of oesophageal involvement. Systemic treatment with an agent such as fluconazole or ketoconazole is generally required. The higher incidence of hepatotoxicity limits the usefulness of ketoconazole and some studies have shown fluconazole to be slightly more effective[8]. Resistance to these agents can develop, although in most cases, severe 'resistant' candidiasis is more usually due to progression of the underlying immunodeficiency, than to the organism. In these cases, a course of intravenous amphotericin B is usually effective, although repeated courses or maintenance treatment may be necessary.

Hairy oral leukoplakia (HOL) (Figure 3a)

Unlike candidiasis which may be widespread in distribution, HOL is characterized by its confinement to the lateral borders of the tongue; it is very rarely painful and cannot be scraped off by a spatula. The causative organism is thought to be Epstein–Barr virus, which has been demonstrated by *in situ* studies[9,10]. A corollary of this is that some patients will respond

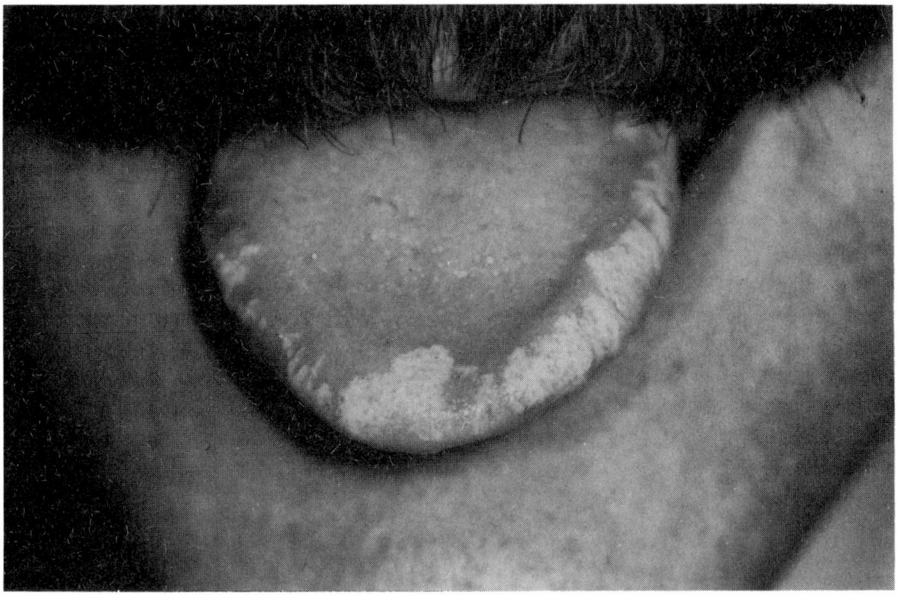

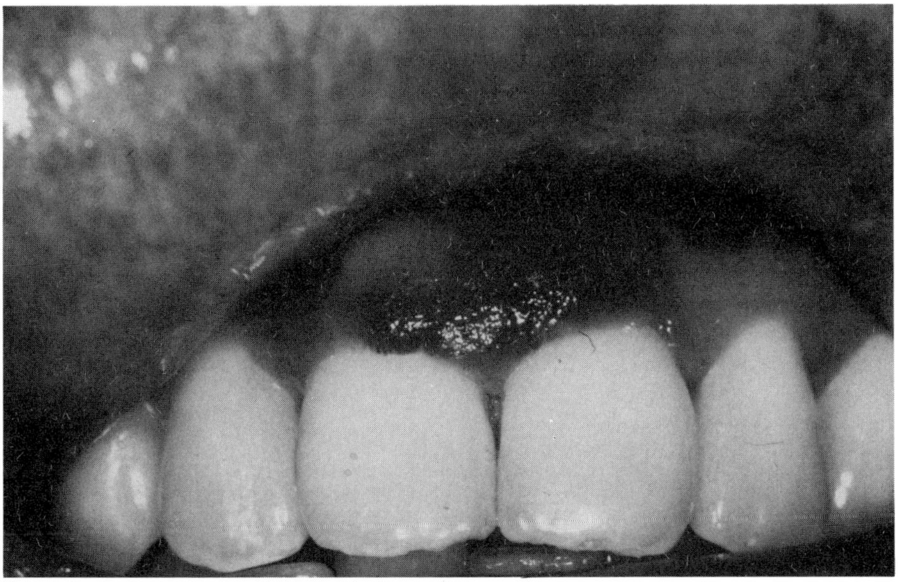

Figure 3 (a) Hairy oral leukoplakia which is very strongly associated with HIV infection. (b) Kaposi's sarcoma affecting the gums, (c) the roof of the mouth and (d) the ear pinna. These lesions are often asymptomatic and first noticed by the doctor
[Figures 3a and 3d courtesy of St. Mary's Hospital Medical School; 3b and 3c courtesy of the Meyerstein Institute of Clinical Oncology, UCL Hospitals.]

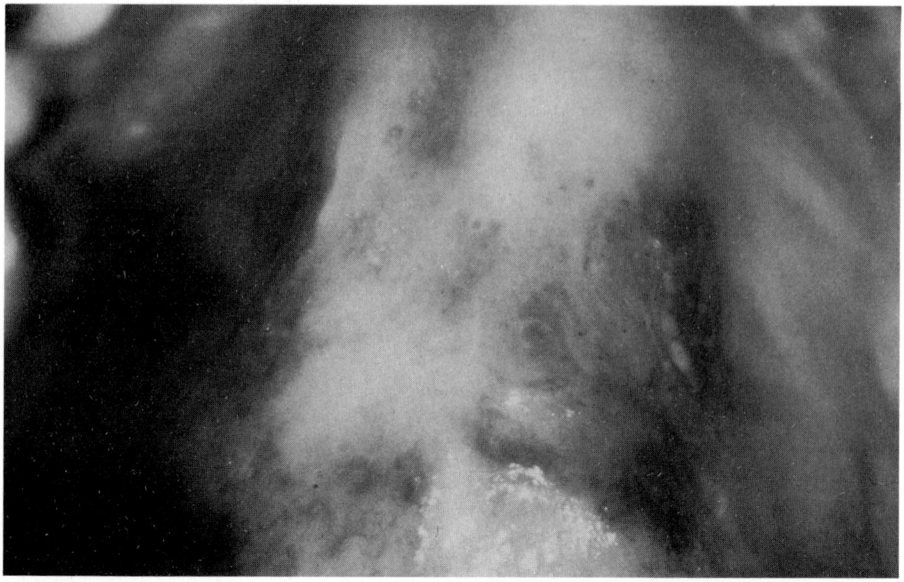

Figure 3c *continued*

to high doses of the anti-herpes virus agent, acyclovir. A histologically similar lesion has also been documented in the oesophagus of patients with HIV infection. The lesion usually presents as a mid-oesophageal ulcer rather than leukoplakia[11].

The lesion does not appear to be premalignant in this group, and it is usually the cosmetic appearance which is distressing.

HOL is very strongly associated with HIV infection. Although a few cases of HOL in congenital cell-mediated immunodeficient states are reported, its presence should alert the physician to the possibility of HIV disease.

Kaposi's sarcoma (Figure 3b,c and d)

Kaposi's sarcoma is a proliferation of the endothelial cells, either of vascular (as demonstrated by the presence of Factor VIII complex by *in situ* hybridization) or lymphatic origin. It is a multifocal tumour that forms spindle-cell-lined vascular spaces, often filled with red blood cells, that give rise to the characteristic purple/red colour. The lesions are commonly asymptomatic, and, particularly in the mouth, more frequently noticed by the examining doctor than by the patient. The most common site is the hard palate, although lesions may occur anywhere in the mouth, tongue and throat (even on the vocal cords[12,13]) and are not always accompanied by cutaneous disease. However, an oral lesion is frequently associated with disease lower down in the gastrointestinal tract, and symptoms suggestive of visceral involvement should be sought.

The lesions may be completely flat. The main problems are mechanical:

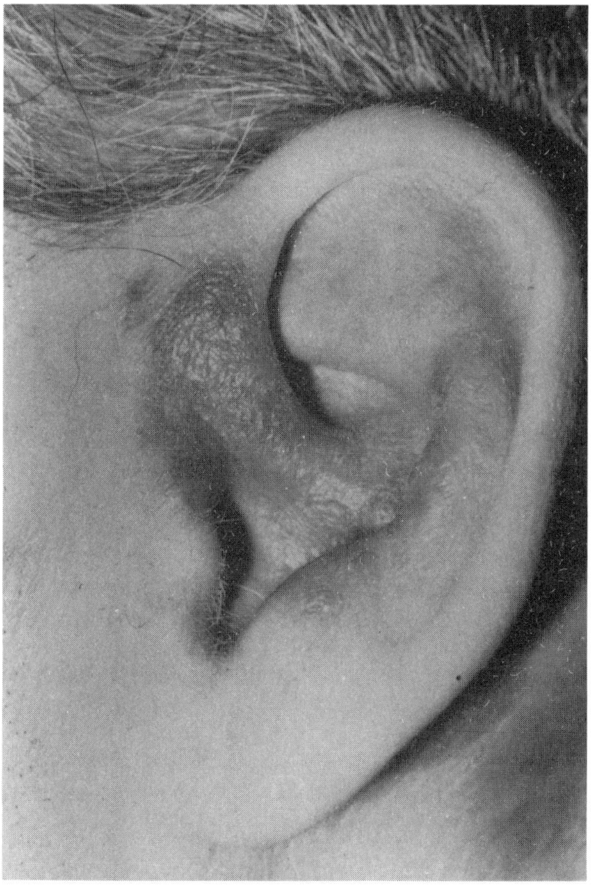

Figure 3d *continued*

if the tumour becomes raised, is around the gum margin, acts as a site for infection, or ulcerates. It is at this stage that treatment (either radiotherapy or chemotherapy, depending on accessibility) is considered.

Ulceration

Oral ulcers are common. Infections such as varicella zoster virus (typically causing gingival ulcers), herpes simplex, and cytomegalovirus[14] are well-described causes, and readily treatable.

Tumours, such as Kaposi's sarcoma and lymphoma, may also ulcerate and, in general, biopsy material is required to exclude these other causes before a diagnosis of aphthous ulceration can be made in persistent disease.

Unfortunately, in many cases, no infection can be found, and the ulcers are termed aphthous. However, it is likely that undiagnosed infection, for example Coxsackie virus, HIV itself (oral ulcers being associated with acute HIV infection[15]) or another opportunist organism may underlie some of these. Symptomatic treatment for resistant, severe oral and oesophageal ulcers of this type is often difficult. There are anecdotal reports of success with thalidomide[16], but the side-effects, neuropathy and teratogenicity, mean it has to be used with caution.

Neutropenia, secondary to drug treatments for HIV-associated conditions is also associated with oral ulceration; it may require cessation of therapy or use of granulocyte-colony stimulating factor (G-CSF). We have recently observed an interesting case of a patient with HIV-associated neutropenia, whose severe persistent oral ulcers healed when the neutrophil count was elevated with G-CSF. Following this, the ulcers consistently returned if the neutrophil count was allowed to drop below even 3.0 × 106/L (Dr Richard Coker, personal communication). Whether this is due to neutrophil function defects is under investigation.

Gingivo-stomatitis

This is another common and distressing problem associated with HIV infection. Specific causes such as *Mycobacterium avium intracellulare* may be identified but, in most cases, no pathogens are isolated, although broad-spectrum antibiotic cover for both anaerobes and aerobes can be helpful. Nutrition is often poor in patients with advanced HIV disease, and vitamin and protein deficiency should be treated.

HIV-positive individuals have an increased rate of allergic drug reactions, common ones being to sulpha drugs (as used in co-trimoxazole treatment for *Pneumocystis carinii* pneumonia) and ciprofloxacin[17]. Stevens–Johnson syndrome is therefore more frequent in this group.

Nose and sinuses

Sinusitis

Disease of the sinuses is the most common presentation in this area, the main cause being allergic disease and infection.

Allergic disorders

Atopic disorders are increased in HIV-infected individuals. This is usually an exacerbation of pre-existing disease, rather than a completely new development[18,19]. In infants, eczema is the most common problem, whereas in adults respiratory tract disease, often allergic sinusitis and rhinitis, present frequently. The increased susceptibility may be a result of poor regulation of IgE synthesis, which is under the control of T helper lymphocytes. It is therefore of interest that some HIV-positive patients with atopic disease have shown a reduction in symptoms with γ-interferon treatment[18]. γ-IFN is normally produced by the subset of T helper cells that downregulate IgE synthesis and its production is diminished in HIV infection.

Standard treatment is used for symptom control. However, it is not advisable that long-term high-dose topical corticosteroids are utilized, as absorption may lead to further systemic immunosuppression.

Infection

Although the 'opportunist' organisms that characteristically cause infection at other sites, for example *Pneumocystis carinii*, *Histoplasma* and *mycobacteria*, or unusual organisms, such as *Legionella pneumophilus*, *Pseudoalleschere boydii*[20] and mycobacteria, can cause infection in the sinuses, these are rare. The infections are generally with the same spectrum of bacteria that cause sinusitis in the immunocompetent host (*Haemophilus influenzae*, *Streptococcus pneumoniae*, and *Staphylococcus aureus*) but with a much higher incidence. Children are particularly susceptible; this is thought to be due to the poor antibody response in this group (see above). In adults with HIV infection, there is characteristically a polyclonal hyper-γ-globulinaemia. However, this hides the common finding of IgG_2 subclass deficiency, which is associated with susceptibility to recurrent pyogenic infection, especially of the respiratory tract[5].

Drug-induced neutropenia increases the risk of invasive fungal infections, such as with *Aspergillus* and *Candida* spp. In our experience, this potential is heightened by the concurrent use of systemic corticosteroids (which are sometimes used to alleviate generalized symptoms associated with late-stage HIV infection, or to reduce raised intracranial pressure). For this reason, they should be avoided if at all possible.

Tumour

In a similar way to the opportunist infections characteristic of HIV-related disease, tumours such as Kaposi's sarcoma and lymphoma only occasionally invade this area. However, their presence in the post-nasal space may lead to obstruction of sinus drainage and therefore secondary infection.

Nasal lesions

Nasal ulcers due to herpes simplex are common. Epistaxis may be due to the autoimmune idiopathic thrombocytopenia associated with HIV infection, or due to drug-induced thrombocytopenia, the presence of local tumour or infection.

Nasopharyngeal lesions

Lymphadenopathy

Benign lymphoid hyperplasia of the adenoids has been reported as a relatively common cause of symptoms[21,22].

Infection

Fungal infections including histoplasmosis, aspergillosis, mycobacterial disease and mucormycosis, may all cause erosive granulomatous disease in the nasopharynx.

Tumour

Kaposi's sarcoma appears to have a particular predilection for the nasopharynx in African patients, having an increased incidence at this site in patients compared with other groups with Kaposi's sarcoma. Patients may present with hearing loss, recurrent sinusitis and otitis media or pain due to sinus or eustachian tube obstruction.

Apart from Kaposi's sarcoma, non-Hodgkin's lymphoma (NHL) is the most common tumour observed. It is often extranodal, favouring the CNS, gastrointestinal tract and nasopharyngeal space. Short non-protein coding EBV transcripts have been demonstrated in a high proportion of CNS NHL[23]. Whether this will also be the case for nasopharyngeal disease is yet to be addressed. Tumours commonly erode through the palate. Necrosis and secondary infection lead to fetor. Despite the increased mucosal sensitivity to radiotherapy reported in AIDS patients[24], this treatment can give excellent results with both tumours.

Ear

The main problems to involve the outer ear are otitis externa, due to seborrhoeic dermatitis, and infections which are similar to those observed in non-HIV-infected patients (with *Aspergillus* or *Pseudomonas* spp.). Kaposi's sarcoma commonly involves the auricle but disease does not usually affect the inner ear. Acute bacterial otitis media is common in children[25].

Sensorineural hearing loss is documented in up to 50% of AIDS patients. There are several causes including drugs such as the chemotherapeutic agent, vincristine, aminoglycoside antibiotics and the antifungal agent, amphotericin. Inadequately treated syphilis may reactivate and is a cause of deafness that needs to be excluded. HIV itself has also been proposed as a cause[26].

The conditions discussed above represent the bulk of HIV-related disease affecting the ENT area. There are case reports of many other unusual presentations of opportunist infections but these are rare. Examples would be CNS infections, such as cryptococcal meningitis leading to nerve lesions secondary to inflammation, direct infection of nerves such as by CMV leading to laryngeal nerve paralysis[27], and acute HIV infection causing transient cranial nerve lesions. Other tumours such as Hodgkin and Burkitt lymphoma[28], and squamous cell carcinomas[29] may be increased in HIV infection, and present atypically in the immunosuppressed patient.

CONCLUSION

Infections can present in an atypical form in the immunocompromised, and organisms usually considered to be non-pathogenic can cause significant disease in such individuals. The inflammatory response is often lacking so that histological appearances are atypical (for example the lack of granuloma formation in mycobacterial infections) and appropriate antibody responses cannot be produced during acute infections, making serological diagnosis difficult. This means that, for diagnosis, direct identification of organisms by culture or histology is necessary. Multiple infections are very frequent and, if a patient does not respond to the treatment of a proven infection or tumour, then concurrent disease should be searched for before deciding that the initial treatment was not effective.

Many of the signs (both early and late) of HIV infection can present to the ENT clinic. It is important to recognize these as it may be the first time that HIV infection is suspected. As the available treatments for HIV[30] and its associated disorders improve, it becomes more important that infection is diagnosed early and appropriate treatment instigated.

References

1. Seligman M, Pinching AJ, Rosen FS, Fahey JL, Khaitov RM, Klatzmann D, Koenig S, Luo N, Ngu J, Reith-Muller G, Spria TJ. Immunology of HIV infection and AIDS – an update. Ann Intern Med. 1987;17:234.
2. Pinching AJ, Nye KE. Defective signal transduction – a common pathway for cellular dysfunction in HIV infection? Immunol Today. 1990;11:256.
3. Ammann AJ, Schiffman G, Abrams D, Volberding P, Zeigler J, Conent M. B-cell immunodeficiency in acquired immunodeficiency syndrome. J Am Med Assoc. 1984;251:1447.
4. Rogers LA, Forster SM, Pinching AJ. IgD production and other lymphocyte functions in HIV infections; immaturity and activation of B-cells at different clinical stages. Clin Exp Immunol. 1989;75:7.
5. Parkin JM, Helbert M, Hughes C, Pinching AJ. Association of IgG subclass deficiency and pyogenic infections in patients with AIDS. AIDS. 1989;3:37.
6. Peters BS, Beck EJ, Coleman DG, Wadsworth MJH, McGuinness O, Harris JRW, Pinching AJ. Changing disease patterns in patients with AIDS in a referral centre in the United Kingdom: the changing face of AIDS. Br Med J. 1991;302:203.
7. Northfelt DW. Extrapulmonary pneumocystosis in patients taking aerosolised pentamidine. Lancet. 1989;2:1454.
8. Kibbler CC, Odds FC. Fluconazole versus ketoconazole in oropharyngeal candidiasis in AIDS. Lancet. 1989;1:1130–1.
9. Greenspan JS, Greenspan D, Lennette ET, Abrams DI, Conant MA, Petersen V, Freese UK. Replication of Epstein–Barr virus within the epithelial cells of oral hairy leukoplakia, an AIDS-associated lesion. N Engl J Med. 1985;313:1564–71.
10. DeSouza YG, Greenspan D, Felton JR, Hartzog GA, Hammer M. Localization of Epstein–Barr virus DNA in the epithelial cells of oral hairy leukoplakia by in situ hybridisation on tissue sections. N Engl J Med. 1989;320:1559–60.
11. Logan RPH, Polson RJ, Kitchen VS, Harris JRW, Baron JH, Pinching AJ. Oral leukoplakia and HIV. Lancet. 1990;335:170.
12. Stafford ND, Herdman RC, Forster S, Munro AJ. Kaposi sarcoma of the head and neck in patients with AIDS. J Laryngol Otol. 1989;103:379–82.
13. Levy FE, Tansek KM. AIDS-associated Kaposi's sarcoma of the larynx. Ear Nose Throat J. 1990;69:182–4.
14. Lalwani AK, Snyderman NL. Pharyngeal ulceration in AIDS patients secondary to

cytomegalovirus infection. Ann Otol Rhinol Laryngol. 1991;100:484–7.
15. Gaines H, Pehrson PO, Lundbergh P, von Sydow M. Clinical picture of primary HIV infection presenting as a glandular fever-like illness. Br Med J. 1988;297:1363–8.
16. Youle M, Hawkins D, Gazzard B. Thalidomide in hyperalgic pharyngeal ulceration of AIDS. Lancet. 1990;335:1591.
17. Peters B, Pinching AJ. Fatal anaphylaxis associated with ciprofloxacin in a patient with AIDS-related complex. Br Med J. 1989;298:605.
18. Parkin JM, Eales L-J, Galazka AR, Pinching AJ. Atopic manifestations of the acquired immunodeficiency syndrome. Response to interferon gamma. Br Med J. 1987;194:1185.
19. Lim DT, Enright T, Shetty R, Park L. Asthma, recurrent sinopulmonary disease and HIV infection (clinical conference). Ann Allergy. 1988;61:175–6.
20. Schlanger G, Lutwick LI, Kurzman M, Hoch B, Chandler FW. Sinusitis caused by Legionella pneumophila in a patient with the acquired immunodeficiency syndrome. Am J Med. 1984;77:957–60.
21. Fairley JW, Dhillon RS, Weller IVD. HIV, glue ear and adenoidal hypertrophy. Lancet. 1988;2:1421–2.
22. Barzan L, Carbone A, Saracchini S, Vaccher G, Tirelli U, Comoretto R. Nasopharyngeal lymphatic tissue hypertrophy in HIV-infected patients. Lancet. 1989;1:42–3.
23. MacMahon EME, Glass JD, Hayward SD, Mann RB, Becker PS, Charache P, McArthur JC, Ambinder RF. Epstein–Barr virus in AIDS-related primary central nervous system lymphoma. Lancet. 1991;2:969.
24. Watkins EB, Findlay P, Gelmann E, Lane HC, Zabel A. Enhanced mucosal reactions in AIDS patients receiving oropharyngeal irradiation. Int J Radiat Oncol Biol Phys. 1987;13:1403–8.
25. Principi N, Marchisio P, Tornaghi R, Onorato J, Massironi E, Picco P. Acute otitis media in human immunodeficiency virus-infected children. Pediatrics. 1991;88:566–71.
26. Timon CI, Walsh MA. Sudden sensorineural hearing loss as a presentation of HIV infection. J Laryngol Otol. 1989;103:1071–2.
27. Small PM, McPhaul LW, Sooy CD, Wofsy CB, Jacobson MA. Cytomegalovirus infection of the largyngeal nerve presenting as horseness in patients with acquired immunodeficiency syndrome. Am J Med. 1989;86:108–10.
28. Schoem SR, Morton AL. Paranasal sinus Burkitt's lymphoma in a human immunodeficiency virus (HIV) positive male. Ear Nose Throat J. 1990;69:844–6.
29. Alhashimi MM, Krasnow SH, Johnston EA, Cohen MH. Squamous cell carcinoma of the epiglottis in a homosexual man at risk for AIDS. J Am Med Assoc. 1985;253:2366.
30. Volberding PA, et al. Zidovudine in asymptomatic human immunodeficiency virus infection. N Engl J Med. 1990;322:941.

Further reading

Herdman RC, Forster S, Stafford ND, Pinching AJ. The recognition and management of the otolaryngological manifestations of AIDS. Clin Otolaryngol. 1989;14:323–32.
Rubin MS, Prasad S. Otologic disease in the acquired immunodeficiency syndrome. Ear Nose Throat J. 1990;69:451–3.

3
The Immunology of the Tonsil

G. K. SCADDING

INTRODUCTION

The tonsil forms part of Waldeyer's ring of lymphoid tissue at the entrance to the respiratory and gastrointestinal systems. It functions as part of the mucosal associated lymphoid tissue (MALT), providing lymphocytes to identify and reject pathogenic organisms. The major function of the tonsil appears to be that of a recognition site where immature B lymphocytes meet antigen and undergo the initial stages of differentiation towards antibody-producing plasma cells.

THE LYMPHOID SYSTEM

This is organized into primary and secondary organs (Table 1).

Primary lymphoid organs

Lymphocytes develop in the bone marrow. From here, T lymphoctes migrate to the thymus where they become educated to recognize foreign antigens in

Table 1 Primary and secondary lymphoid organs

Primary	*Secondary*
Bone marrow	Spleen
Thymus	Lymph nodes
	Mucosal-associated lymph tissue (MALT) including: Gut-associated lymphoid tissue (GALT) Bronchial-associated lymphoid tissue (BALT) Tonsil Urinogenital tract lymphoid tissue Mammary lymphoid tissue Salivary lymphoid tissue

the context of self-histocompatibility antigens. Millions of lymphocytes die in the thymus, possibly because they are auto-reactive; the survivors are then spread throughout the blood and lymphoid system.

Secondary lymphoid organs

B lymphocytes pass from the bone marrow to the secondary lymphoid organ where they contact antigen and other lymphoid tissues. The immune response to antigen is made in the secondary lymphoid tissues and is disseminated from them.

The MALT is a secondary lymphoid organ concerned with immunity at mucosal surfaces. It generates antigen-sensitized B cells which, after some second signal (S) can differentiate into plasma cells capable of antibody secretion. Antibody responses at mucosal surfaces are largely separate from those occurring systemically. The nasal mucosa has been investigated immunohistologically and found not to contain organized lymphoid structures of maturing B lymphocytes, only their terminal form: antibody-producing plasma cells. The palatine tonsil, however, demonstrates a typical lymphoid structure and contains all activation and differentiation stages of B lymphocytes from premature to plasma cells. This suggests that the human nasal mucosa is not itself capable of providing a local immune response, but is dependent on lymphoid organs, like the tonsils, as the regional mucosal lymphoid tissue.

ANTIGEN CONTACT

The tonsils receive antigen through their crypt epithelium, unlike the majority of lymph nodes which receive it via the blood stream. At the base of the palatal tonsillar crypts are specialized M (micropore) cells with an antigen transport system. These were first described in Peyer's patches and have recently been seen in the nasopharyngeal tonsillar epithelium. Micropores are also found on crypt wall but these could be artefacts rather than physiological. The epithelial covering of the various MALT organs does vary: the oral palatine and lingual tonsils have squamous epithelium, the pharyngeal and laryngeal tonsils have ciliated epithelium, whereas the Peyer's patches and appendix have columnar epithelium. There are also differences in the relationship between the small salivary glands adjacent to the various tonsils, e.g the crypts of the lingual tonsils are washed through by saliva, but those of the palatine tonsils are not.

TONSILLAR IMMUNOHISTOLOGY

Using monoclonal antibodies directed against B cell, T cell and macrophage cell surface receptors, it has been shown that there are OK T6+ cells, probably representing Langerhans cells, which are capable of antigen presentation, in the crypt epithelium. The cells in the germinal centres are B cells, those in the outer mantle zone being immature: dense, with surface IgM and IgD. More central B cells show maturation changes, losing first their IgD and then surface IgM, and are less dense. Both populations express Class II HLA antigens: DR, DP and DQ. T cells are mainly present in interfollicular areas, although there are a few within germinal centres in a linear distribution on the capsular side; the majority are of the helper phenotype, with some suppressor/cytotoxic T cells seen between follicles. In the germinal centre there are also large dendritic cells with membrane and or cytoplasmic staining for HLA Class II antigens.

The likely fate of antigen within the tonsils is as follows. It is probably taken up and processed by HLA Class II positive antigen-presenting cells, which are either macrophages or Langerhans cells, or even epithelial cells. Antigenic fragments are then presented in association with HLA DR molecules to T helper cells which have the correct receptor to recognize the combination. B lymphocytes bearing the relevant antigen receptor (antibody) on their surface are activated by this combination of T cell/macrophage and antigen and start to divide. These events take place in the germinal centres which are found in large numbers in tonsillar tissue (Figures 1 and 2). Immature B lymphocytes move from the mantle zone to the middle of the germinal centre. Subsequently the majority of these B cells migrate through blood and lymphatics, maturing meanwhile, to colonize various secretory structures, such as respiratory tract, mammary glands and salivary glands. At these sites various second signals, which could include further antigen contact, T cell cytokines, local hormones or mitogen, cause terminal differentiation of the maturing B cells into immunoglobulin-secreting plasma cells. A proportion of these cells do not undergo this differentiation but remain as memory cells, capable of being stimulated on a further occasion.

HOMING OF B LYMPHOCYTES

It seems that the majority of B lymphocytes home or return to the organ of the site of their initial stimulation. For example, gut-derived lymphocytes appear to home selectively to gut. Tonsillar lymphocytes probably return to both upper and lower respiratory tract, including the tonsil. Mammary and salivary glands appear to derive lymphocytes from both gut and respiratory tract.

In addition, there is continuous lymphocyte traffic between lymphoid organs via blood and lymphatics; approximately 1–2% of the lymphocyte pool recirculates hourly. This permits lymphocytes to meet their appropriate antigen, since there is a finite number of lymphocytes capable of reacting with any particular antigenic epitope.

IMMUNOGLOBULIN SECRETION

Immunoglobulin A (IgA) is the major immunoglobulin secreted by MALT lymphocytes. It acts as 'mucosal antiseptic paint', being able to combine

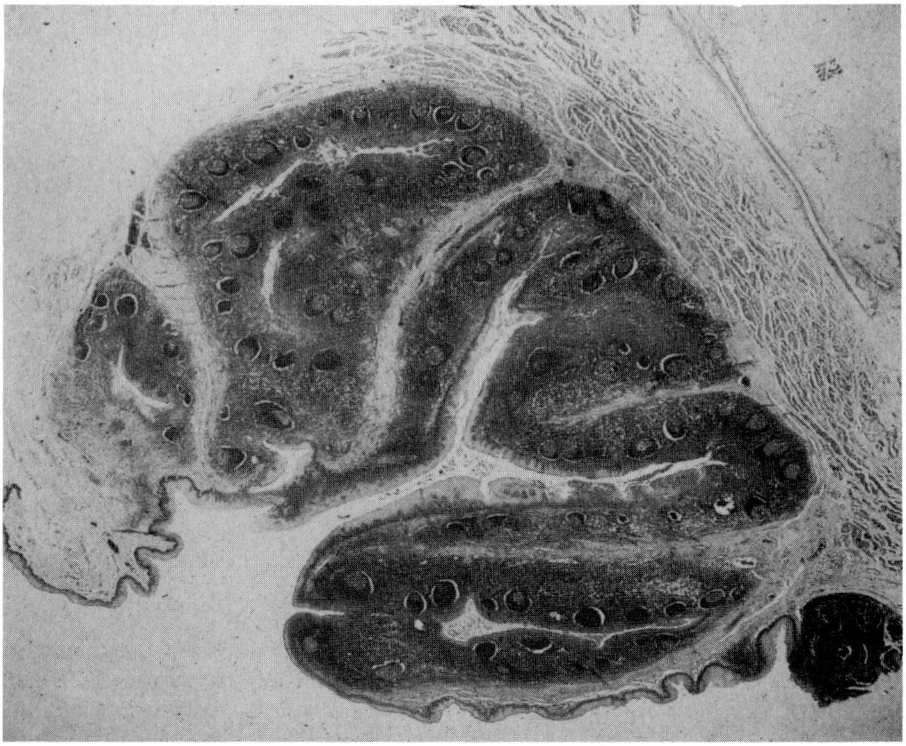

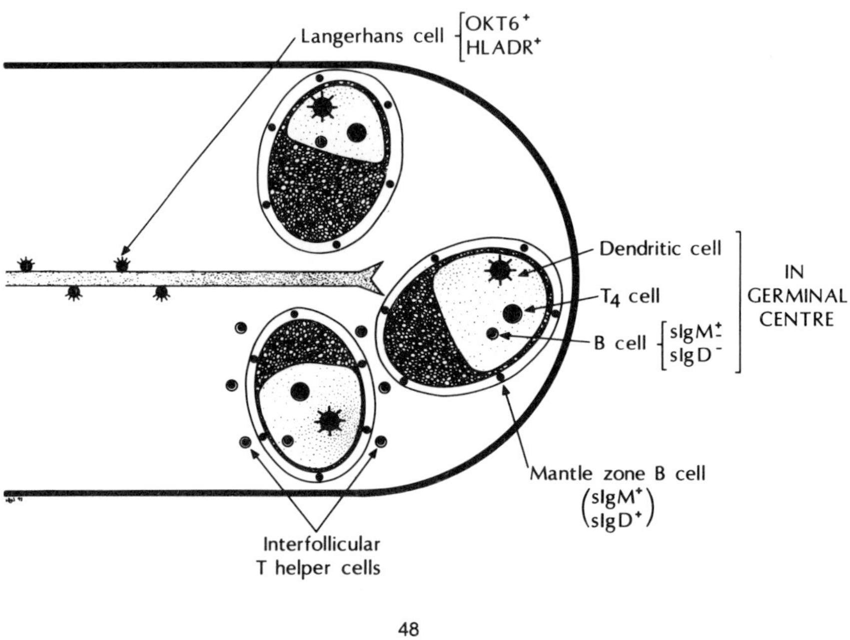
Langerhans cell
OKT6⁺
HLADR⁺
Dendritic cell
T4 cell
B cell
sIgM⁺
sIgD⁻
IN GERMINAL CENTRE
Mantle zone B cell
(sIgM⁺
sIgD⁺)
Interfollicular
T helper cells

Figure 1 Opposite. (a) Section of human tonsil to show MALT. The crypts are seen with, beneath them, large numbers of germinal centres. (Reprinted with kind permission of Gower Medical, London from Roitt, Brostoff, Male, eds. Immunology, 2nd edn, 1989). (b) Diagrammatic representation to show cell population of this tissue as assessed by immunohistology

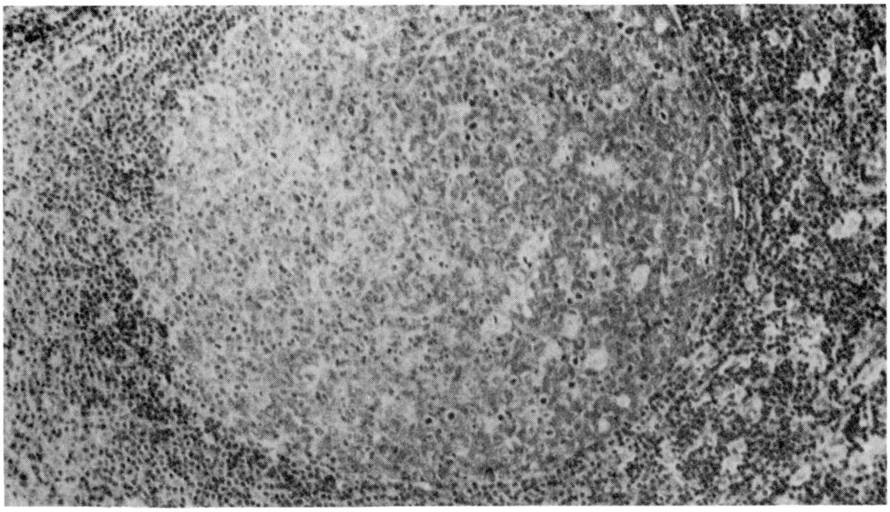

Figure 2 Germinal centre. This contains actively proliferating B lymphocytes, the most active, together with macrophages, being in the darker portion. The outer or mantle zone contains smaller denser resting B cells. (Reprinted with kind permission of Gower Medical, London from Roitt, Brostoff, Male, eds. Immunology, 2nd edn, 1989)

with pathogens, toxins or other molecules, either preventing attachment and absorption or rendering them harmless. Immune complexes thus formed are transported to the liver and dealt with by the reticuloendothelial system. Human IgA occurs in polymeric and monomeric forms and in two subclasses, IgA_1 and IgA_2, which show differential distribution between the mucosal and circulatory parts of the immune system. Secretory IgA is a dimeric immunoglobulin molecule, the two individual molecules being held together by a J chain, which is also formed by the plasma cell. IgA dimers bind to membrane receptors on the internal surface of the epithelial cells. They are endocytosed and transported across the cell to the luminal surface where the vesicle fuses with the plasma membrane, releasing dimeric IgA and a secretory component derived from cleavage of the poly-Ig receptor. This secretory component probably protects the immunoglobulin from enzymic digestion in the lumen of the gut (Figure 3).

In comparison to monomers, polymeric immunoglobulins, even if of low intrinsic affinity for antigenic determinants, possess high avidity for multivalent or solid-phase antigens due to the presence of 4–10 antigen-binding sites per molecule. Polymeric IgA is thus more effective in virus neutralization than corresponding monomeric IgA and is also bound more effectively by receptors on phagocytes, T cells and hepatocytes, probably

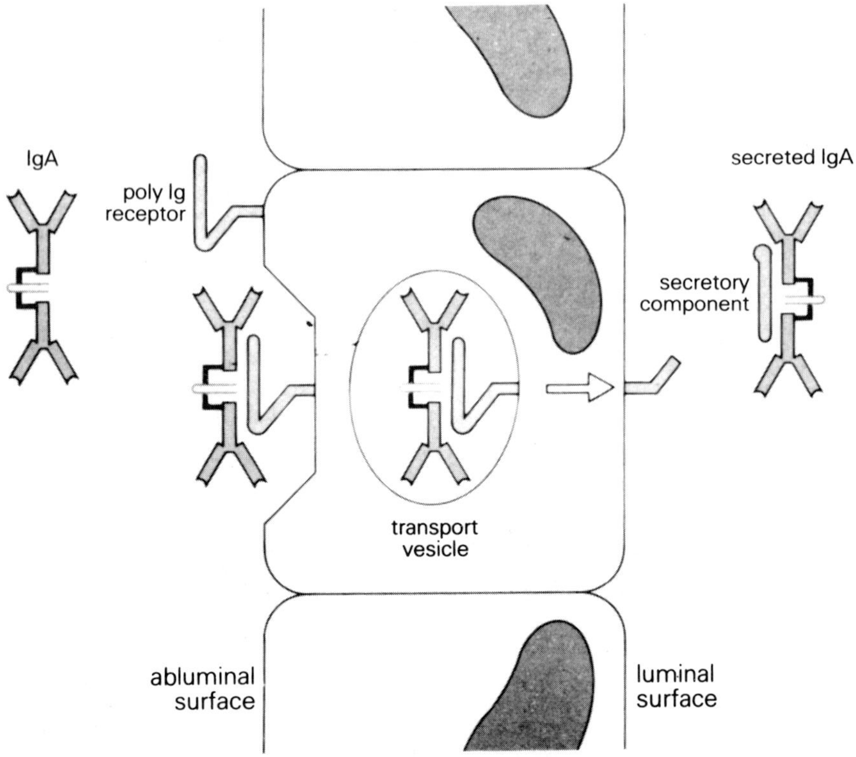

Figure 3 IgA transport across mucosal epithelium. Dimeric IgA molecules, joined by a J-chain are secreted by plasma cells. They are bound by the poly-immunoglobulin receptor on the mucosal surface of the epithelial cell, endocytosed and transported in a vesicle to the luminal surface. Here the vesicle fuses with the cell surface membrane, releasing dimeric IgA and a secretory component, derived from the poly-Ig receptor, which may provide protection against enzymic digestion in the lumen. (Reprinted with kind permission of Gower Medical, London from Roitt, Brostoff, Male, eds. Immunology, 2nd edn, 1989)

reflecting greater functional activity.

Functional differences between IgA_1 and IgA_2 have not been fully elucidated, but some differences exist. IgA_1 binds more effectively to hepatocytes and to fibronectin; IgA_2 is a more efficient inhibitor of carbohydrate (mannose)-dependent bacterial adherence. The distribution of IgA_1 and IgA_2 differs between tissues: the upper aerodigestive tract is populated by IgA_1-producing cells, while the lower digestive and female genital tracts contain equal numbers of IgA_1- and IgA_2-producing cells. This is interesting in view of the fact that several important mucosal pathogens elaborate IgA_1 proteases which cleave one of the Pro—Thr or Pro—Ser bonds of the hinge region to yield Fab and Fc fragments. These proteases appear to be virulence factors since non-pathogenic strains do not make them. It is possible that the Fab antibody fragments coat the organism harmlessly, rendering it invulnerable to other defence mechanisms.

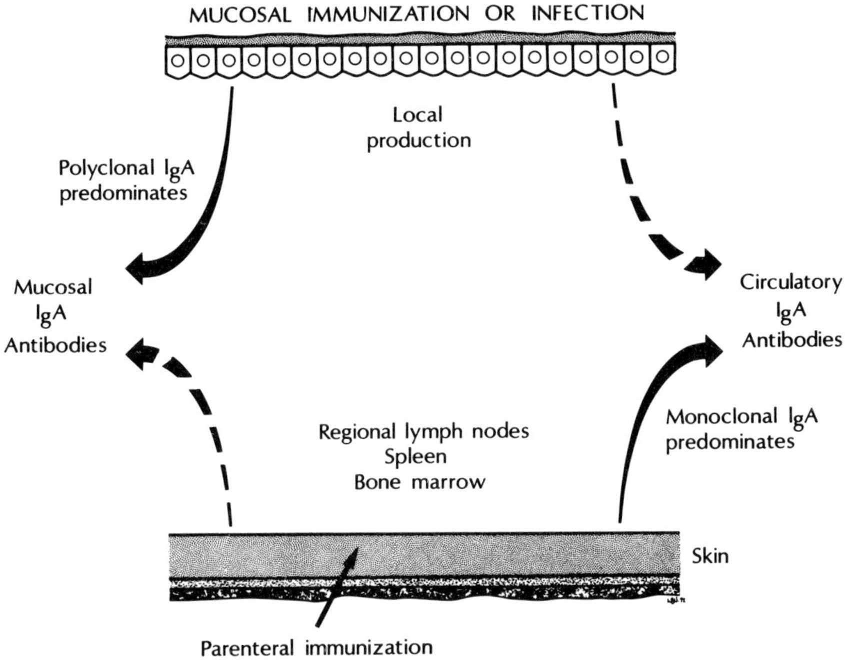

Figure 4 IgA produced by mucosal immunization is polyclonal. The subclass depends on the nature of the antigen (proteins induce predominantly IgA_1 and polysaccharides IgA_2). A systemic response does not usually occur unless the antigen is live. Parenteral immunization induces a circulatory IgA response, but is an inefficient route of immunization for the mucosal component. Serum IgA is predominantly monoclonal and of the IgA_1 subclass. Diagram modified from Russell Maw et al. Clin Immunol. 1992;87:1–6, with kind permission from Blackwell Scientific Publications

Plasma IgA is predominantly monomeric and of the IgA_1 subclass. It is probably derived from bone marrow, regional lymph nodes and spleen, but there is evidence for a small contribution from mucosal tissue, especially following mucosal presentation of live organisms. The IgA-producing cells in the mucosal compartment mature earlier so that secretory IgA reaches adult levels before systemic IgA. Systemic immunization probably contributes little to mucosal immunity (Figure 4).

Tonsillar immunoglobulin secretion differs in several respects from the usual MALT pattern. Immunoglobulin G (IgG)-producing cells predominate in nasopharyngeal and palatine tonsils, with only 30–35% IgA immunocytes present. There is no tonsillar secretory piece production, both IgA and IgG passing out directly between epithelial cells into pharyngeal secretions. This process is enhanced when there is inflammation present. The adenoids, however, do produce secretory piece.

IgD-producing cells are more common than in gut lymphoid tissue, although they form only 1–3% of tonsillar immunocytes. Bacteria which inhabit the upper respiratory tract, but not the gut, have IgD receptors and these probably stimulate the multiplication and division of IgD-bearing B lymphocytes, thus causing the increased proportions present in tonsil. IgE-producing cells also occur in tonsils, being more common in tonsillectomy specimens than is atopy in the population, suggesting that atopic individuals are more likely to undergo tonsillectomy. Studies on immunoglobulin synthesis by pokeweed mitogen-stimulated tonsillar lymphocytes showed that lymphocytes of 12 out of 18 donors secreted IgE; all 18 secreted IgG. Radiosensitive T cells were found to exert a suppressive influence.

OTHER IMMUNE FUNCTIONS OF THE TONSIL

Tonsils contain elements of the innate immune system (see Chapter 1); natural killer cells are present in close relationship with blood vessels (Figure 4). These can kill tumour cells and virally infected cells, presumably by detecting surface alterations.

Of the 10^9 lymphocytes present in tonsil, about half are T cells. Many of these are helper T lymphocytes, which aid B lymphocyte antibody secretion as described above. Other T lymphocytes (T suppressor cells) may be involved in preventing or terminating unwanted antibody responses. Further T lymphocytes (Tdth) are involved in cell-mediated immune (delayed hypersensitivity) reactions to larger organisms, such as fungi and mycobacteria. Cytokines from stimulated Tdth cells can keep macrophages in the vicinity of the stimulating organism, activate them to increase phagocytosis and enhance their cytotoxic powers. Cytotoxic T cells can kill virus-infected cells. In these cases, the T cell antigen receptor, which is structurally similar to the antigen-combining site of antibody, is used to recognize the cell or organism. Tonsillar lymphocytes, as well as those from the adenoids, are capable of producing α-interferon (IFN) in amounts comparable to that produced by peripheral blood lymphocytes. The IFN-producing potential is constant in humans between the ages of 3 and 38 years and is not adversely affected during the first trimester of pregnancy.

IMMUNE DEFICIENCY

The commonest humoral immune deficiency, which involves about 1 in 500 to 1 in 700 of the population, is a selective deficiency of IgA. This may be a transient situation in children, in whom normal levels of IgA are not reached until about 7 years of age (Figure 5). About half of the individuals deficient in IgA suffer from an increase in respiratory tract and other mucosal surface infections; the remainder appear unaffected. There are two possible reasons for this: in the unaffected individuals IgM replaces IgA as protective secretory antibody; in the affected group there is an excess of IgD-producing plasma cells. IgD cannot act as secretory antibody and thus these individuals are prone to infection. Recently, it has become apparent that, in a proportion of IgA-deficient patients, there is a concomitant deficiency of an IgG subclass, usually IgG_2. These individuals, with a joint deficiency, are most likely to suffer repeated infections. There is also an association between IgA deficiency

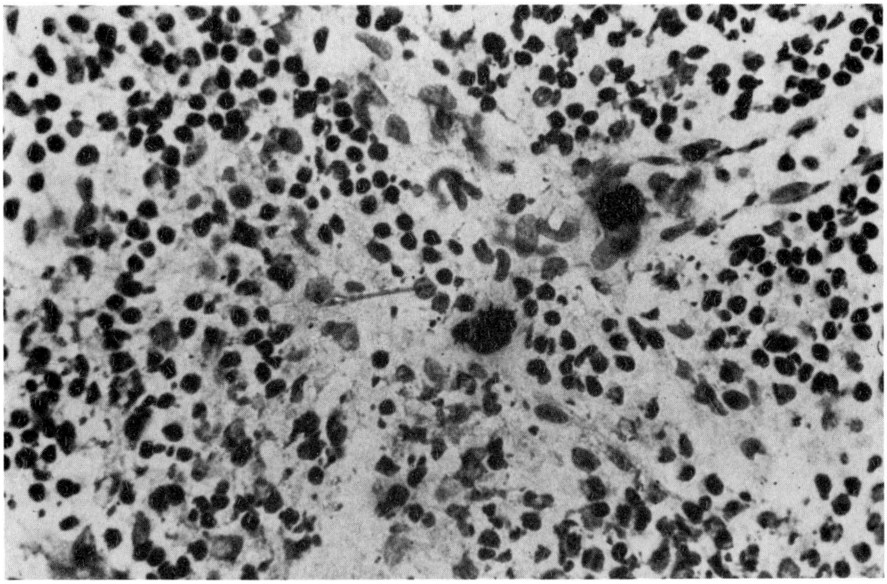

Figure 5 Two natural killer (NK) cells are shown in close approximation to blood vessels in this human tonsil section stained with HNK-1 monoclonal antibody conjugated with horseradish peroxidase. NK cells can kill cells with surface alterations due to neoplasia or viral infection. (Photograph courtesy of Ms H Wang, St Mary's Hospital)

and atopy, and, in some patients, with autoimmune disorders.

Absence of tonsillar tissue in small boys with recurrent infections suggests the possibility of more severe dysglobulinaemia, such as Bruton's disease.

INFLAMMATION OF THE TONSILS

The continuous presence of antigen on the tonsillar epithelium, followed by its presentation to lymphocytes, results in an amount of physiological inflammation.

Studies of the histological differences between chronically inflamed tonsillectomy specimens and 'normal' tonsils have been few in number. The former contain fewer activated lymphoid cells and immunoglobulin-containing cells, but this could be a primary defect. IgD-bearing cells are relatively increased in tonsillectomy specimens, possibly due to stimulation by bacteria. There are epithelial cell changes connected with chronic inflammation. Normally, reticulated epithelium covers only the follicles; in inflamed tonsils, this becomes continuous, with the later development of squamous epithelium over the follicles. There are no M cells present in this: thus antigen entry is probably decreased.

When organisms are trapped on or in the tonsil, but are able to multiply despite the immune mechanisms present, tonsillitis occurs. This is often polymicrobial. In one study[13], tonsil swabs were collected from 248 children who presented with acute tonsillitis. A β-haemolytic streptococcus was grown from over 50%, being especially common in children over 6 years (68%) and rare under 4 years (18%). The majority were Type A and 47% of typable isolates contained the potentially nephritogenic serotypes 8 and 12. Younger children showed a high isolation rate of viruses, with echo- and adenoviruses being common. There was no clinical difference between those with viral isolates and those with streptococci.

It is probable that several predisposing factors are involved, including virulence of the organisms, failure of host defence and possible local β-lactamase production by other bacteria within the tonsil. Histamine release from tonsillar mast cells can be caused by bacteria; this will add to the inflammation present. Chronic viral infection, e.g. with Epstein–Barr virus can reduce host resistance via alteration of T cell functions.

Not all tonsillitis is infective. Nasal challenge with allergen can result in sore throats and tonsillar inflammation after several hours. This is probably related to the late allergic reaction, consisting of inflammatory cell infiltration, oedema of the mucosa, and hyperreactivity. When allergen exposure is chronic, the initial immediate reaction is not always obvious. Therefore a detailed history and skin prick testing or RAST testing are necessary to identify the responsible allergens. Cows' milk ingestion has been postulated as a causative factor in the increased incidence of tonsillitis in European children compared with African children in Rhodesia. Symptoms can result from allergy alone or by infection which follows the mucosal oedema and obstruction. Treatment of the underlying allergy should reduce the number of episodes of 'tonsillitis'. A recent paper[7] showed that children presenting for ENT operations were far more likely to be atopic than those attending hospital for orthopaedic problems. They were far more likely to respond to medical treatment (90%) than surgical treatment (40%).

TONSILLECTOMY

Although tonsillectomy has been practised since classical times, knowledge of the exact function of the tonsil and of the effect of tonsillectomy is incomplete. In the human, the tonsils are most active during childhood with some involution occurring after puberty. However, there is still evidence of B cell activity in adults as old as 80.

The indications for tonsillectomy remain controversial. Obviously, malignant disease and obstructive sleep apnoea caused by hypertrophic tonsils are definite indications for tonsillectomy. There is little evidence that tonsillectomy and/or adenoidectomy have an influence on the natural history of upper respiratory tract infections. In particular, there is no evidence for prevention of the recurrence of streptococcal hypersensitivity diseases, such as rheumatic fever. A controlled study over 11 years involving twelve authors[6] showed that the benefit from tonsillectomy in rigorously selected patients presenting with recurrent severe tonsillitis was modest. The operated group showed some advantage over the non-operated group over the first 2 years. However, the latter suffered less than three infections a year and these were mostly minor. Conversely, there was a 14% incidence of complications related to surgery. These results are similar to those of an earlier study[5] which also noted a decrease in sore throats for the first 2 years post-operation.

There is, however, some evidence that adenoidectomy has a prolonged influence upon recurrent secretory otitis media.

Immunological effects of tonsillectomy

Children undergoing tonsillectomy were studied by Donovan et al.[11]. They showed a decrease in the activated B cell population, decreased secretory IgA and low normal levels of other immunoglobulins. Sequential studies pre- and post-tonsillectomy are few.

There does not appear to be a postoperative general increase in infections. However, resistance to polio viruses is reduced. Previously orally immunized children showed a three- to four-fold fall in antipoliovirus titre following tonsillectomy and adenoidectomy. Seronegative children who had tonsils and adenoids removed prior to immunization showed delayed and lowered secretory IgA responses to polio virus in nasopharyngeal secretions.

Theoretically, the increased meningococcal carrier state after tonsillectomy could increase the risk of meningococcal meningitis. This has only been noted in Russia, where there have been five reports since 1959 (reviewed in 10).

In 1971, an increased incidence of Hodgkin's disease in tonsillectomized children in New York was reported[9]. This has been further investigated by several authors with conflicting results[10]. It seems that the association could be between Hodgkin's disease and tonsillitis, rather than tonsillectomy.

The immune defects post-tonsillectomy are slight, but could well be relevant in an area where polio virus is endemic. This, and the possibility that other treatable underlying defects, such as allergic disease and immune deficiency, may be responsible for a patient's symptoms, should be considered before proceeding to tonsillectomy for recurrent tonsillitis.

References and further reading

Tonsillar immunoglobulins

1. Brandtzaeg P. Immunobarriers of the mucosa of the upper respiratory and upper digestive pathways. Acta Otolaryngol (Stockh). 1988;105:172–80.
2. Brandtzaeg P, Surgan L, Berdal P. Immunoglobulin system of human tonsils. I. Control subjects of various ages: quantification of Ig-producing cells, tonsillar morphometry, and serum Ig concentrations. Clin Exp Immunol. 1978;31:367–75.
3. Surjan L Jr, Brandtzaeg P, Berdal P. Immunoglobulin systems of human tonsils. II. Patients with chronic tonsillitis or tonsillar hyperplasia: quantification of Ig-producing cells, tonsillar morphometry and serum Ig concentrations. Clin Exp Immunol. 1978;31:386–90.
4. Brandtzaeg P, Karlsson G, Petruson B, Bjorkander J, Hanson LA. The clinical condition of IgA-deficient patients is related to the proportion of IgD- and IgM-producing cells in their nasal mucosa. Clin Exp Immunol. 1987;67:626–36.

Surgery

5. Mawson SR, Adlington P, Evans M. A controlled study evaluation of adeno-tonsillectomy in children. J Laryng. 1967;81:777–90.
6. Paradise JL, Bluestone CD, Bachmann RN, et al. Efficacy of tonsillectomy for recurrent throat infection in severely affected children. Results of parallel randomized and non-randomized clinical trials. N Engl J Med. 1984;310:674–84.
7. Sanderson J, Warner JO. Previous ENT surgery in children presenting with allergic perennial rhinitis. Clin Allergy. 1987;17:113–17.

Immunological studies pre- and post-tonsillectomy

8. Ogra PL. Effect of tonsillectomy and adenoidectomy on nasopharyngeal antibody responses to poliovirus. N Engl J Med. 1971;284:59–64.
9. Vianna NJ, Greenwald P, Davis JNP. Tonsillectomy and Hodgkin's disease. Lancet. 1971;2:168–9.
10. Langman AW, Kaplan MJ. Hodgkin's disease and tonsillectomy. Otolaryngol Clin N Am. 1987;20:399–404.
11. Donovan R, Soothill JF. Immunological studies in children undergoing tonsillectomy. Clin Exp Immunol. 1973;14:347–57.

IgA

12. Russell MW, Lue C, Van Den Wall Bake AWL, Moldoveanu Z, Mestecky J. Molecular heterogeneity of human IgA antibodies during an immune response. Clin Exp Immunol. 1992;87:1–6.

Tonsillitis

13. Douglas RM, Miles H, Hansman D, et al. Acute tonsillitis in children: microbial pathogens in relation to age. Pathology. 1984;16:1:79–82.

Tonsillar immunohistology

14. Yamanaka N, Sambe S, Harabuchi Y, et al. Immunohistological study of tonsil. Distribution of T cell subsets. Acta Oto-laryngol. 1983;96:509–16.
15. Feller AC, Parwaresh MR, Wacker HH, et al. Combined immunohistochemical staining for surface IgD and T-lymphocyte subsets with monoclonal antibodies in human tonsils. Histochem J. 1983;15:557–62.
16. Ledbetter JA, Clark EA. Surface phenotype and function of tonsillar germinal centre and mantle zone B cell subsets. Hum Immunol. 1986;15:30–43.

M-cells

17. Owen R, Jones A. Scanning electron microscopic evaluation of Peyer's patches in rats and humans. Anat Rec. 1973;175:404–5.
18. Owen R, Nemanic P. Antigen processing structures of the mammalian intestinal tract: an SEM study of lymphoepithelial organs. Scanning Electron Microsc. 1978;2:367–78.
19. Karchev T, Kabakchiev P. M cells in the epithelium of the nasopharyngeal tonsil. Rhinology. 1984;22:201–10.

4
Fungal Infections

R. J. HAY

TYPES OF FUNGAL INFECTION

The pathogenic fungi include many of the most prevalent causes of human disease, such as the ringworm fungi or *Candida* species, as well as rare and exotic infectious agents. The commonest are a group of organisms which only invade epithelial or mucosal surfaces, causing superficial mycoses. The principle infections amongst these are the dermatophytoses, or ringworm, superficial candidiasis, or thrush, and pityriasis versicolor. In the ear, otomycosis, an infection usually caused by moulds such as *Aspergillus niger* and confined to the surface of the external auditory meatus, is an example of a superficial fungal infection.

The second group, the subcutaneous fungal infections, are generally rare and are usually only found in the tropics and subtropics. They normally affect sites on the peripheries as they are infections which are introduced transcutaneously, often as a result of traumatic injury. Examples include mycetoma and sporotrichosis. While these may affect the region of the head and neck they are more commonly associated with lesions on the legs or arms. The subcutaneous disease conidiobolomycosis, previously known as rhinoentomophthoromycosis, however, involves the facial tissue and originates from the region of the inferior turbinates. It is a rare infection, mainly seen in the tropics and has been most often reported from West Africa.

Finally, certain fungi may cause deep invasive infections. These may occur in otherwise healthy patients (endemic systemic mycoses) or develop as a result of host predisposition (opportunistic mycoses). The first of these are common in certain parts of the world and are usually respiratory infections which may spread to other sites. The infection paracoccidioidomycosis, or South American blastomycosis, is an example which may involve the head and neck region by affecting the oral mucosa and hard palate in the course of systemic dissemination. The opportunistic infections include candidiasis

Table 1 Fungal infections in ENT disease

Infection	*Organism(s) – genus*	*ENT relevance*
Superficial mycoses		
Dermatophytosis (ringworm)	*Trichophyton* *Microsporum* *Epidermophyton*	Rarely affect the auricle
Superficial candidiasis	*Candida* spp.	May infect the external meatus, paranasal sinuses, pharynx
Pityriasis versicolor, *Pityrosporum* infections	*Pityrosporum*	Colonize external meatus
Subcutaneous mycoses		
Mycetoma	Many	Invasion of skull – rare
Sporotrichosis	*Sporothrix*	May infect face
Chromomycosis	Many	May infect face
Conidiobolomycosis	*Conidiobolus*	Infects subcutis of face
Systemic mycoses		
Opportunists		
Candidiasis	*Candida* spp.	ENT involvement – rare
Aspergillosis	*Aspergillus* spp.	Important (see text)
Mucormycosis	Many	Rhinocerebral mucormycosis
Cryptococcosis	*Cryptococcus*	ENT involvement – rare
Pathogens		
Histoplasmosis	*Histoplasma*	Oral ulcers in some forms
Blastomycosis	*Blastomyces*	ENT involvement – rare
Coccidioidomycosis	*Coccidioides*	ENT involvement – rare
Paracoccidioidomycosis	*Paracoccidioides*	Oral, palatal ulcers

Table 2 Pathogenesis of fungal disease

Tissue invasion
Toxin production, e.g. aflatoxin A from *Aspergillus flavus*
Allergy, e.g. *Aspergillus*, sinusitis, ?*Trichophyton*-sensitive perennial rhinitis

and aspergillosis as well as the less common infections, mucormycosis and cryptococcosis. These infections are a particular problem in immunocompromised patients, such as those with neutropenia or AIDS. However, they may also develop if there are abnormalities of organ structure or drainage and, for this reason, may localize in the paranasal sinuses.

Examples of these infections and their significance in diseases of the ear, nose and throat are shown in Table 1. This table is by no means comprehensive and for more detailed information the reader is referred to references 1, 2 and 3.

PATHOGENESIS OF DISEASE

While invasion of tissue is a feature of most mycoses, fungi may also contribute to the pathogenesis of disease in two other ways – by the formation of toxins (mycotoxicosis) and hypersensitivity or allergy. Toxin production is a property of a number of fungi, including some common aspergilli. For

Table 3 Host defence against fungal invasion

Innate	
	Ciliary activity
	Serum factors, e.g. transferrin
	Phagocytes – neutrophils, macrophages
	Natural killer (NK) cells
Acquired	
	Cell-mediated immunity
	Antibody

example *A. flavus* may elaborate mycotoxins such as aflatoxin A which is potentially hepatotoxic. Certain fungi are also common allergens and hypersensitivity may develop after exposure to inhaled particles, such as airborne spores or during the process of colonization or invasion. Immunological reactions are a particular feature of aspergillosis of the lung and there is some evidence to suggest that the same may occur in the paranasal sinuses. However, it is always difficult to separate which of the pathogenic properties of a particular organism can be attributed to invasion and which to an immunologically mediated reaction or even toxin production.

HOST DEFENCE AGAINST FUNGAL INVASION

Host resistance to fungal attack depends on two main mechanisms – those that do not require sensitization or prior exposure (natural or innate resistance) and acquired resistance or immunity. Neither function in isolation and defence depends on the interaction of both types of response.

Innate resistance to fungal infection

Natural resistance mechanisms include the direct participation of inhibitory serum factors and phagocytosis by neutrophils and macrophages, amongst others, in the destruction of fungi. Many fungi can be shown to be inhibited by non-immune human serum. For some time, the nature of these inhibitory substances has remained unknown, but one potential candidate is unsaturated transferrin[4]. This has been shown to interact directly with certain mycelial fungi, such as dermatophytes or zygomycetes to cause inhibition of their growth. The interaction involves binding of transferrin to the cell wall and the kinetics of the inhibition suggests that the mode of control is not solely dependent on competition for iron. Other potential inhibitory factors are probably only relevant in the skin[5], such as the presence of medium-chain-length fatty acids or in ciliated epithelium where clearance of inhaled fungal spores by ciliary activity is an important elimination mechanism.

Generally, fungi are susceptible to attack by phagocytic cells although many elaborate a catalase which may act as a defensive mechanism against respiratory burst products[6]. This also depends on the nature of the fungal propagule and whether it is in resting (spore) or hyphal phase. Airborne spores produced by organisms such as *Aspergillus* species or zygomycetes such as *Rhizopus* can penetrate to different parts of the upper respiratory tract. The first point of contact between the fungus and host defences is often a tissue macrophage. There is evidence from experimental animal work that aspergilli are highly susceptible to ingestion by macrophages in the lungs of rabbits but that zygomycete spores appear to resist destruction[7]. Rabbits with experimentally induced diabetes mellitus, on the other hand, are susceptible to both. In the case of *Aspergillus* spores, these are more easily destroyed if they are incubated in vitro for one or two hours prior to challenge, a phenomenon associated with swelling of the cell wall[8]. Other fungi can be similarly destroyed by such mechanisms. It appears, in the case of alveolar macrophages, that killing of aspergilli depends on both oxidative and non-oxidative mechanisms[9]. However, this does not involve myeloperoxidase which is not present in macrophages. The same is probably true of monocytes isolated from blood. One intriguing observation is that monocytes from patients with chronic granulomatous disease can kill aspergilli even though they cannot form reactive oxygen[10].

While the spore is probably the first fungal element, in many cases, to contact human epithelial surfaces, many fungi form chains of cells, hyphae or mycelium, which are too large to be ingested. In the case of aspergilli, some zygomycetes, *Candida* and dermatophytes, fungal cells can be destroyed without ingestion. The mechanism involves attachment of the fungus to the phagocyte cell surface. Once again, both oxidative and non-oxidative mechanisms are involved[11], although, in the case of *Rhizopus*, a zygomycete, non-oxidative mechanisms appear to play little part.

Polymorphonuclear leukocytes (PMN) are mobile sources of defence against fungal attack. For some time, it has been known that neutropenic patients are particularly susceptible to fungal infection with a variety of pathogens from *Candida* to *Aspergillus* species. The main exception amongst opportunistic fungi is *Cryptococcus*. These observations can be confirmed in animal models. Both aspergilli and zygomycete spores are susceptible to human neutrophils in vitro if they are metabolically active, but not if they are in the resting phase[12]. The mechanisms of killing depend on oxidative mechanisms, particularly the formation of reactive oxygen, such as single oxygen, as well as the myeloperoxidase halide system[13]. Other non-oxidative paths, such as the generation of cationic proteins, are also important effector mechanisms. Both systems appear to work on hyphal forms of these organisms as well as spores.

There is good evidence that many fungi are leukocyte attractants and that this may involve the mediation of the alternative pathway of complement activation[14,15]. Complement-independent attraction has also been demonstrated[16]. A further difference between the metabolically active spore and its resting phase can be seen in the observation that intranasally inoculated spores of *Rhizopus* will not attract neutrophils if they are in resting phase but will if they have been preincubated[16].

Natural killer (NK) cells have been shown to play a part in the destruction of some fungi, such as *Cryptococcus neoformans* and *Paracoccidioides brasiliensis*.

Immune defence against fungi

Antibody

The immune system also has an important part to play in defence against most fungi. Generally, the role of antibody in host defence against fungi is controversial. In the case of *Candida*, there is evidence that, in some animals, passive transfer of antibody can be protective[17] but this is not the experience of all workers and, indeed, most have found that antibody is ineffective in defence, as it is in dermatophytosis and aspergillosis[18]. Antibody may, however, play a role in some other forms of immunological defence, such as antibody-dependent cell-mediated cytotoxicity[19]: it may also be involved in the immunomodulation of cellular immunity.

Cell mediated immunity

This plays an important role in defence against many fungi. In the case of dermatophytes, *Cryptococcus* and *Histoplasma*, transfer of immunity can be correlated with the transfer of lymphocytes bearing the T helper phenotype from immune animals[20]. Infection is modified and may be more common in patients with defects in T lymphocyte numbers and function, such as AIDS. However, this is not universally true and some infections, such as systemic candidiasis and aspergillosis, are not common in AIDS patients, although they may occur. In aspergillosis, the role of cell-mediated immunity is particularly confusing. Some patients with defects in cellular immunity, such as recipients of renal and heart transplants appear to be susceptible to aspergillosis[21], whereas, in the absence of neutropenia, AIDS patients generally are not. Nu/nu mice which are congenitally defective in T lymphocytes are no more susceptible to experimental *Aspergillus* infections than their normal litter mates[22]. But it can be shown that resistance to infection can be transferred to naive animals by lymphocytes with the characteristics of T cells. Likewise, nu/nu mice are also no more susceptible to zygomycete infections. These observations suggest that, in these infections, T cell-mediated responses are less important in limiting penetration.

The effector mechanisms for fungal killing after T cell activation are also not well understood. The process may involve the recruitment of macrophages and production of the cytokine, MIF. Production of this factor had been found in candidiasis and dermatophytosis as well as other infections[23]. γ-Interferon produced by T lymphocytes may play a complicated role here as it not only arms monocytes to kill fungi, but also appears to enhance the capacity of neutrophils to kill *Candida* and possibly other fungi[24]. This is an example of collaboration between the immune and non-immune defence systems.

FUNGAL DISEASES OF THE EAR, NOSE AND THROAT

While the fungal infections described earlier may occasionally affect the ear, nose and throat, most are uncommon. There are, however, a small number

Table 4 Factors predisposing to *Candida* infection

Physiological: age, pregnancy	
Endocrine: diabetes mellitus, hypothyroidism, hypoparathyroidism, hypoadrenalism (CMC only)	
Immunological: neutrophil defects associated with cancer, leukaemia, drugs, congenital disease	
	T lymphocyte defects associated with cancer, leukaemia, drugs, HIV and congenital disease
Antibiotic therapy	
Presence of foreign material (dentures, IV cannulae)	
Local epithelial defects	
Miscellaneous: iron or zinc deficiency, malnutrition	

of infections which more commonly pose problems in ENT practice. These are discussed below.

Oropharyngeal candidiasis

Yeasts of the genus *Candida* are common commensals of the oral mucosa, gastrointestinal tract and vagina[25]. They are less frequently found on the healthy skin surface. The commonest of these organisms is the species *C. albicans* but other related species such as *C. tropicalis*, *C. parapsilosis* and *C. guilliermondii* may also be isolated, as well as *Candida* (*Torulopsis*) *glabrata*. The frequency of oral carriage may be very high in certain groups, such as hospitalized patients where up to 70% may have oral colonization. Generally, at least 18% of the population appear to be colonized at any time. While *Candida* species are normally commensals, they can also change status to become invasive pathogens. They are therefore endogenous opportunistic pathogens. A number of factors are known to play a role in the conversion of these yeasts from commensal to pathogen. These are listed in Table 4. In many cases, the underlying abnormalities, such as neutropenia and T lymphocyte dysfunction, are directly related to defective immunity. On other occasions, factors affecting the ability of the organism to adhere to underlying epithelium or compete with local bacteria (the effect of antibiotics) play a role by a direct effect on the fungus[26].

Oral candidiasis is the commonest disease caused by this organism. It usually presents in childhood or old age or in the presence of one of the underlying factors listed in Table 4. The commonest of these are denture wearing, antibiotic therapy, neutropenia or immunosuppression affecting T lymphocytes, including AIDS.

The patients present with soft white plaques on the buccal or palatal mucosa. These may coalesce to form a sheet of erythema and white debris. The affected area is often sore and the patients may be unable to tolerate hot foods. In chronic cases, the oral lesions may appear hyperplastic or atrophic with minimal plaque formation. A further variant, denture sore mouth or chronic atrophic candidiasis, presents with erythematous patches without a white pseudomembrane. The corners of the mouth often show cracking, angular cheilitis.

In the presence of retrosternal discomfort on swallowing in a patient with oral candidiasis, the possibility of oesophageal candidiasis should be considered[27]. Some patients, including those with HIV infections, may have asymptomatic oesophageal candidiasis[28]. This complication is more commonly seen in patients with the more profound forms of immunological disturbance. In these individuals, the presence of oesophageal infection may be associated with herpes simplex virus infection of the mucosa. Chronic oesophageal infection may occur in the rare syndrome of chronic mucocutaneous candidiasis and can result in the formation of oesophageal strictures.

Chronic mucocutaneous candidiasis (CMC)

This is a rare syndrome where there is a combination of oral and cutaneous candidiasis, often involving the finger nails, skin and scalp[29]. As mentioned above, oesophageal candidiasis may also occur in severely affected patients. Usually, these patients have an underlying medical or immunological abnormality. The commonest is the polyendocrinopathy syndrome which usually presents with either hyperparathyroidism and hypoadrenalism, or hypothyroidism, but other autoimmune abnormalities may occur, such as the coexistence of pernicious anaemia and alopecia areata. Other patients have a genetic predisposition to this condition inherited as either an autosomal dominant or recessive trait. Patients with CMC also appear to have difficulty in combatting other skin infections, such as dermatophytosis and viral warts. A host of different immunological abnormalities have been associated with CMC. These include *Candida*-specific defects in lymphocyte transformation, more general depression of lymphocyte blastogenesis, defective production of MIF, absent or reduced phagocytosis or intracellular killing of yeasts. These may be associated with cutaneous anergy to intradermally administered *Candida* antigen. There is, however, doubt as to which, if any, of these abnormalities is a primary defect and, in some patients, reversal of these immunological defects can be seen with the institution of successful therapy.

The diagnosis of *Candida* infections depends on the demonstration of the organism in culture and direct microscopy of swabs or smears. However, as the organism is also a commensal, it is important for the investigator to show that the presence of the fungus is likely to be associated with disease. For instance, in oesophagitis, endoscopy or demonstrating the presence of characteristic radiological findings with multiple filling defects on barium swallowing are both helpful.

Dermatophyte infections and hypersensitivity diseases

Reports have occurred associating urticaria, rhinitis and asthma with the combination of dermatophyte infections, such as tinea pedis, and specific IgE antibodies. The first of these was in the 1930s when Sultzberger and his colleagues[30] recommended that trichophytin skin tests should be routinely performed on allergic patients. More recently, a RAST test has been developed[31] and patients suffering from asthma[32] and perennial rhinitis[33] due to trichophytin sensitivity have been described. Trichophytin-sensitive asthmatic patients frequently also have chronic sinusitis with or without nasal polyposis[34]. These patients and those with perennial rhinitis give positive nasal provocation tests to extracts of dermatophyte fungi including trichophytin.

Dermatophytosis is common, but is probably more frequent and more severe in hotter climates. Anecdotal evidence suggests systemic antifungal treatment may be helpful in hypersensitive patients but double-blind placebo-controlled trials are needed. Some caution should be exercised in interpreting these data as dermatophytosis is more common in atopic individuals and because there is extensive cross-reactivity between airborne mould fungi which are allergenic and dermatophytes.

Aspergillosis

The range of *Apsergillus* infections of the ear, nose and throat extends from otitis externa to paranasal aspergillosis. Other sites of involvement include secondary invasion of mastoid cells by aspergilli and oesophageal aspergillosis in the neutropenic patient. The commonest pathogen amongst the aspergilli is *A. fumigatus*, but *A. niger* (otitis externa) and *A. flavus* (paranasal aspergillus granuloma) are also implicated in infections of the head and neck. Aspergilli are common saprophytic moulds which are not usually carried on the human body, although, in some instances, they can colonize patients with chronic pulmonary disease or chronic sinusitis. Aspergilli may also colonize sites such as lung cavities and, on some occasions, they develop into a solid mass of fungus or aspergilloma. Alternatively, they may invade tissue, particularly in the presence of neutropenia[35]. Generally, environmental sources of *Apsergillus* may generate large numbers of airborne spores which can be inhaled. Since the spores are ubiquitous, environmental exposure to the organisms rarely plays a part in the epidemiology of the disease unless the patient is severely immunocompromised or allergic[36]. In the former instance, contamination of air in isolation cubicles from hospital building work or blocked ventilation systems is recognized as a cause of outbreaks of infection in severely immunocompromised patients.

Otitis externa

Otitis externa is a superficial infection of the external auditory meatus caused by fungi. In many cases where fungi are isolated from this area, it is probable that they are simply acting as colonizers on an eroded or inflamed area of epithelium. This is likely to be the case, for instance, where *Candida* is isolated and the presence of fungi can be precipitated by use of topical antibacterial antibiotics. The organisms associated with otitis externa include species of the genera *Candida*, *Aspergillus*, *Fusarium*, *Penicillium* and zygomycete fungi[37]. However, their role in causing invasive disease in many cases

Table 5 Classification of diseases caused by *Aspergillus* species in the paranasal sinuses

(Colonization)
Aspergilloma of the paranasal sinuses
Hypersensitivity due to *Aspergillus*:
Allergic rhinitis
Allergic paranasal aspergillosis
Invasive aspergillosis:
Chronic necrotizing paranasal aspergillosis
Acute invasive paranasal aspergillosis
Paranasal *Aspergillus* granuloma

remains in doubt. One organism, *Aspergillus niger*, does appear to be associated with genuine fungal growth in the external auditory canal. This presents with pain, discharge and loss of hearing in one ear and the canal, on examination, can be seen to be partially obstructed with a mat of dark material, growth of *Aspergillus*. This occurs in otherwise healthy patients and the mechanisms of resistance are unknown. Occasionally, the fungus will elicit a severe necrotic response[38] in the epithelium. Infection of the middle ear or even the mastoid cells can also occur. The latter is mainly seen after surgery or in immunocompromised patients[39].

Aspergillosis of the paranasal sinuses

There are a number of different ways in which aspergilli can affect the paranasal sinuses. Most frequently this involves the maxillae, less commonly the ethmoid cells. It also follows the pattern described above in which the organisms can colonize without disease, grow as a solid mass or aspergilloma, cause hypersensitivity reactions or invade tissue. A similar classification to that used for lung infections due to *Aspergillus* can therefore be applied (Table 5).

Colonization by Aspergillus

By definition, colonization implies growth of the organism without pathology. Aspergilli can be isolated from sinus washings in patients with sinusitis or when other diseases are present. They are one of several different fungi, ranging from *Candida* to *Pseudallescheria boydii* and zygomycetes, which may be isolated from this source. In the UK, *A. fumigatus* is the commonest *Aspergillus* species to be isolated from this site, but, in tropical areas such as the Sudan, *A. flavus* is the dominant organism[40]. Once again, there is no evidence in such patients that the organisms are contributing to the pathology.

Aspergilloma

Here there is unrestricted growth of aspergilli in the paranasal sinus, usually the maxillary sinus. The condition is found either on X-ray, where it presents as a rounded opacity sometimes containing flecks of calcification, or at operation. The patient has chronic sinusitis and nasal obstruction with intermittent facial pain, but symptoms may be unilateral. The fungus does not invade the mucosa and, unlike aspergilloma of the lung, bleeding is not a feature of an aspergilloma in this site. Occasionally, other fungi may produce a similar picture and various *Aspergillus* species, such as *A. fumigatus*, *A. flavus* and *A. niger*, may also be involved. Sometimes patients produce strong antibody titres to the organism which can be detected by immunodiffusion or counterimmunoelectrophoresis. However, again, these responses are less predictable than those seen in lung disease where high *Aspergillus* titres are virtually diagnostic of the condition. It is also not clear how this is related to other types of aspergillosis, such as fungal hypersensitivity, or whether pathological damage may follow antibody-mediated damage, for instance through type III hypersensitivity.

Hypersensitivity aspergillosis of the paranasal sinuses

This is a recently described phenomenon in which *Aspergillus* or other fungi in the sinuses causes immunologically mediated damage[41]. In some ways, it is analogous to allergic bronchopulmonary aspergillosis affecting the lungs[42]. Few cases have been described, although it may be more common than these data would suggest. In some cases, the patients have an atopic background and can be shown to have immediate type hypersensitivity to aspergilli on prick testing or *Aspergillus*-specific IgE with RAST tests. Patients also have antibody to the organism and, in aspirated material or in histopathology, there are numerous eosinophils in the infiltrate. Charcot Leyden crystals are also commonly found in sinus material (Figures 1, 2 and 3). While the proof of immunologically mediated damage remains tantalizing, more work needs to be done to confirm the immunological nature of this entity. However, there are sufficient grounds for suggesting that, in some patients, presence of *Aspergillus* can elicit a type 1, or possibly a type III, hypersensitivity response which contributes to symptoms of sinusitis by triggering tissue odema and sinus obstruction. These patients may respond to corticosteroid therapy[43].

Invasive aspergillosis

In contrast to the last few diseases, in this condition, fungi invade the mucosa and can penetrate further into the bone, even reaching the cranial fossa or regional blood vessels[44]. In some patients, this process seems to be more indolent and the invasion occurs over a number of months, possibly longer. The term chronic necrotizing aspergillosis, which is used for a similar form of pulmonary infection, could be applied to this slow-onset type of infection. Patients with this form of infection usually have an underlying disease, such as diabetes mellitus, and may produce low titre anti-*Aspergillus* antibodies. The more common form of paranasal aspergillosis is a rapidly invasive type, acute invasive aspergillosis, which is mainly seen in severely immunocom-

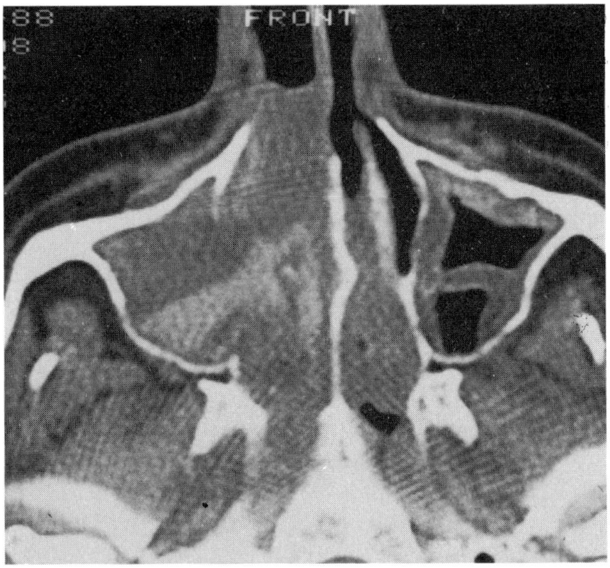

Figure 1 CT scan – axial section through skull to show opacification of L maxillary sinus and thickening of the lining on the R. Calcification is present on the L, suggesting fungal disease. There is some destruction of the medial wall of the left antrum

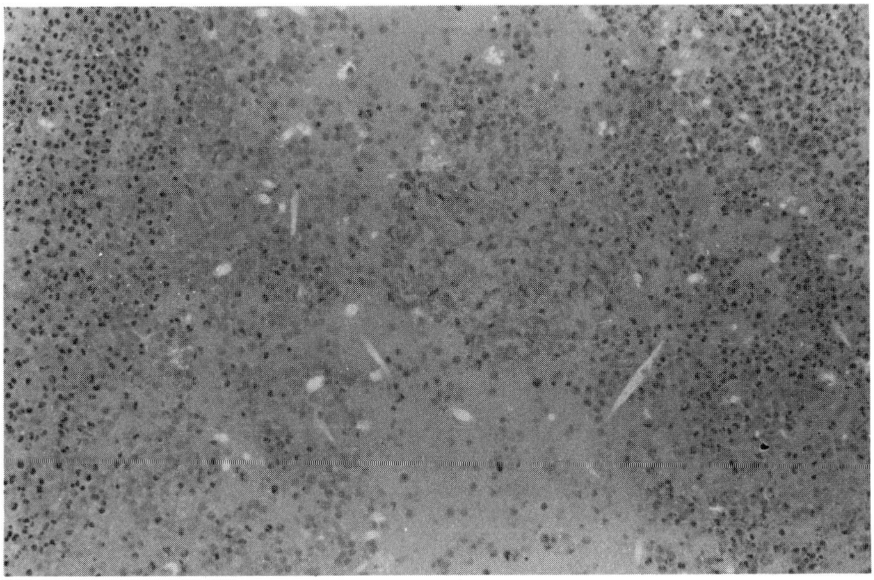

Figure 2 Histology from the same patient as in Figure 1. Fungal hyphae can be clearly seen at higher magnification, especially if a silver stain is used (see Figure 3) (H&E ×180)

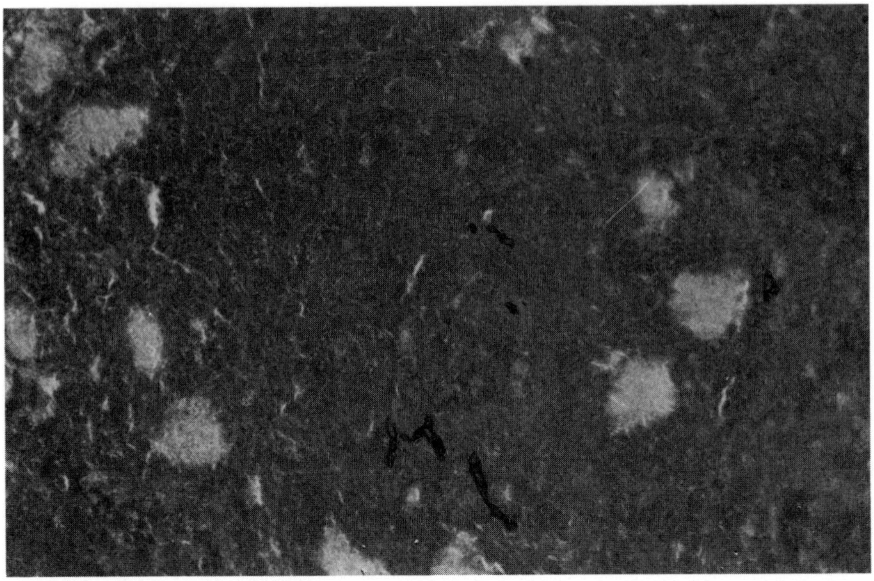

Figure 3 Histology from the same patient as in Figure 1. Fungal hyphae can be clearly seen at higher magnification (Methenamine silver stain ×180)

promised patients. This accords with the observation discussed previously that neutrophil-mediated defence appears to be a key factor in prevention of infection, as the major predisposing cause in this type of invasive disease is neutropenia. Patients with leukaemia or those undergoing treatment for cancer are the main targets[45]. The patient presents with facial pain, nasal obstruction and facial swelling. This may appear as oedema and erythema on facial skin. Proptosis is less common, but palatal invasion may develop. Necrotic lesions may appear in the nose, although, in some cases, this is related to mucosal trauma. The spread is often not as rapid or extensive as rhinocerebral mucormycosis (see below) but the two diseases can appear identical. Invasion is progressive but the process is usually halted if the leukocyte count recovers.

A third form of invasive sinus disease which is more common in the tropics, particularly Sudan, the Arabian peninsula and India or Pakistan, is paranasal *Aspergillus* granuloma[46]. The causative organism is nearly always *A. flavus*. The patients are otherwise well but present with chronic nasal obstruction, headache and facial swelling. Proptosis is a common presenting feature. If left, this infection is progressive and may spread to the brain and orbit. The characteristic of this condition is the formation of sclerosing granulomas containing short fragments of hyphae embedded in giant cells. In some areas of the inflammatory response, there is necrosis. Whether this is a variant of the more indolent forms of sinus invasion is not known but the histology, the epidemiology and the presence of *A. flavus* are typical. Patients often have low titres of antibody to aspergilli. The pathogenesis of paranasal aspergilloma is unknown.

While these conditions have been presented as discrete entities, it is likely that, in many cases, the divisions between them are not so clear cut and, indeed, as with pulmonary aspergillosis, one type may evolve into another. However, they provide a useful way of classifying the disease. All forms, though, are comparatively rare.

Rhinocerebral mucormycosis

Mucormycosis or acute zygomycosis is an infection caused by zygomycete fungi of the genera *Absidia*, *Rhizomucor* and *Rhizopus*[47]. Less commonly other fungi, such as *Cunninghamella bertolletiae* or *Saksenaea vasiformis* are implicated. These fungi are environmental saprophytes which only rarely cause disease in man. The zygomycetes invade in the presence of a number of different host defects, the commonest being neutropenia, uncontrolled diabetes mellitus and burns. They may also cause disease in patients suffering from malnutrition. The immunological features of the zygomycete infections have been discussed above and, from this, it can be seen that the specific predispositions of neutropenia and diabetes are logical.

In the head and neck, the commonest presentation of this infection is rhinocerebral mucormycosis, a rapidly spreading infection which usually starts in the maxillary sinus. Spread involves extensive oedema and infarction across the face, orbit and palate. Invasion of blood vessels is a feature of the infection, hence the severe necrotic reaction. In the acute forms, progression is difficult to halt. The diagnosis is made by growing the organism and by finding the characteristic broad hyphae in biopsy material or impression smears. Serology to a battery of zygomycete fungal antigens is unreliable and is often negative. There are more indolent forms of this infection, although they are generally uncommon, and, with these, the prognosis is better, the infection appearing to respond to antifungal therapy. These are mainly seen in diabetics. One major problem with therapy is that few of the antifungal drugs currently available have sufficient activity against these organisms.

While other fungi, such as *Paracoccidioides brasiliensis*, occasionally affect the mucosa of the mouth or nose, generally, few of the other pathogens invade this region except as part of a general dissemination. In these cases, the main site of infection is usually the bone, mucosa or skin and lesions seldom involve other structures.

References

1. Rippon JW. Medical mycology. Philadelphia: W.B. Saunders Co. 1982.
2. Vanden Bossche H, Mackenzie DWR, Cauwenberg G, eds. *Aspergillus* and aspergillosis. New York: Plenum Press: 1988.
3. Warnock DW, Richardson MD, eds. Fungal infection in the compromised patient. Chichester, UK: John Wiley & Sons; [In press].
4. Artis WM, Patrisky E, Rastinejard F, Duncan RL. Fungistatic mechanisms of human transferrin for *Rhizopus oryzae* and *Trichophyton mentagrophytes*: alternative to simple iron

depletion. Infect Immun. 1983;41:290–5.
5. Svejgaard E. Immunologic investigations of dermatophytes and dermatophytosis. Semin Dermatol. 1985;4:201–21.
6. Schonheyder L, Storgaard L, Andersen P. Variation of a 470,000 daltons antigen complex and catalase antigen in clinical isolates of *Aspergillus fumigatus*. J Med Vet Mycol. 1985;23:339–49.
7. Merkow LP, Epstein SM, Sidransky H, Verney E, Pando M. The pathogenesis of experimental pulmonary aspergillosis. An ultrastructural study of alveolar macrophages after phagocytosis of *Aspergillus flavus* spores in vivo. Am J Pathol. 1971;62:57–74.
8. Levitz SM, Selsted ME, Ganz T, Lehrer RI, Diamond RD. In vitro killing of spores and hyphae of *Aspergillus fumigatus* and *Rhizopus oryzae* by rabbit neutrophil cationic peptides and bronchoalevolar macrophages. J Infect Dis. 1986;154:483–90.
9. Shaffner A, Douglas H, Braude AI, Davis CE. Killing of *Aspergillus* spores depends on the anatomical source of the macrophages. Infect Immun. 1983;42:1109–15.
10. Schaffner A. Therapeutic concentrations of glucocorticoids suppress the antimicrobial activity of human macrophages without impairing their responsiveness to gamma interferon. J Clin Invest. 1985;76:1755–61.
11. Diamond RD, Huber E, Haudenschild CC. Mechanisms of destruction of *Aspergillus fumigatus* hyphae mediated by human monocytes. J Infect Dis. 1983;147:474–83.
12. Levitz SM, Diamond RD. Mechanisms of resistance of *A. fumigatus* conidia to neutrophil killing in vitro. J Infect Dis. 1985;152:33–42.
13. Lehrer RI, Jan RG. Interaction of *Aspergillus fumigatus* spores with human leukocytes and serum. Infect Immun. 1970;1:345–52.
14. Waldorf AR, Diamond RD. Neutrophil chemotactic responses induced by fresh and swollen *Rhizopus oryzae* spores and *Aspergillus fumigatus* conidia. Infect Immun.1985;48:458–63.
15. Davies RR, Denning TJV. *Candida albicans* and the fungicidal activity of the blood. Sabouraudia. 1972;10:301–12.
16. Chinn RYW, Diamond RD. Generation of chemotactic factors by *Rhizopus oryzae* in the presence and absence of serum: relationship to hyphal damage mediated by human neutrophils and effects of hyperglycaemia and ketoacidosis. Infect Immun. 1982;381: 1123–9.
17. Pearsall NN, Adams BL, Bunni R. Immunologic responses to *Candida albicans*. III. Effect of passive transfer of lymphoid cells and serum on murine candidiasis. J Immunol. 1978;120:1176–80.
18. Monga DP. Studies on experimental aspergillosis in immunodeficient mice. Zentralbl Bakteriol Parasit Infekt Hyg Abt 1 A. 1983;254:552–60.
19. Kurup VP, Nair MPB, Schwartz SA, Fink JN. Serum antibodies and their role in antibody-dependent cell mediated cytotoxicity in aspergillosis. Immunobiology. 1985;169:362–8.
20. Khardori N, Chaudhary S, McConnachie P, Tewari RP. Characterization of lymphocytes responsible for protective immunity to histoplasmosis in mice. Mykosen. 1983;26:523–32.
21. Gustafson TL, Schaffner W, Lavely GB, Stratto CW, Johnson HK, Hutcheson RH. Invasive aspergillosis in renal transplant recipients: correlation with corticosteroid therapy. J Infect Dis. 1983;148:230–8.
22. Williams DM, Weiner MH, Drutz DJ. Immunologic studies of disseminated infection with *Aspergillus fumigatus* in the nude mouse. J Infect Dis. 1981;143:726–33.
23. Bice DE, Lopez M, Rothschild H, Salvaggio J. Comparison of Candida delayed hypersensitivity skin test size with lymphocyte transformation, migratory inhibitory factor production and antibody titer. Int Arch Allergy Appl Immunol. 1974;47:54–62.
24. Djeu JY, Blanchard DK, Halkias D, Friedman H. Growth inhibition of *Candida albicans* by human polymorphonuclear neutrophils: activation by gamma interferon and tumour necrosis actor. J Immunol. 1986;137:2980–4.
25. Odds FC. Candida and candidosis. 2nd ed. London: Bailliere Tindall Co.; 1988.
26. Kennedy M. Adhesion and association mechanisms of *Candida albicans*. Curr Top Med Mycol. 1988;2:73–169.
27. Kodsi BE, Wickremesinghe PC, Kozinn PJ, Iswara K, Goldberg PK. Candida esophagitis. A prospective study of 27 cases. Gastroenterology. 1976;71:715–9.
28. Tavitian A, Raufman JP, Rosenthal LE. Oral candidosis as a marker of oesophageal candidiasis in AIDS. Ann Intern Med. 1986;104:54–9.

29. Kirkpatrick CH, Rich RR, Bennett JE. Chronic mucocutaneous candidiasis: Model building in cellular immunology. Ann Intern Med. 1971;74:955–78.
30. Sultzberger MB, Vaughan WT. Experiments in silk hypersensitivity and inhalation of allergen in atopic dermatitis (neurodermatitus disseminatus). J Allergy. 1934;5:544–60.
31. Platts-Mills TAE, Fiocco GP, Hayden ML, Guerrant JL, Pollart SM, Wilkins SR. Serum IgE antibodies to Trichophyton in patients with urticaria, angioedema, asthma and rhinitis: development of a radioallergosorbent test. J Allergy Clin Immunol. 1987;79:40–5.
32. Gumowski P, Lech B, Chaves I, Girard JP. Chronic asthma and rhinitis due to Candida albicans, Epidermophyton and Trichophyton. Ann Allergy. 1987;59:48–51.
33. Kivity S, Schwarz Y, Fireman E. The association of perennial rhinitis with Trichophyton infection. Clin Exp Allergy. 1992;22:498–501.
34. Platts-Mills TAE, Call RS, Devell BA, Karlsson G, Ward GW. The association of hypersensitivity diseases with dermatophyte infections (Editorial). Clin Exp Allergy. 1992;22:427–8.
35. Walsh TJ, Pizzo PA. Fungal infections in granulocytopenic patients: current approaches to classification, diagnosis and treatment. In Holmberg K, Meyer RD, eds. Diagnosis and therapy of systemic fungal infections. New York: Raven Press; 1989:47–70.
36. Aisner J, Schimpff SC, Bennett JE, Young VM, Wiernik PH. *Aspergillus* infections in cancer patients. Association with fireproofing material in a new hospital. J Am Med Assoc. 1976;86:539–43.
37. Grigoriou D, Font N. Les otomycoses. Dermatologica. 1970;141:138–42.
38. Cunningham M, Yu VL, Turner J, Curtis H. Necrotising otitis externa due to *Aspergillus* in an immunocompetent patient. Arch Otolaryngol Head Neck Surg. 1988;114:554–6.
39. Stanley RJ, McCaffery TV, Weiland LH. Fungal mastoiditis in the immunocompromised patient. Arch Otolaryngol Head Neck Surg. 1988;114:198–9.
40. Gentles JC. Mycotic infections of the paranasal sinuses. Mykosen. 1978:(Suppl 1):94–7.
41. Katzenstein AA, Sale SR, Greenberger PS. Allergic aspergillus sinusitis: a newly recognised form of sinusitis. J Allergy Clin Immunol. 1983;72:89–93.
42. McCarthy DS, Pepys J. Allergic bronchopulmonary aspergillosis: clinical immunology. 1) Clinical features. Clin Allergy. 1971;1:261–72.
43. Dunlop IS, Billson FA. Visual failure in allergic *Aspergillus* sinusitis: a case report. Br J Ophthalmol. 1988;72:127–30.
44. Viollier A, Peterson DE, de Jongh CA, Newman KSA, Gray WC, Sutherland JC. *Aspergillus* sinusitis in cancer patients. Cancer. 1986;58:366–71.
45. Schubert MM, Peterson DE, Meyers JD, Hackman R, Donnall Thomas E. Head and neck aspergillosis in patients undergoing bone marrow transplantation. Cancer. 1986;57:1092–5.
46. Milosev B, Mahgoub El S, Aal OA. Primary aspergilloma of the paranasal sinuses in the Sudan. Br J Surg. 1969;56:132–7.
47. Meyer RD, Rosen P, Armstrong D. Phycomycosis complicating leukaemia and lymphoma. Ann Intern Med. 1972;77:871–9.

5
Immunocytochemistry in the Diagnosis of Pathological Conditions of the Ear, Nose and Throat

L. MICHAELS

Immunological methods have recently been applied with success to the problems of diagnosis in histopathology. Although pathological anatomy has been a foundation of medical diagnosis for hundreds of years, strengthened over the past century by the addition of microscopy of diseased tissues, a serious deficiency in modern medicine has been the inability of pathologists to ascribe a molecular basis to morphological tissue changes. Because of this, by the 1960s, the reputation which pathologists had built up for their science in medical diagnosis had become diminished. This loss appeared magnified by notable advances in other medical diagnostic fields, notably radiology and biochemistry. Immunology was gaining importance in clinical medicine and, by the early 1970s, sufficient technical expertise had developed in this field for molecular identifications to be made within cells through the specificity of the antigen–antibody combination. In subsequent years, the efficiency of this method was much improved and its application to histopathological diagnosis was now possible. The last ten years have witnessed an outpouring of pathological discoveries utilizing antigen–antibody methods for identification of diagnostic substances in pathological tissues. Pathological changes in the ear, nose and throat have participated in this resurgence. It was fortunate that this came about at a time when clearer ideas had been developed using routine staining methods for the classification of pathological conditions of the ear, nose and throat, as a result of which the new immunological methods could be applied to entities whose places in the nosology of otolaryngic diseases were now accepted.

In the first part of this chapter, a brief review will be given of the immunological methods particularly available for use in the histopathology laboratory, i.e. those involving immunocytochemistry (IMC). In the second part of this chapter, the applications of these methods to some pathological conditions of the ear, nose and throat will be discussed. The content of this chapter is not geared to the needs of histopathologists and so deals very briefly with the techniques and the histopathological changes. For more detailed discussions of the methods in use, see Reference 1.

IMMUNOLOGICAL METHODS IN DIAGNOSTIC HISTOPATHOLOGY

The basis of identification of molecular changes in tissue cells through antigen–antibody reactions was provided by Coons and his colleagues[2]. At first, the antibody to a particular antigen in the tissues was labelled with a fluorescent dye. Later, to improve sensitivity, the specific antibody from one animal species was first applied and the antibody to the protein of the first one, prepared in another animal species and labelled with fluorescein isocyanate, was then applied[2]. Thus the antigen molecules being tested for could be identified in the tissues when observed in ultraviolet light. The disadvantages of this method are that it requires a fluorescence microscope, that it cannot be carried out in paraffin sections and that the preparations are not permanent, the fluorescent attachment to the antibodies not being able to withstand dehydration. Nevertheless, for reasons probably concerned with the abundance of collagen in skin tissue, this method is still the standard one in dermatopathology, in most cases when IMC needs to be used[3]. Dermatological conditions often present in the ear, nose and throat region, but, through limitations of space, this aspect will not be discussed.

The ability to utilize IMC methods in paraffin sections produced an upsurge in histopathological research and this method is now in the forefront of new studies in histopathology, including that of the ear, nose and throat. Although polyclonal antibodies are used in paraffin sections, it was the development of the highly specific monoclonal antibodies which provided the crucial technique for the current utilization of IMC in such routine preparations.

Monoclonal antibodies

The use of monoclonal antibodies is so important in ear, nose and throat IMC that a brief account of the method of production of these substances is included.

1. A mouse or rat is immunized against the antigen to which an antibody is required. Sometimes this is a crude antigen injected ‘blind’ in the hope that it will be possible to obtain monoclonal antibodies against hitherto undescribed cellular antigens.
2. The immunized mouse or rat is killed and a suspension of spleen cells is added in tissue culture to those of mutant mouse myeloma cells, which lack an enzyme for synthesizing DNA (pathway 1). In order to grow and proliferate, these cells use an alternative method (pathway 2). About 1% of the spleen cells fuse with the mouse myeloma cells.

3. Immediately after mixture and fusion of the two groups of cells, aminopterin is added to the cell culture. This stops pathway 2, so that cells which have not fused (the majority) will not grow. Also, hypoxanthine and thymidine (HAT medium) are added so that cells which have fused can grow by pathway 1, and, because they are partly composed of immunoglobulin-synthesizing plasma cells from the spleen, they will produce the characteristic antibody to the original antigen in a pure state.
4. Antibodies produced from the cultures are extracted and assayed by a standard method.
5. Cultures producing interesting antibodies are 'cloned', i.e. subcultured so that each individual cell culture is derived from a single fused cell.

IMMUNOCYTOCHEMICAL STAINING TECHNIQUES

Three immunocytochemical methods are in frequent use for the diagnostic detection of the antigens in paraffin sections to which specific antibodies have been affixed.

Peroxidase–antiperoxidase method (PAP)

In this method, the first stage is to apply a specific antibody derived from a rabbit to combine with the antigen in question in the deparaffinized section. The second layer is an anti-rabbit IgG antibody derived by immunizing a goat. This is applied in excess so that one of the two identical sites (Fab portions) is free to combine in the third part of the test. In this part, the antiperoxidase in the mixture of peroxidase–antiperoxidase is derived from a rabbit so that the goat–antirabbit antibody binding sites left over in the second layer can unite with the free binding sites on the third layer. Peroxidase is then developed by a histochemical method, such as one involving the use of diaminobenzidine and hydrogen peroxide, giving a brown colouration wherever antigen had been present in tissue cells.

Avidin biotin method

Avidin and biotin have a very high affinity for each other. These are proteins derived from egg white and yolk, respectively. Biotin also binds strongly to immunoglobulin.

A commonly used method is to apply rabbit antibody primarily, and then to apply, as the second layer, goat antirabbit IgG combined with biotin. The third layer is an avidin–biotin complex, the avidin having been reacted with biotinylated peroxidase to such a degree that some biotin binding sites on the avidin are available to react with the biotin on the second layer antibody. The peroxidase is then developed in the same way as in the PAP method.

Alkaline phosphatase–antialkaline phosphatase

This method is essentially the same as the PAP method with the substitution of alkaline phosphatase–antialkaline phosphatase for peroxidase–antiperoxidase. The alkaline phosphatase is then developed to produce a red colouration by the use of naphthol phosphate and new fuchsin.

TISSUE ANTIGENS

A wide variety of tissue antigens are commonly tested for by immunocytochemical methods. There are two important groups, intermediate filament proteins and membrane antigens. In addition, other proteins to which antisera are commonly applied are S-100 protein, seen in neuroectodermal derivatives, such as schwannoma and melanoma, factor VIII-related antigen, expressed by megakaryocytes and endothelial cells, and a variety of enzymes including neurone-specific enolase and lysozyme.

Intermediate filament proteins

Each of the cells of the body contains a fine skein of proteins, the chemical composition of which varies according to the type of tissue in which the cell in question is found. There are five classes of these substances, known as intermediate filament proteins:

1. Cytokeratins, found in epithelial cells. In this group, there are individual antibodies by which subclasses of keratin can be recognized, depending on their molecular weight.
2. Vimentin, found in all mesenchymal cells.
3. Desmin, found in both smooth and skeletal muscle cells.
4. Neurofilament protein, observed in neuronal and neuroendocrine cells.
5. Glial fibrillary acidic protein, found only in glial cells.

The specificity of these proteins enables the diagnostic pathologist to utilize their presence in the identification of the corresponding cell types when he is dealing with tumours and other pathological processes.

Membrane antigens

There are some proteins that are restricted to the membranes themselves and their detection often provides valuable diagnostic information. These include epithelial membrane antigen (EMA), expressed by most epithelia and occasional mesenchymal cells; leukocyte common antigen (LCA), found in the vast majority of both reactive and neoplastic leukocytes; carcinoembryonic antigen (CEA) expressed by many epithelial cells and occasional mesenchymal elements; blood group isoantigens A, B and H, expressed by epithelial and endothelial cells.

PATHOLOGICAL CONDITIONS OF THE EAR, NOSE AND THROAT

In this section, some pathological conditions of the ear, nose and throat will be surveyed from the point of view of the usefulness of immunocytochemical methods in their diagnosis and prognosis. In some conditions, IMC provides concepts useful to an understanding of aetiology rather than diagnosis. Such conditions will also be mentioned. At the present time, most use has been obtained from IMC in neoplasms of the ear, nose and throat. Occasionally, infective conditions, viral or bacterial, may be identified by IMC.

The ear

Adenoma of the middle ear

A benign glandular neoplasm confined to the middle ear and originating from its epithelium was not recognized until 1976[4]. The epithelium of the middle ear has a propensity for gland formation in otitis media and adenoma would seem to represent a benign neoplastic transformation of this epithelium along the same lines.

Adenoma of the middle ear is easily recognized histologically, being formed by closely apposed small glands with a 'back to back' appearance. Lysozyme has been found in each of five adenomas stained for this enzyme by an immunochemical method[5]. We have examined four adenomas for lysozyme using the same antiserum as reported in that study, but have been unable to find this enzyme in any of them.

Since the first descriptions of a benign glandular tumour arising in the middle ear, there have been reports of 'carcinoid tumours' arising in the middle ear. Essentially, these are glandular neoplasms with neuroendocrine features, i.e. the presence of positivity to neurone-specific enolase, chromogranin and any of a variety of polypeptide substances in the cytoplasm of the tumour cells shown by IMC[6]. There is also seen, by electron microscopy, neurosecretory granules in the same location, and Grimelius staining, a silver staining method observed by light microscopy, is also found to be positive. Such carcinoid tumours of the middle ear have the same morphological pattern as the adenomas which do not possess these neuroendocrine features, but, nevertheless, are often felt to possess a 'low-grade malignancy'[7]. Thus, an ill-defined concept has grown up that there is a *benign* mucous type adenoma and a neoplasm of *low-grade malignancy* which has neuroendocrine features. It is very doubtful whether there are two such types of glandular middle neoplasm. Recent studies show that many, perhaps a majority of, adenomas may differentiate in both directions[8] so that the presence of IMC features of neuroendocrine differentiation in an adenoma of the middle ear is no indication of a tendency to aggressiveness of the neoplasm.

Jugulotympanic paraganglioma

Jugulotympanic paragangliomas arise most frequently from paraganglia situated in the wall of the jugular bulb; a minority of the tumours arise from the paraganglion situated near the middle ear surface of the promontory. The distinction between jugular and tympanic paragangliomas can easily be made by modern methods of imaging. The jugular neoplasm shows evidence of invasion of the petrous bone. The tympanic neoplasm is confined to the middle ear.

The neoplasm in a typical histological section shows some resemblance to the carotid body tumour. Epithelioid, uniform cells are separated by numerous blood vessels. The tumour cells often form clusters or 'Zellballen'. Neurone-specific enolase, chromogranin and polypeptides, as demonstrated by IMC, are always present in the cells of this neoplasm – a useful diagnostic feature. IMC for cytokeratins is usually negative.

The normal paraganglionic tissues of the carotid body (and presumably also the smaller ones) contain two types of cell: chief or type I cells, which are neuroendocrine cells, and sustentacular or type II cells, which are not neuroendocrine, but contain S-100 protein. The clue that the S100-protein-containing sustentacular cells are diminished in hyperplasia and neoplasia of the adrenal medulla[9] has led to investigations of the status of the sustentacular cells in benign as opposed to malignant neoplasms of paraganglionic tissue at other sites[10]. Sustentacular cells were identified by their positivity to S-100 protein and glial fibrillary acidic protein (GFAP). Low-grade tumours, i.e. those which were not recurrent, locally aggressive or metastatic, contained sustentacular cells. The majority of intermediate-grade paragangliomas, i.e. those which were recurrent or locally aggressive, had diminished or absent reactivity to S100-protein and GFAP. All malignant paragangliomas were devoid of sustentacular cells except in one case, and that one showed only rare S-100 protein-positive cells. Immunostaining, particularly for neuron-specific enolase and chomogranin of chief cells in the tumour was also inversely related to tumour malignancy. Jugulotympanic paragangliomas usually have sparse, but not absent, S-100 protein-staining sustentacular cells, implying a rather aggressive, but not fully malignant, activity.

Meningioma

Meningiomas are usually intracranial neoplasms. Extracranial meningiomas are, however, not uncommon. The commonest temporal bone site for primary meningioma is the middle ear cleft. Intranasal meningiomas are less rare. Microscopically, the neoplasm takes the same forms as any of the well-described intracranial types of meningioma. The commonest variety seen in the middle ear is the meningothelial type, in which the tumour cells form masses of epithelioid regular cells, often disposed as whorls. Fibroblastic and psammomatous varieties are also sometimes seen in the middle ear.

Histological diagnosis of meningioma is often difficult because the above features are indistinct. Under these circumstances, IMC may be of some diagnostic value. Most of the markers are negative, including those for cytokeratins. Epithelial membrane antigen is, however, positive in the majority of meningiomas.

Nose

Scleroma

Scleroma (often termed 'rhinoscleroma') is a chronic inflammatory condition in which large deforming masses of tissue distend the nasal cavity. It is likely that *Klebsiella rhinoscleromatis* is the causative agent of this infection. Plasma cells are prominent and Russell bodies are numerous. The specific cell of the lesion is the Mikulicz cell, which is large with clear cytoplasm containing bacilli, and the characteristic feature of the histology of scleroma is the presence of clusters of these cells among the plasma cells. The organisms in the Mikulicz cells are difficult to identify in conventionally stained sections, but may be displayed by IMC, using an antibody to mixed types of *Klebsiella rhinoscleromatis*.

Wegener's granulomatosis

Wegener's granulomatosis is a systemic inflammatory condition affecting the nose (often with the paranasal sinuses), lung and kidneys in all cases and other organs in some cases. Biopsy sections of the nose and paranasal sinuses frquently show only a non-specific chronic inflammatory infiltration of the nasal mucosa with some necrosis, Langerhans and foreign body giant cells and a moderate infiltration of eosinophils. The renal changes in Wegener's granulomatosis are those of focal segmental necrotizing glomerulonephritis. Weiss and Crissman[11] failed to demonstrate evidence of an immune-complex pathogenesis for this condition in the renal glomeruli. Serum autoantibodies against neutrophils and monocytes – the ANCA (antineutrophil cytoplasmic antibody) test – have been discovered to be largely specific for Wegener's granulomatosis (see Chapter 8), providing an accurate marker of disease activity[12], but there is, as yet, no technique involving IMC for tissue diagnosis of the condition.

Midline granuloma

I do not believe that 'midline granuloma' exists as a pathological entity[13]. Lymphoma, occurring usually in the nose in its T cell variety, is only one of the many pathological conditions that may give rise to severe ulceration of the nose to which the term 'midline granuloma' has been attached.

Papilloma

Nasal papillomas can be separated into two distinct categories: everted squamous papilloma and cylindric cell papilloma. The use of IMC has not yet led to any significant advance in the diagnosis or understanding of the aetiology of these neoplasms.

Carcinoma

Carcinomas of the nose and paranasal sinuses are stratified squamous, adenocarcinoma or adenoid cystic in type. No significant advances in the diagnosis or understanding of the aetiology of these neoplasms has yet resulted from the use of IMC.

Neuroectodermal tumours

Cerebral tissue 'tumours'

Deposits of cerebral tissue are occasionally seen in the nose. If they are not in direct communication with the brain, they are called gliomas. If they are, they are known as encephaloceles. Neither group is, strictly speaking, a neoplasm. The gliomas may be confirmed on IMC by the use of antibody to glial fibrillary acidic protein, since the component cells are usually astrocytes. Encephaloceles often contain nerve cells which may be demonstrated by a positive reaction for neurofilament protein and S-100 protein.

Neurogenic tumours

Neurogenic tumours, probably all derived by proliferation of Schwann cells, occur in four varieties in the nose: neurilemmoma, neurofibroma, plexiform neurofibroma and neurogenous sarcoma (malignant schwannoma). Each of these neoplasms is likely to show a positive reaction for S100-protein (Figure 1).

Malignant melanoma

Malignant melanomas are tumours arising from melanin-producing cells. Malignant melanomas of the nose often contain large bizarre, polygonal or giant cells. Large eosinophilic nucleoli are present in the nuclei of about half the cases, situated mainly in the polygonal cells. In the majority of cases, the tumour cells are heavily pigmented; in a few pigment is scanty or absent. Mitotic figures are always frequent in nasal and paranasal sinus malignant melanomas. Junctional activity is an important feature of malignant melanoma of the skin, but this change is unusual in the nasal variety of the tumour because, unlike the skin neoplasm, only small amounts of normal epithelium are removed with the tumour.

When diagnosis is in doubt, especially in the amelanotic variety of malignant melanoma of the nose, the identification of S100-protein by IMC is an important adjunct in malignant melanoma, since almost every case gives a positive reaction. Another marker determined by IMC, known as HMB-45, has been recently introduced and is valuable in the diagnosis of melanoma, being far more specific than the S-100 protein.

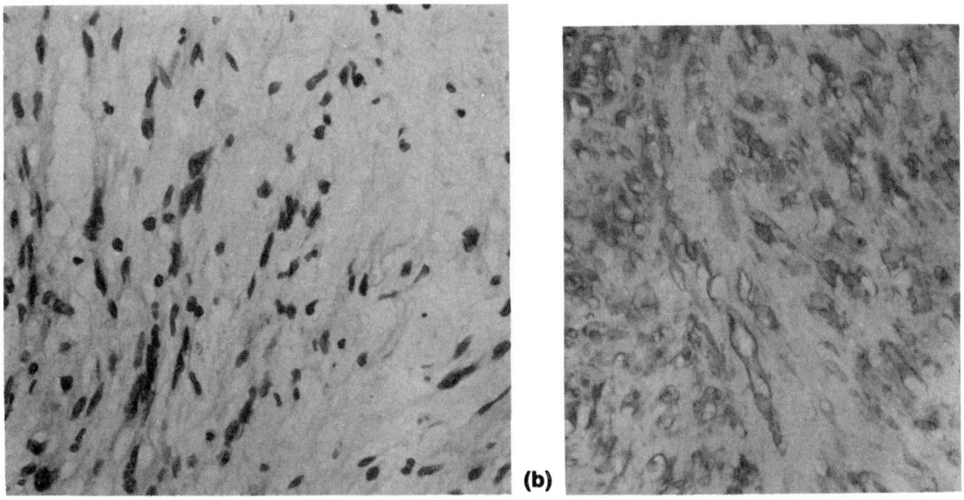

(a) (b)

Figure 1 (a) Histological section of schwannoma (neurilemmoma) of maxillary antrum. The neoplasm is composed of benign spindle cells, the nuclei of which are arranged together in a palisade fashion (Antoni A areas), as seen on the left. In other places, there is a looser formation (Antoni B areas) as seen on the right. Haematoxylin and eosin. (b) Immunoperoxidase stain of schwannoma shown in (a) using antibody against S-100 protein. The cytoplasm of the spindle cells of the neoplasm is stained positively for the antigen (brown in the original)

Olfactory neuroblastoma

Olfactory neuroblastoma is a tumour which arises from olfactory neuroepithelium. Its site of origin is the usual location of that structure, high up in the nasal cavity. Unlike neuroblastoma derived from abdominal sympathetic ganglia or adrenal medulla, which occurs principally in young children, olfactory neuroblastoma occurs in adults, with a mean age of onset of 41 years. The olfactory neoplasm is, moreover, slow growing with only a moderate tendency to recur, and a small tendency to metastasize, unlike the childhood abdominal form of neuroblastoma which possesses decidedly aggressive tendencies.

The neoplasm has two histological features which enable the pathologist to make an unequivocal diagnosis[13]: (a) well-demarcated lobules of uniform tumour cells showing nuclei which are oval and finely granular with uniformly distributed chromatin and without prominent nucleoli; and (b) congeries of blood vessels in close apposition to the tumour lobules.

It should be stressed that IMC should be relegated to a secondary place in the diagnosis of olfactory neuroblastoma. Immunochemical reactions for neurone-specific enolase are positive. This marker is of low specificity since it has a tendency to stain background tissues as well as the neuroendocrine cells of the tumour. Thus, only a strong reaction can be considered as positive. Other markers for neuroendocrine cells are often positive, notably chromogranin, but these reactions are variable. Cytokeratin markers are negative in about 50% of tumours.

The histological pattern of olfactory neuroblastoma has diagnostic characteristics which are important since the tumour can usually be cured by surgery and irradiation. IMC can be misused, with the production of an erroneous diagnosis if this basic tenet is ignored. Thus, a case of purported olfactory neuroblastoma has been described in which skeletal muscle fibres (identified by desmin IMC) were present as well as neuroblast rosettes[14]. The characteristic pattern of olfactory neuroblastoma was not, however, identified and it seems possible that the neoplasm belonged to a different, more malignant, category, namely teratocarcinoma[15], in which these constituents may be seen and identified by IMC, but the neoplasm does not show the essential morphology of olfactory neuroblastoma.

Another neoplasm which often occurs in the nasal region and which is characterized by collections of neuroblasts, but which is *not* olfactory neuroblastoma is the melanotic neuroectodermal tumour of infancy (melanotic progonoma). Two cell populations are present: cuboidal cells which contain large amounts of melanin granules in their cytoplasm; and small dark cells arranged in an alveolar pattern, which resemble neuroblasts and which show neuroendocrine features by IMC. This neoplasm is benign.

These last two entities exemplify a point which has not perhaps received enough attention in the rightful acclaim with which the use of IMC to identify molecules useful in diagnosis has been greeted. IMC is but an aid in diagnosis. Different pathological entities may share the same molecules and their relevant tissue types. The whole picture must be assessed in diagnosis, not just what is revealed by IMC.

Nasopharynx

Nasopharyngeal carcinoma

In a classification proposed by the World Health Organization[16], there are two histological types of nasopharyngeal carcinoma:

1. Squamous-cell carcinoma (keratinizing squamous-cell carcinoma);
2. Non-keratinizing squamous-cell carcinoma:
   (a) Differentiated non-keratinizing carcinoma,
   (b) Undifferentiated carcinoma.

It is type 2(b) that is particularly important because of its great frequency in the southern Chinese. There is some relationship to infection with Epstein–Barr virus, since high titres of antibody to this virus are usually found in patients with the disease. This neoplasm often presents problems in histological diagnosis, particularly in differentiation from malignant lymphoma of large cell type, notably the centroblastic form and, in this area, IMC is of particular value.

Undifferentiated carcinoma of the nasopharynx is composed of groups of or scattered individual tumour cells in a stroma which is often largely composed of lymphocytes and plasma cells. This is why it has been frequently described in the past as 'lymphoepithelioma'. The cellular appearance of undifferentiated carcinoma presents rather distinct features. Nevertheless, the histological separation of this condition from malignant lymphoma is often difficult.

The use of immunochemical markers has served to increase the accuracy of diagnosis of this tumour by providing an objective means of differentiation from lymphoma. To do this, two types of marker are used: one for cytokeratins and one for leukocytes in general (leukocyte common antigen). Staining of tumour cells for keratin antigen gives a positive result, while that for leukocyte common antigen gives a negative result[17]. An antigen which is normally present in certain populations of bone marrow-derived cells involved in humoral and specific cell-mediated immune responses, HLA-DR, has also been found in the tumour cells of the majority of nasopharyngeal carcinomas[18]. This antigen requires frozen sections for its determination by monoclonal antibody. So far, it has not been possible to use IMC for the detection of Epstein–Barr virus in relation to this neoplasm.

Angiofibroma (juvenile nasopharyngeal angiofibroma)

Angiofibroma, or juvenile nasopharyngeal angiofibroma, is a fibrous and vascular tumour-like swelling of the nasopharynx which occurs only in young males. There is, at present, no important contribution from IMC to its diagnosis or the understanding of its aetiology.

Embryonal rhabdomyosarcoma

Malignant tumours of the skeletal muscle are the commonest sarcoma in the head and neck. Most cases are of the embryonal type. The nasopharynx is the second most frequent situation for this tumour within the head and neck, the orbit being the most frequent. The average age at presentation is seven years. Embryonal rhabdomyosarcoma is a largely undifferentiated 'small blue-cell' neoplasm. The cells of embryonal rhabdomyosarcoma are round or somewhat elongated and the nuclei are usually hyperchromatic, irregularly shaped and showing numerous mitotic figures. The cytoplasm in many areas shows vacuolation due to a high glycogen content. Cross-striations are not usually observed and morphological diagnosis of the tumour is frequently difficult. Antibodies to fast myosin and skeletal muscle actin are said to be more diagnostic for poorly differentiated rhabdomyosarcomas than antibodies to myoglobin, which is generally only present in cytoplasm-rich well-differentiated tumour cells[19]. We have found the presence of desmin to be the most valuable marker for this neoplasm; almost all cases can be identified with the aid of this antibody.

Chordoma

Chordoma is a neoplasm which is derived from the primitive notochord and resembles it histologically. The largest proportion of chordomas (about 45%) occurs in the sacrococcygeal region, with a rather smaller number (39%) in the cranio-occipital region, and it is members of this latter group that involve the nasopharynx. Three constant features may be recognized in the histology of this tumour: the formation of large lobules or alveoli of tumour; strands of tumour cells; and 'physaliferous' (bubble) cells. A characteristic growth pattern is the formation of strands of tumour cells within a mucoid ground substance. Nevertheless, such histological features may be shown by several other tumour entities. IMC gives valuable assistance in the diagnosis of this condition.

Immunochemical markers for cytokeratins and S-100 protein are positive. Chordomas, however, stain negatively for lysozyme, unlike chondrosarcomas in which it is present[20].

Chordomas seen in the base of skull (but not the sacrococcygeal variety) have been observed in about one third of cases to possess a chondroid appearance. The separation of this chondroid group is important because patients with chondroid chordoma have a much longer survival time than those with typical chordoma. It is naturally even more important to distinguish them from chondrosarcomas and it is here that the presence of cytokeratin, as shown by IMC, is particularly helpful.

Infectious mononucleosis

Infectious mononucleosis is an infection caused by the Epstein–Barr virus. Changes are mainly in the mononuclear cells of the blood and in the lymph nodes and an antibody against sheep red cells is present in the blood. Complete recovery from the infection is the rule. In a few cases, the tonsils become markedly enlarged during the course of the infection and even impede swallowing and breathing[21]. Microscopic appearances are those of massive replacement of crypt epithelium and follicles by lymphoid cells of blast cell appearance. Immunohistochemical studies carried out on paraffin sections[22] show both λ and κ light chains (i.e. immunoglobulin polyclonality) in the proliferated cells. Such an investigation is now used in doubtful cases to exclude the monoclonal immunoglobulin secretion of malignant lymphoma.

Malignant lymphoma

Malignant neoplasms derived from cells of the reticuloendothelial system are common in the tonsils and other parts of the upper air and food passages, the tonsil being the commonest site. In lymph nodes, diagnosis of malignant lymphoma is made by noting a disturbance of the overall normal architecture, and recognizing the predominant cell type as being specifically of lymphoid origin, e.g. centrocytes, centroblasts or immunoblasts. In the upper air and food passages, although the classification of malignant lymphomas is similar to that of comparable lesions in lymph nodes, histological diagnosis presents different problems. The normal structure of mucosae is quite different, even in the palatine tonsil, from that of lymph nodes. Biopsy material in the nose and throat usually consists of small fragments and there is a greater difficulty

Table 1 Classification of non-Hodgkin lymphomas[24]

B-cell
Low-grade malignant lymphomas
Lymphocytic
Chronic lymphocytic leukaemia
Prolymphocytic leukaemia
Hairy-cell leukaemia
Lymphoplasmacytic/lymphoplasmacytoid (immunocytoma)
Plasmacytic
Centroblastic–centrocytic, follicular ± diffuse, or diffuse
Centrocytic
Monocytoid
High-grade malignant lymphomas
Centroblastic
Immunoblastic
Large cell, anaplastic (Ki-l antigen +)
Burkitt lymphoma
Lymphoblastic
T-cell
Low-grade malignant lymphomas
Lymphocytic
Chronic lymphocytic leukaemia
Prolymphocytic leukaemia
Small cell, cerebriform
Mycosis fungoides, Sézary syndrome
Lymphoepithelioid (Lennert lymphoma)
Angioimmunoblastic
T-zone lymphoma
Pleomorphic, small cell (HTLV-1 ±)
High-grade malignant lymphomas
Pleomorphic, medium-sized and large cell (HTLV-1 ±)
Immunoblastic
Large cell, anaplastic (Ki-l antigen +)
Lymphoblastic

in obtaining representative material from the deeper mucosae than is the case with lymph nodes.

The diagnosis of malignant lymphoma in the tonsil, other parts of Waldeyer's ring and in the upper respiratory tract in general has been greatly enhanced by IMC. Malignant lymphoma is divided into the Hodgkin and non-Hodgkin types. It is now generally agreed that Hodgkin's disease hardly ever affects the upper respiratory tract. A currently used classification of non-Hodgkin lymphoma is given in Table 1. The details of the application of IMC to the diagnosis of these conditions in the ear, nose and throat is beyond the scope of this book. It is often necessary first to identify the neoplastic cells as lymphoid in type by recognizing the leukocyte common antigen using IMC. The next step, after confirming the lymphoid nature of the cells, is to determine whether they are T or B cells using the corresponding antibodies. If they are B cells, it is possible that they may be non-neoplastic rather than those of malignant lymphoma. An additional criterion, which can be of great value in distinguishing benign from malignant exudates, is the clonal nature of the B cells. Using the immunoperoxidase method for detection of κ and λ light chains in these cells, lymphoma cells are monoclonal (exhibit either κ or λ light chains, but not both) (Figure 2), whereas, in benign reactive infiltrates, B cells are polyclonal (exhibit κ and λ light chains)[23]. No such method exists for determination of the malignant nature of a T cell infiltrate. For this purpose, the methods of molecular biology rather than IMC have been applied.

Larynx

Infection

Bacterial and fungal infection

Infections of the larynx are infrequent, mainly because few infecting organisms settle in the larynx and those that do are efficiently eliminated. Bacterial and fungal infections are most important and are recognized by culture. IMC plays little part in their detection.

Viral

Some antigens of viruses causing infection in the larynx may be detected by IMC. A frequent form of virus infection in the larynx is that of human papilloma virus associated with papillomas. The infection may be detected by IMC but it is not possible to determine antigen type by this method. The latter procedure may be successfully performed by the molecular biological technique of *in situ* hybridization[25].

Herpes virus infection of the larynx is seen occasionally, when it is usually of the herpes simplex rather than zoster type. The vocal cord may be affected and, in that region, the epithelial cells show inclusions in the nuclei and cell fusion with formation of syncytia. IMC allows confirmation that the basis of the lesion is herpes virus by the detection of the antigen (Figure 3).

Squamous carcinoma

In contrast to the ear, nose, nasopharynx and tonsil, the lesion of surpassing diagnostic importance in the larynx is squamous cell carcinoma. IMC is of minor importance in the diagnosis of this condition. Like all epithelial lesions, benign or malignant, squamous carcinoma displays positive staining by IMC for a variety of cytokeratins. This fact is occasionally of diagnostic importance

Figure 2 Opposite. (a) Supraglottic neoplasm of larynx composed of mature plasma cells, presumably a low-grade B cell lymphoma known as plasmacytic lymphoma. Haematoxylin and eosin. (b) Immunoperoxidase stain of sections of the neoplasm shown in (a) using antibody against κ light chains. Most of the neoplastic plasma cells have stained positively for the antigen (brown in the original). (c) Immunoperoxidase of the same tumour using antibody to λ light chains. In contrast to the κ light chains, the plasma cells are negative for this antigen, indicating that they are monotypic, and therefore neoplastic

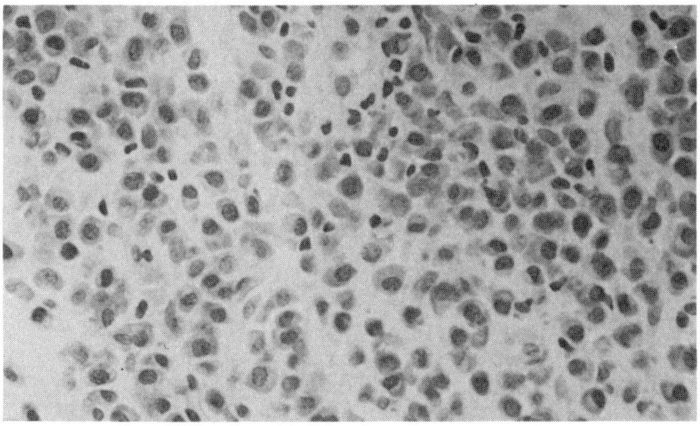

(a)

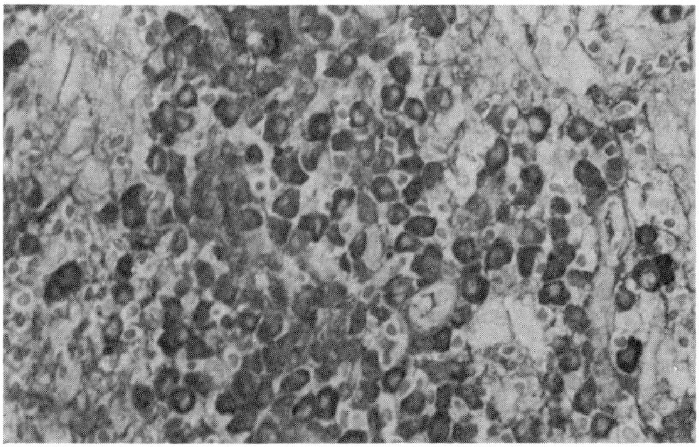

(b)

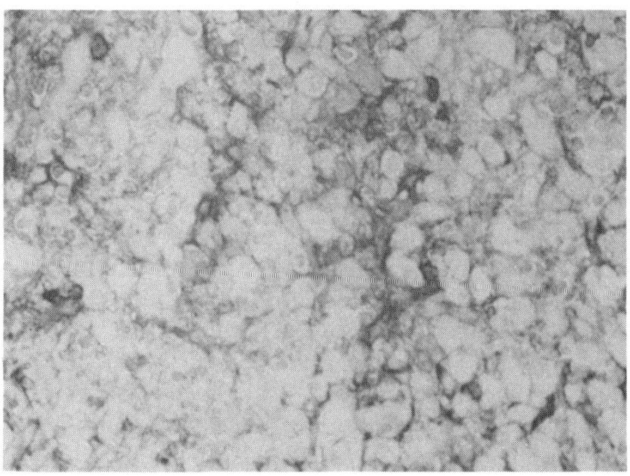

(c)

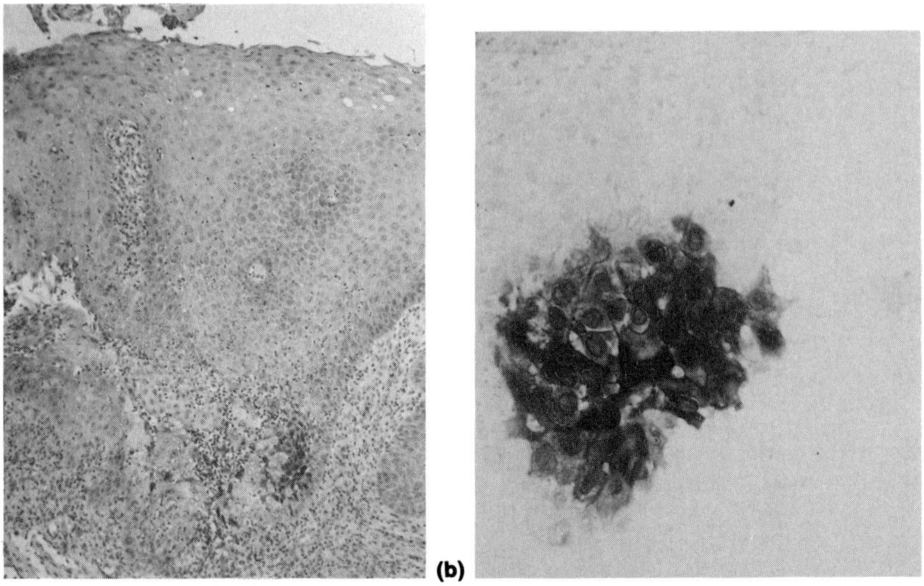

(a) (b)

Figure 3 (a) Biopsy of vocal cord of an 18-month-old child with an inflammatory lesion. The stratified squamous epithelium is hyperplastic. At the bottom of the figure, a collection of epithelial cells near the basement membrane appears basophilic due to expansion of their nuclei by basophilic inclusions, and the cells have fused together to form a syncytial like structure. Haematoxylin and eosin. (b) Immunoperoxidase of cell collection from (a) using antibody against herpes virus type 1. The cells exhibit marked positive staining (brown in the original), indicating herpes virus type 1 infection of the epithelium

when it is necessary to identify the carcinomatous character of apparently undifferentiated cells.

Spindle cell carcinoma

Spindle cell carcinomas are those in which carcinoma cells have taken on a mesenchymal appearance. The tumour has been encountered most frequently in the larynx but it also occurs in the maxillary antrum, oral cavity, hypopharynx, oesophagus, skin and breast. Most of the lesions of spindle cell carcinoma are present on the vocal cord. The diagnosis of spindle cell carcinoma requires identification of squamous cell carcinoma in some part of the tumour. In many cases, however, a diligent search with multiple sections is required since, frequently, malignant epithelium is scarce and may be absent from the surface in many areas. Sometimes, only carcinoma in situ without an invasive component is present, and a diagnosis of spindle cell carcinoma can only be suspected. Immunochemical findings in spindle cell carcinoma indicate that the spindle cells usually stain for vimentin alone, being negative for cytokeratin markers. In a smaller number of cases, the spindle cells coexpress keratin and vimentin in the same cells, but this is in situations near the origin of the spindle cells from the carcinoma cells, where the former appear in groups and are more rounded.

Neuroectodermal tumours

Granular cell tumour ('myoblastoma')

Granular cell tumour, which is commonly seen in surgical histology practice in such sites as the subcutaneous tissue and the tongue and other mucosal surfaces, also presents quite frequently in the larynx. The histological characteristic of the lesion is the presence of rows of cells with granular eosinophilic cytoplasm. The nuclei are usually small and inconspicuous. The cytoplasmic granules are eosinophilic by ordinary staining and positive by the periodic acid–Schiff method. In the larynx, as in other mucosal surfaces, pseudo-epitheliomatous hyperplasia of the overlying squamous epithelium commonly, but not always, takes place. The only useful feature of IMC in this neoplasm is the positivity for S-100 protein, appearing to confirm a relationship between this tumour and nerve sheaths, which has been suggested previously.

Neuroendocrine carcinoma

Carcinoid tumours constitute a well-defined group of tumours that characteristically grow in the small intestine and vermiform appendix. On light microscopy, they show a regular solid or trabecular arrangement of epithelial cells, and, on ultrastructural examination, there are neuroendocrine granules in the cytoplasm. A direct reducing effect on silver nitrate solution – the argentaffin effect – is produced by the tumour cells to give black cytoplasmic granules. Soluble substances, notably serotonin, 5-hydroxytryptamine, are characteristically produced by the tumour cells and often cause symptoms when released into the bloodstream.

A morphologically similar neoplasm, which also has a tendency to produce hormonal substances, grows in the bronchi, where it is usually regarded as one of the 'adenomas' in spite of a slight propensity for metastases to develop. These bronchial tumours do not usually show the argentaffin reaction, but frequently they are argyrophilic, i.e. they will reduce silver solutions with the help of a reducing agent. Cells containing neuroendocrine granules may be normally found among both the surface epithelial cells and the deep mucous glands of the bronchi, and it is possible that the carcinoid tumour arises from these cells.

Small round and oat cell carcinoma is a frequent poorly differentiated malignant tumour of the bronchus in which the tendency to tubule formation and the presence of neurosecretory cytoplasmic granules on electron microscopy indicates an origin similar to carcinoid tumour of the bronchus. Intermediate forms between carcinoid tumour and oat cell carcinoma are well known in the bronchus[26].

A concept of 'endocrine' or 'neuroendocrine' carcinoma has arisen in recent years and includes carcinoid tumours of intestine and lung and a wide variety of other tumours of endodermal or neuroectodermal origin, including oat cell carcinoma. These tumours have an epithelial structure and are usually argentaffin or argyrophil positive. IMC reveals the presence of neurone-specific enolase and inappropriate hormone secretion within the tumour cells, such as adrenocorticotrophic hormone or calcitonin.

In the larynx, two forms of neuroendocrine carcinoma have been described: (a) large cell neuroendocrine carcinoma, which is a less differentiated form of the carcinoid type of tumour, and (b) small cell neuroendocrine carcinoma, which is histologically similar to oat cell carcinoma. A third type of tumour, paraganglioma, which is said to be derived from laryngeal paraganglia, has some features in common with large cell neuroendocrine carcinoma.

It has been indicated recently that neuroendocrine carcinomas, often highly malignant neoplasms, may have been mistaken for paragangliomas in the larynx[27,28]. The use of the S-100 protein and glial fibrillary acidic protein techniques for sustentacular cell identification in paragangliomas (see above) has clarified the difference between the benign paraganglioma and the neuroendocrine carcinoma[29]. The latter study has allowed, for the first time, the distinction of a benign paragangliomatous tumour, a rare entity, from other more malignant neuroendocrine tumours of the larynx.

References

1. Polak JM, Van Noorden S. Immunochemistry. Modern methods and applications in pathology and biology. Bristol: Wright; 1986.
2. Coons AH, Leduc EH, Connolly JM. Studies on antibody production. A method for the specific demonstration of specific antibody and its application to the hyperimmune rabbit. J Exp Med. 1955;102:49–60.
3. Marks R, Knight A, Laidler P. Atlas of skin pathology. Lancaster: MTP Press Ltd; 1986.
4. Hyams VJ, Michaels L. Benign adenomatous neoplasms (adenoma) of the middle ear. Clin Otolaryngol. 1976;1:17–26.
5. Mills SE, Fechner RE. Middle ear adenoma. A cytologically uniform neoplasm displaying a variety of architectural patterns. Am J Surg Pathol. 1984;8:677–85.
6. Polak JM, Bloom SR. Endocrine tumours. Edinburgh: Churchill Livingstone; 1985.
7. Krouse JH, Nadol JB, Goodman ML. Carcinoid tumors of the middle ear. Ann Otol Rhinol Laryngol. 1990;99:547–52.
8. Wassef M, Panagiotis K, Polivka M, Nemeth J, Monteil J-P, Frachet B, Huy PTB. Middle ear adenoma. A tumor displaying mucinous and neuroendocrine differentiation. Am J Surg Pathol. 1989;13:838–47.
9. Lloyd RV, Blaivas M, Wilson BS. Distribution of chromogranin and S-100 protein in normal and abnormal adrenal medullary tissues. Arch Pathol. 1985;109:633–5.
10. Kliewer KE, Wen D-R, Cancilla PA, Cochran AJ. Paragangliomas: assessment of prognosis by histologic immunohistochemical and ultrastructural techniques. Hum Pathol. 1989;20: 29–39.
11. Weiss MA, Crissman JD. Renal biopsy findings in Wegener's granulomatosis: segmental necrotizing glomerulonephritis with glomerular thrombosis. Hum Pathol. 1984;15:943–56.
12. van der Woude FJ, Rasmussen N, Lobatto S et al. Autoantibodies against neutrophils and monocytes: tool for diagnosis and marker of disease activity in Wegener's granulomatosis. Lancet. 1985;1:425–9.
13. Michaels L. Ear, Nose and throat histopathology. London: Springer; 1987.
14. Slootweg L, Lubsen H. Rhabdomyoblasts in olfactory neuroblastoma. Histopathology. 1991;19:182–4.
15. Heffner DK, Hyams VJ. Teratocarcinoma (malignant teratoma?) of the nasal cavity and paranasal sinuses: a clinicopathologic study of 20 cases. Cancer. 1984;53:2140–54.

16. Shanmugaratnam K, ed. Histological typing of upper respiratory tract tumours. 2nd ed. Berlin: Springer; 1991.
17. Gusterson BA, Mitchell DP, Warburton MJ, Carter RC. Epithelial markers in the diagnosis of nasopharyngeal carcinoma. J Clin Pathol. 1983;36:628–31.
18. Thomas JA, Iliescu V, Crawford DH, Ellouz R, Cammoun M, de The G. Expression of HLA-DR antigens in nasopharyngeal carcinoma: an immunohistochemical analysis of the tumour cells and infiltrating lymphocytes. Int J Cancer. 1984;33:813–9.
19. Roholl PJ, de Jong AS, Ramaekers FC. Review. Application of markers in the diagnosis of soft tissue tumours. Histopathology. 1985;9:1019–35.
20. Salisbury J, Isaacson PG. Demonstration of cytokeratins and an epithelial membrane antigen in chordomas and human fetal notochord. Am J Surg Path. 1985;9:791–7.
21. Buchanan G. Infectious mononucleosis. Ear Nose Throat J. 1982;61:557–61.
22. Sosa-Melgarejo J. Vergleichende immunozytochemische Untersuchungen zur rezidivierenden Tonsillitis und Mononucleosis Infectiosa. HNO. 1985;33:75–83.
23. Knowles DM, Jacobiec FA. Cell marker analysis of extranodal lymphoid infiltrates: to what extent does the determination of mono- or polyclonality resolve the diagnostic dilemma of malignant lymphoma v pseudolymphoma in an extranodal site. Sem Diagnos Pathol. 1985;2:163–8.
24. Lennert K, Feller AC. Histopathology of Non-Hodgkin-lymphomas (according to the updated Kiel-classification). 2nd ed. Berlin: Springer; 1991.
25. Quiney RE, Wells M, Lewis FA, Terry RM, Michaels L, Croft CB. Laryngeal papillomatosis: correlation between severity of disease and prsence of HPV 6 and 11 detected by in situ DNA hybridisation. J Clin Path. 1989;42:694–8.
26. Spencer H. Pathology of the lung, vol. 2. 4th ed. Oxford: Pergamon Press, 1985.
27. Woodruff JM, Huvos AG, Erlandson RA, Shah JP, Gerold FP. Neuroendocrine carcinomas of the larynx. A study of two types, one of which mimics thyroid medullary carcinoma. Am J Surg Pathol. 1985;9:771–90.
28. Wenig BM, Hyams VJ, Heffner DK. Moderately differentiated neuroendocrine carcinoma of the larynx. A clinicopathologic study of 54 cases. Cancer. 1988;62:2658–76.
29. Milroy CM, Rode J, Moss E. Laryngeal paraganglioma and neuroendocrine carcinomas. Histopathology. 1991;18:201–9.

6
Allergic Rhinitis

G. K. SCADDING

INTRODUCTION

Straightforward nasal allergy, with symptoms of sneezing, itch and rhinorrhoea, is usually simple to recognize and diagnose, and frequently responds to adequate medical treatment. However, unsuspected allergic disease may be the underlying factor in many other rhinological and otological problems and its treatment may obviate the need for surgery or potentiate its effects.

This chapter attempts to explain the immunological mechanisms that are, at present, thought to be involved in allergic disease; how these relate to clinical problems; and how they are affected by various therapeutic approaches. The rapidly increasing prevalence of allergic disease (Figure 1) means that it is a common factor in ENT patients.

MECHANISMS

The basic mechanism of allergic rhinitis is the degranulation of cells (usually mast cells or basophils) which have been rendered sensitive to allergen by specific antibody (IgE) which is held upon their surface. Release of various mediators, including histamine, occurs with resultant clinical effects (Figure 2).

A similar mechanism operates in immunity against worms, such as schistosomes. IgE-coated schistosome larvae can be killed by eosinophils which are attracted into the reaction site. Eosinophils are also seen in allergic rhinitis, both in the nasal mucosa and in nasal secretions. It seems as though a sensitive basic immunological mechanism is misapplied to various harmless protein molecules, such as those of pollens, danders and droppings of *Dermatophagoides pteronyssius*. Recently, it has become appreciated that

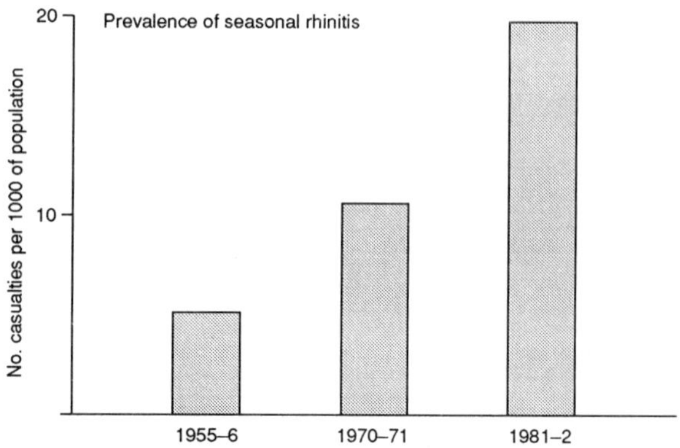

Figure 1 There is an increase in the incidence of seasonal rhinitis despite the lower grass pollen counts in recent years due to to silage production. Other allergic disorders, such as asthma and eczema are also increasing (Data from Fleming DM, Crombie DL. BMJ. 1987;294:279.)

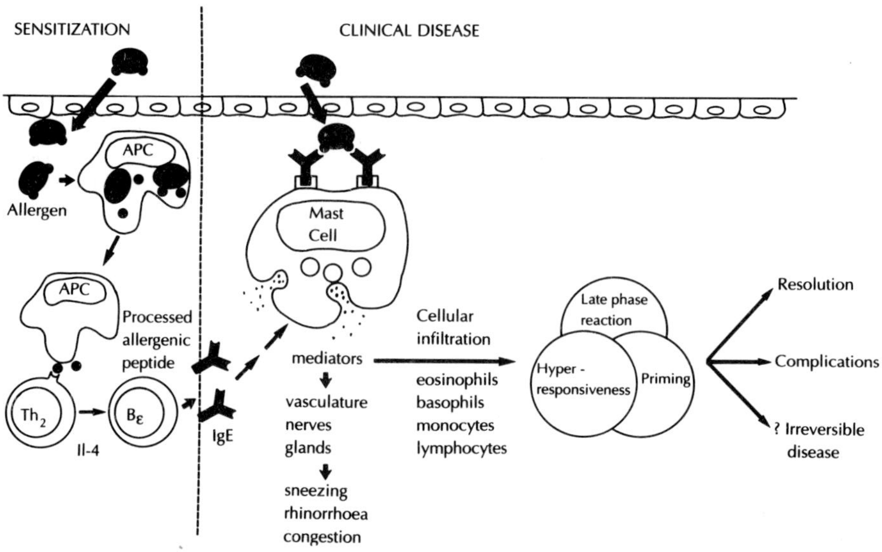

Figure 2 Mechanism of allergic rhinitis. Inhaled allergen is processed by antigen-presenting cells (which may be Langerhan's cells, macrophages or nasal epithelial cells) and presented to T helper cells and to B cells. The latter become IgE antibody-producing plasma cells. The IgE is rapidly and avidly taken up and held by mast cell and basophil Fc receptors. Subsequent allergen contact causes the sensitized mast cell to degranulate, releasing mediators which cause rhinorrhoea, itch and sneeze and nasal obstruction. This same mechanism (Type 1 hypersensitivity) underlies other allergic diseases, such as asthma and anaphylaxis. APC = antigen presenting cell; IL-4 = interleukin 4; Th_2 = helper T cell (type 2); B_ε = B cell capable of IgE production. Reproduced with permission from Naclerio RM. N Engl J Med. 1991;325:860–9

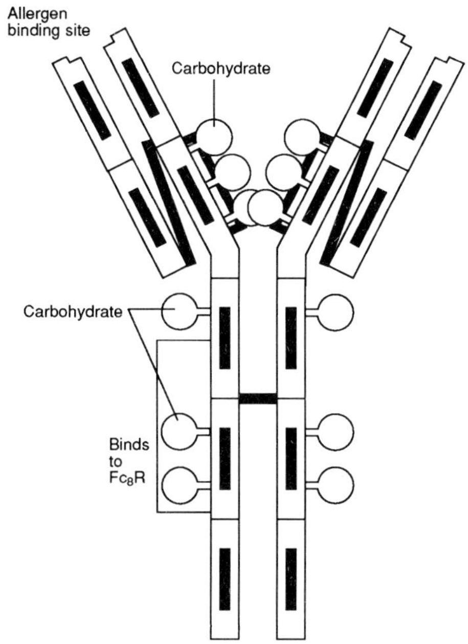

Figure 3 Structure of IgE. IgE has the basic 4-chain structure of all immunoglobulins, with 2 heavy and 2 light chains. The allergen binding sites are at the hypervariable ends of the chains as shown. A part of the Fc portion (tail piece) is involved in the binding to mast cells and basophils. This is heat-labile, being destroyed by 30 minutes at 56°C. IgE differs from IgG in several respects: it is more glycosylated, has 5 heavy chain domains rather than 4, does not cross the placenta, and has a very short serum half life of 2.5 days, compared with 21 days for IgG. IgE should probably be regarded as a secretory immunoglobulin. [Adapted from Brostoff J, Male D, Roitt IM. Immunology, 2nd Edn. London: Gower Medical Publishing; 1989, by kind permission]

other cells, such as T lymphocytes, cytokines and adhesion molecules are also important in the allergic reaction.

Immunoglobulin E

IgE is an immunoglobulin of similar structure to the other four classes, that is it contains two heavy chains and two light chains (Figure 3). The antigen-binding capacity resides in the Fab portion where the amino acid composition is at its most variable. The Fc or tail piece of the molecule is bound by high-affinity receptors ($Fc_{\varepsilon}RI$) on mast cells and basophils. There are also lower affinity IgE receptors, $Fc_{\varepsilon}RII$, on other cell types, including alveolar macrophages, monocytes, T and B lymphocytes, platelets and Langerhans cells. The Fc portion of the molecule is heat labile: 30 minutes at 56°C will abrogate the cytophilic capacity.

The serum half life of IgE is only 2.5 days, but, once cell bound, this is extended up to 12 weeks. Serum levels of IgE are much smaller than those of IgG, being measured in nano- rather than milligrams. The ability to make

IgE is universal, but certain individuals form IgE in response to harmless environmental allergens and tend to suffer from allergic diseases, such as asthma, eczema, hay fever, urticaria and food allergy. Such individuals are called atopic, (from the Greek 'out of place').

Atopy

In 1923, Coca and Cooke[6], noted that allergy ran in families and that allergic patients showed positive wheal and flare skin reactions to common inhalant allergens. The incidence of atopy is closely related to the serum IgE concentration: less than 5% of individuals with levels less than 60 IU/ml (1 IU = 2.4 ng), but over 95% of those with values over 450 IU/ml being affected. There is also an obvious genetic influence, over 50% of individuals having two allergic parents being atopic, compared with 15% in the normal population.

There are at least three genetic influences determining IgE production: an autosomal dominant gene codes for low IgE levels; HLA-linked genes control IgE and IgG production against specific allergenic proteins (most noticeable for minor determinants when total IgE is low); and HLA-B8 and DRW3 are associated with general immune hyper-responsiveness, possibly via decreased T suppressor activity. A recent study[7] suggests that there may be a major autosomal dominant gene on chromosome 11 controlling IgE responsiveness. This is being further investigated.

Environmental factors

Studies of identical (monozygotic) and non-identical (dizygotic) twins show that the concordance for atopic disease in dizygotic twins is slightly greater than in the general population; however, the concordance in monozygotic twins is well below the 100% expected if genotype were the sole determining factor. This suggests that the environment must also be involved in the expression of atopy. Environmental factors fall into two major groups: specific allergen exposure and non-specific trigger factors.

Early contact with highly allergenic substances is more likely to result in an allergic response. This is possibly related to the failure of mucosal protective mechanisms, such as IgA, in early life. Sensitization to food allergens, such as cow's milk proteins and ovalbumin, may occur during fetal life. Small quantities of IgE are detectable in cord blood in children of atopic parents and are regarded as a risk factor for the development of allergic disease.

There appears to be a window of opportunity for allergic sensitization during the first year or so of allergen contact, even in adult life. Certain factors increase the likelihood of allergic sensitization.

Disruption of mucosal surfaces, by pollutants like sulphur dioxide or during viral infections, allows increased allergen entry. Repeated exposure to minute quantities of protein favours an IgE, rather than an IgG, response.

Environmental pollutants, such as sulphur dioxide, nitrogen oxide, diesel

Table 1 Environmental factors in the development of childhood allergic diseases. Early exposure to inhalant or ingested allergens before mucosal defence mechanisms are fully developed increases the likelihood of allergic sensitization

Pregnancy	smoking β-blocking drugs month of birth
Perinatal	stress early operations gastroenteritis
Childhood	low IgA levels viral infections inhalant allergens smoke diet position in family

[From Brostoff J, Scadding GK, Male D, Roitt IM. Clinical immunology. London: Gower Medical Publishing; 1991, with permission]

fumes and fly ash, can increase mucosal permeability and therefore enhance antigen entry and IgE responsiveness. The effect of smoking is biphasic: IgE levels are enhanced with low cigarette consumption and suppressed with high consumption. Smoking also causes a reduction in the IgG immune response to inhaled antigens. Diesel exhaust particulates act as an adjuvant for IgE production. They are less than 1 μm in diameter, are buoyant in the atmosphere of polluted districts (with concentrations in urban air of 2–500 $\mu g/m^3$ being recorded) and are inhaled. Their adjuvant effect is seen experimentally with low-dose antigen exposure, simulating that which occurs naturally. The increase in allergic rhinitis and asthma in the last three decades parallels an increase in air pollution and diesel exhaust.

Other important factors in the development of allergic disease in childhood are seen in Table 1.

Control of IgE production

The alterations responsible for the dysregulation of IgE production in human allergic disorders are still not fully known despite several decades of research. Early studies in rodents suggested that antigen-specific helper and suppressor T lymphocytes were involved. In man, there are several clinical conditions with an association between low T suppressor cell numbers and high levels of IgE, supporting this hypothesis. Some of this control is exerted by IgE-binding factors: an IgE-potentiating factor (IgE-PF) and an IgE-suppressor actor (IgE-SF), which differ only in glycosylation. The relative amounts of these are controlled by glycosylation-enhancing, or glycosylation-inhibiting factors produced by T helper and T suppressor cells respectively.

More recently, another pathway of IgE regulation, based on the reciprocal activity of the cytokines, interleukin-4 (IL-4) and interferon-γ (IFN-γ), has been discovered in both mice and man. IL-4 is the essential mediator for the synthesis of IgE, and IFN-γ exerts a negative regulatory effect. A prior physical interaction with helper T cells is required by B cells to synthesize IgE in response to IL-4; this interaction can be either cognate or non-specific. The increased production of IgE antibodies against common environmental allergens in atopic individuals could occur because allergens differ from other antigens in their ability to select helper T cells able to produce IL-4 (Th2 cells) but not inhibitory amounts of IFN-γ. Several groups have investigated the profile of cytokine production by allergen-specific T cell clones[12,13]: most are usually high producers of IL-4, but there is no complete agreement with regard to the production of IFN-γ. However, T cell clones specific for bacterial antigens, particularly PPD, consistently produced IFN-γ, whereas production of IL-4 was not the rule. Recently, T cell clones derived from the conjunctival infiltrates of patients with allergic conjunctivitis demonstrated high IL-4 production with little or no IFN-γ. This suggests that helper cells with Th2-like functional profiles of cytokine production accumulate in the target organs of patients suffering from allergic diseases. Although experiments in mice suggest that, in principle, every B cell can switch to IgE production, in practice, only about 1 in 33 human B cells does so under experimental IL-4 stimulation. This is a lower frequency than the switch from IgM to other isotypes and always occurs directly from IgM, not via an IgG-producing step. The IgE clone tends to be smaller than those producing IgG, though individual cell production is similar to that of other isotype-producing cells. Interestingly, and opposite to IgG, switch to IgE occurred only at low B cell densities, with an optimum of 1000 cells/well. This may have physiological relevance: IgE-mediated allergic reactions leading to cell influx could decrease further local switching to IgE production. However, there is evidence of spontaneous IgE production in vitro without the need for IL-4 in cells taken from atopic individuals, suggesting that IgE-committed cells may persist in vivo.

Recent evidence suggests that mast cells may have an autocrine function, secreting cytokines IL-3, 4, 5 and 6 several hours after degranulation. IL-4 has been demonstrated in tryptase-positive cells from the subepithelial region of human lung and nose. It is conceivable that T cells initiate IgE production and that mast cells maintain it until autonomy sets in.

CD23

The $Fc_{\varepsilon}RII$ is also known as CD23 and is a 45 kDa integral membrane protein, expressed primarily on B cells and monocytes, that binds IgE with low affinity. Functionally, CD23 has been linked to the regulation of IgE synthesis[14] as well as to other immune mechanisms. CD23 is rapidly processed at the cell surface to yield a variety of cleavage products (soluble CD23), most of which retain IgE-binding activity. Soluble CD23 can, in synergy with IL-4, upregulate IgE synthesis and promote the growth of CD23-positive B cells.

The amount of CD23 on the cell surface is itself upregulated by IL-4 and tempered by interferons. Interestingly, a monoclonal antibody to another

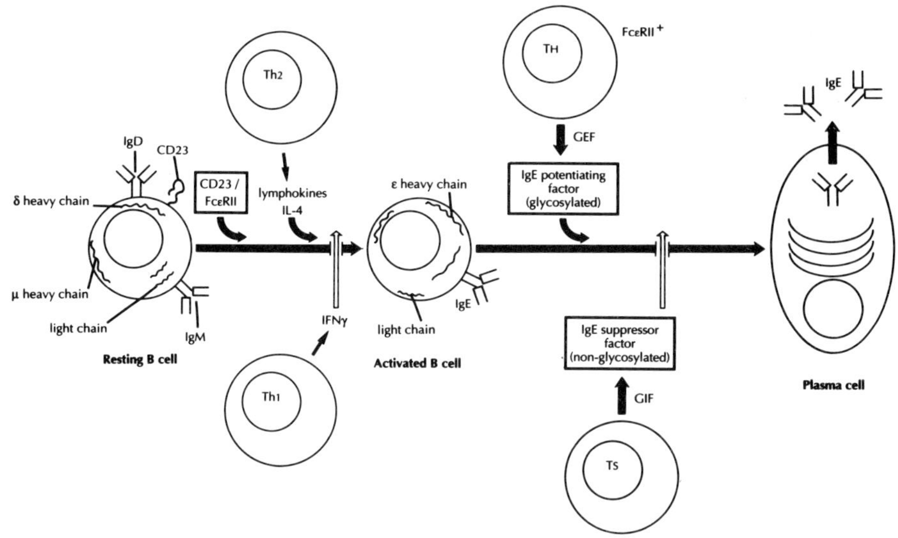

Figure 4 Different helper T cells produce IL-4 (Th2 cells) and IFN-γ (Th1 cells); the former promotes IgE synthesis, the latter is inhibitory. Soluble CD23 (a part of the lower affinity IgE receptor which enters the serum) potentiates IL-4. There is also evidence for binding factors produced by human T cells which can enhance or inhibit IgE production and which differ only in glycosylation [From Brostoff J, Scadding GK, Male D, Roitt IM. Ciinical immunology. London: Gower Medical Publishing; 1991, with permission]

cell surface receptor, CD40, has recently been shown to override all the usual inhibitors of IL-4-promoted CD23 induction, including interferons and corticosteroids. This may be of relevance in steroid-resistant asthma and rhinitis. (Figure 4 attempts a diagrammatic representation of these controlling influences.)

CELLS INVOLVED IN THE ALLERGIC RESPONSE

Mast cells

More than 100 years ago, Paul Ehrlich first described mast cells and basophils as granular cells that stained metachromatically with basic dyes. There are similarities between mast cells and basophils but they are distinct cell types. Both synthesize and store histamine, proteoglycan and proteases in their granules and have surface receptors that bind IgE with high affinity ($Fc_{\varepsilon}RI$). Cross-linking of this surface IgE leads to a calcium-dependent activation with degranulation.

Neutral proteases have been used to distinguish two populations of human mast cells. Most mast cells found at mucosal surfaces, such as in the nose, contain tryptase, whereas those in connective tissue contain chymase and tryptase. Drug sensitivity and the pattern of mediator release differ between mast cells and basophils and between these different types of mast cells.

The allergic response in the nose

The initial event is inhalation of allergen followed by its solubilization in the watery nasal mucus. In this form, allergen probably first contacts basophilic cells present on or in the nasal surface layer. The basophilic cells present in nasal secretions have been studied by Okuda[19]. They are of two types: one resembles the basophil leukocyte of human peripheral blood, being characterized by the lobulated nucleus with peripheral condensation of chromatin, and small in size with minimum microphyllae (Figure 5). The other is similar to the mucosal mast cells which were demonstrated by Enerback in rat intestine. These are small and round with few granules. In contrast, the classical mast cells found in connective tissue, deeper in the lamina propria, are larger with many dark scrolled granules (Figure 5b and c). Differences exist between these cell types, both in their mediator contents and in their reactions to drugs. For example, basophils do not contain prostaglandin D_2 and classical mast cells are not cromoglycate sensitive, unlike mucosal mast cells. These factors may be important in determining symptomatology and responses to treatment.

If allergen cross-links the IgE molecules on the mast cell or basophil surface, a sequence of events occurs with an increase in cyclic AMP and free calcium in the cell cytosol. The preformed granules are moved to the cell periphery and their contents are discharged. At the same time, the cell membrane arachidonic acid is acted upon by an enzyme, phospholipase A_2, and is converted by two major pathways: the cyclo-oxygenase pathway to prostaglandins and thromboxanes, and the lipoxygenase pathway to the leukotrienes (previously called slow-reacting substance of anaphylaxis). Recent research suggests that a third phase of cytokine production takes place in the mast cell during the hours after degranulation. This involves synthesis of protein from messenger RNA and results in the generation of interleukins 3, 4 and 6.

Degranulation of mast cells and basophils can also occur following cross-linking of adjacent membrane-bound IgE molecules by anti-IgE, by anti-idiotype or by lectins. Fab portions of anti-idiotype could occupy IgE antigen-binding sites without causing cross-linking and degranulation and could thus theoretically act to prevent mast cell degranulation.

Pseudoallergy

Certain substances can affect mast cell membranes directly, allowing calcium ion influx and release of granule contents. These include the anaphylatoxins, C3a and C5a, mellitin (a component of insect venom) and drugs, such as

Figure 5 The three types of basophilic cells in the nose. (a) The basophil leukocytes which are mainly in nasal mucus, (b) atypical mast cells found in the epithelium and (c) typical mast cells found in the lamina propria. In allergic rhinitis, the basophilic cells increase in the mucus and epithelial layers and produce symptoms by reacting to allergen. The role of the lamina propria mast cells is unknown. From Okuda M. Mast cells and the nose. Allergy Today. 1987;2(4):4–6, by permission from Fisons Pharmaceuticals

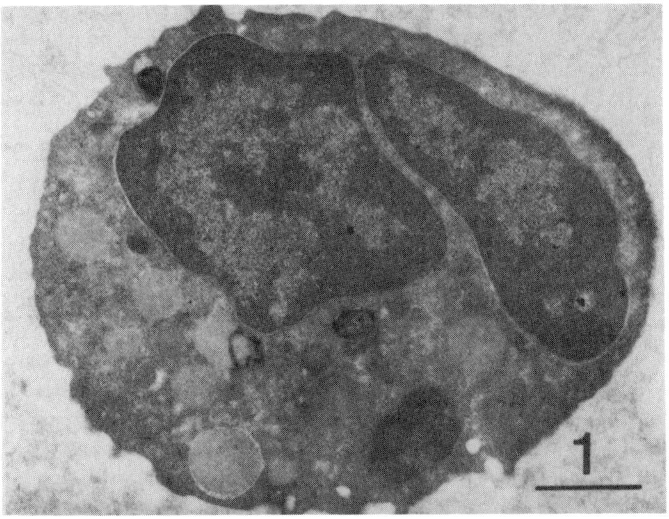

(a)

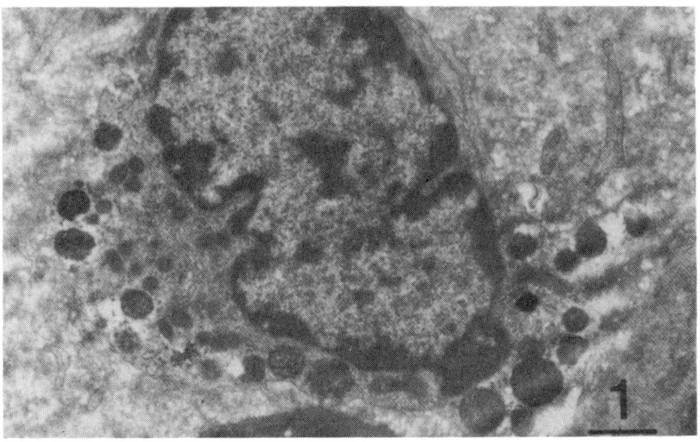

(b)

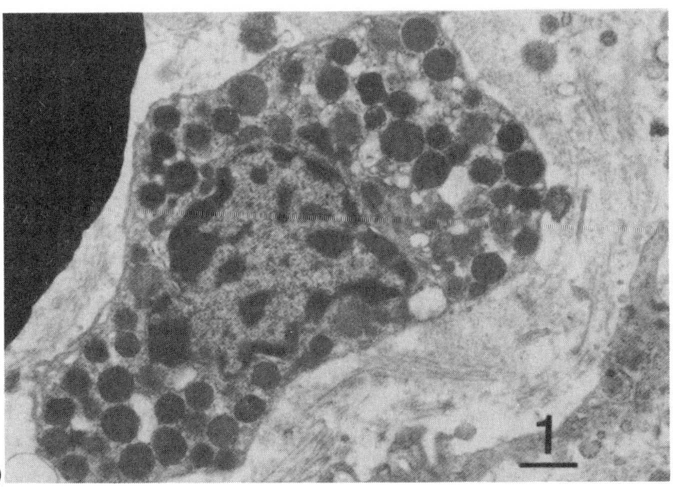

(c)

codeine, morphine and synthetic ACTH. Physical stimuli, such as pressure, heat, cold and sunlight, can cause mast cell degranulation in certain individuals.

Other cells involved in the allergic response

For many years, allergists have focused on mast cells as the responsible cell type in the allergic reaction. More recently, the importance of other cells, such as T lymphocytes and eosinophils, has begun to be appreciated.

T cells

The exquisite sensitivity of the T lymphocyte to therapeutic doses of corticosteroids in vitro, in contrast to the relative resistance of mast cells and eosinophils, suggests that T lymphocytes may be a controlling influence. CD3-positive (T) cells can be seen in the skin 24 hours after allergen infiltration; CD4-positive (helper T) cells are seen in the nasal late-phase response and are decreased in patients pretreated by immunotherapy compared with a placebo group[20]. There is a correlation between the number of eosinophils present in the late phase and the numbers of CD4+ve T cells.

Autoradiography, after the addition of labelled antisense (complementary) mRNA for various cytokines, shows increases in IL-3, IL-4, IL-5 and GM-CSF. There is also a correlation, in biopsy samples several hours after allergen exposure, between activated eosinophils and IL5 mRNA+ cells. Recently, patients with steroid-resistant asthma have been shown to improve on treatment with cyclosporin[29], which is known to have major effects on T cell function.

Eosinophils

These bone-marrow-derived granulocytes develop under the influence of various lymphokines, including IL-5. They are both secretory and phagocytic and are associated with parasitic infestation as well as with allergy. When recruited into allergic reactions by chemotactic factors, including GM-CSF, they are 'activated', with increased oxidative metabolism, enhanced cytotoxicity and elevated membrane receptor expression for IgG and complement.

As in mast cells, there are two groups of eosinophil mediators: granule-associated (e.g. MBP, ECP) and membrane-derived (e.g. LTC4 and platelet activating factor).

The role of the eosinophil in allergy is disputed. It was thought to be a 'switch off and repair cell' deactivating mediators and phagocytosing allergen–IgE complexes and mast cell granules. However, the finding of eosinophilic infiltrates in mucus plugs, in epithelia and beneath the basement membrane of bronchi in patients dying with asthma, the capability of eosinophil

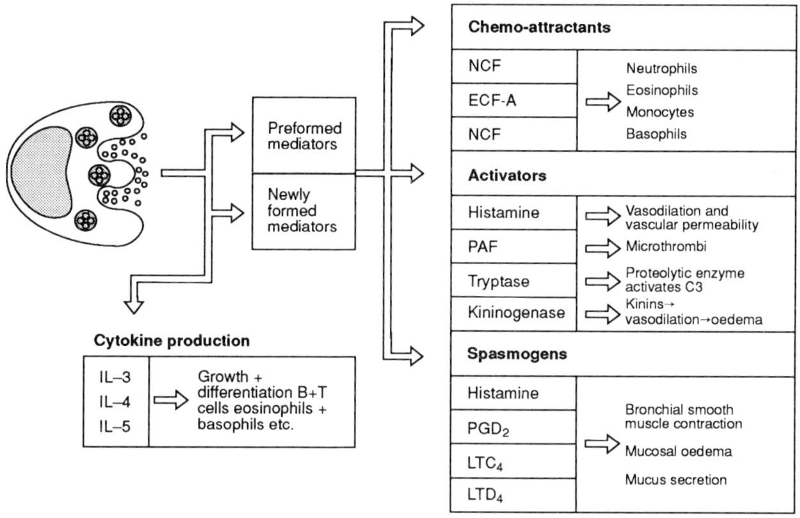

Figure 6 Physiological effects of mast-cell-derived mediators. These have three main functions. Chemoattractants draw other cells to the site of mast cell activation, including eosinophils, basophils, neutrophils and mononuclear cells (including lymphocytes). Inflammatory activators cause vasodilatation and increase vascular permeability, leading to oedema. They also activate other inflammatory systems, such as the complement and kinin cascades. In the nose, the major effect of the spasmogens is to increase mucus secretion. Histamine also irritates nerve endings in the mucosa causing reflex sneezing. Cytokine production by mast cells probably amplifies inflammation [Adapted from Brostoff J, Male D, Roitt IM. Immunology, 2nd Edn. London: Gower Medical Publishing; 1989, with permission]

mediators to damage tissues, together with the demonstration of ECP in the late-phase response, has given rise to the idea that it is an important pathogenic cell.

PHYSIOLOGICAL EFFECTS OF MEDIATORS

Mast-cell-derived mediators fall into three main groups according to their physiological effects: spasmogens, activators and chemoattractants. In man, histamine is the major vasoactive amine; this causes vasodilation, increased capillary permeability and bronchoconstriction. The physiological effects of the major mast cell and basophil mediators in man are shown in Figure 6.

The evidence for the role of various mediators in nasal allergy has been reviewed by Pipkorn[15]. Table 2 shows the putative mediators identified in nasal secretions, either after allergen challenge or during natural allergen exposure. In such experiments, levels of n-tosyl-L-arginine methyl esterase (TAME-esterase), a plasma-derived non-specific marker of inflammation, best reflects symptomatology. This suggests that plasma leakage plays a crucial part in the production of nasal allergic symptoms by bringing peptide mediators from the kinins, complement and coagulation systems into contact

Table 2 Putative mediators identified in nasal secretions

Mediator	*Origin*
Histamine Prostaglandin D_2 (PGD_2) Tryptase	Mast cells/basophils
Eosinophil cationic protein (ECP) Major basic protein (MBP)	Eosinophils
Myeloperoxidase (MPO)	Neutrophils
Platelet activating factor (PAF) Serotonin	Platelets
Platelet activating factor Leukotrienes B_4, C_4, D_4 Prostaglandins D_2, F_2, E 5-Keto prostaglandin F_1 Thromboxane	Various cells
Kinins Complement factors	Plasma
Substance P Vasoactive intestinal polypeptide (VIP)	Neural cells

Taken from Pipkorn U. Mediators and nasal allergy. Clin Exp Allergy. 1989;19:586, with kind permission from Blackwell Scientific Publications

with the site of reaction, thus augmenting inflammation.

Nasal challenge with a number of putative mediators has been attempted and the effects of specific mediator antagonists are being investigated. However, the redundancy of the systems involved, with more than one mediator being able to produce a given effect, means that lack of inhibition by an antagonist does not rule out a role for its agonist.

Histamine is still the only mediator which behaves consistently in terms of release at appropriate challenge and production of all major rhinitic symptoms (secretion, sneezing and blockage) on local administration. These are influenced by specific antagonists: both H_1 and H_2 receptor antagonists decrease the amount of secretion, H_1 receptor antagonists decrease sneezing, but neither effects blockage, which may be mediated via H_3 receptors. Unfortunately, the very variable baseline level of histamine in nasal secretions makes the lavage procedure unsuitable for demonstration of changes in this mediator during natural exposure. However, tissue levels of histamine in nasal mucosa do correlate well with symptom scores.

Other possible contributors to nasal obstruction are leukotrienes C_4 and D_4 and prostaglandin D_2. LTC_4 and D_4 on nasal application produce a dose-dependent sustained nasal blockage and increased secretion, but no itch or sneeze. PGD_2 infusions give rise to complaints of nasal stuffiness. Evidence suggests that kinins may be mediators of allergic rhinitis, since bradykinin and kallidin are found in the nasal secretions of patients with naturally occurring allergic rhinitis[17], and application of bradykinin to the nasal airway has been shown to induce symptoms of rhinitis[18]. Recent studies (Austin, Foreman and Scadding, data in press) indicate that the BK_2 receptor antagonist, [D-Arg^0,Hyp^3,Thi^5,D-Tic^7,Oic^8]bradykinin, is an effective antagonist of the BK-induced response in the human nasal airway, and of the nasal response to allergen challenge. A further contribution to nasal obstruction could be the infiltration of cells, such as eosinophils, drawn by chemoattractants, such as eosinophil chemotactic factor (ECF) and leukotriene B_4 (LTB_4).

LATE-PHASE RESPONSES

Although the symptomatic response to nasal allergen exposure occurs within minutes and is usually over by 1 hour, studies have demonstrated that a late response occurs in about 50% of patients. This phenomenon, which can also be seen following allergic reactions in the skin and bronchi, involves the ingress of inflammatory cells and is associated with hyper-reactivity to allergen or non-specific challenge.

Studies on the nasal mucous membrane in the hours following challenge have demonstrated the ingress of neutrophils, eosinophils and, later, mononuclear cells. Levels of eosinophil-derived proteins, such as eosinophil cationic protein (ECP), eosinophil-derived neurotoxin (EDN) and major basic protein (MBP) are elevated in nasal secretions some hours post-challenge. These cause epithelial damage and may cause hyper-reactivity via exposure of nerve endings. There is a strong correlation between the number of basophils and the level of histamine in the late reaction, suggesting that basophils not only enter the nasal mucosa at this stage, but also degranulate. The absence of PGD_2 in late-phase nasal secretions also suggests basophil involvement since these cells do not, unlike mast cells, contain PGD_2.

The number of mast cells and eosinophil progenitors in nasal scrapings increases after exposure to allergens and correlates with the severity of seasonal disease. About half the individuals with allergic rhinitis show increased sensitivity to allergen after repeated daily exposure. This is associated with the cellular influx of basophils and increased release of some mediators, such as histamine. In the nose and sinuses, the thickened mucosa may be a predisposing factor to chronic or recurrent rhinosinusitis.

CYTOKINES

These are substances which are made by one cell and act locally to influence further cells of the same or different types. The role of various cytokines in allergic inflammation is under investigation; the effect of IL-4 on B cell development and differentiation has already been mentioned. Other pro-inflammatory interleukins, such as IL-4, IL-3, IL-5 and IL-6, are probably involved in the regulation of cell development. mRNA coding for TNFα (tumor necrosis factor) has recently been demonstrated in allergic inflammation in nose, skin and lungs. This potentiates inflammation by making endothelial cells express ICAM-1 (an adhesion molecule) so that granulocytes stick to the vessel wall. It also has a direct action on eosinophils and

Table 3 Cytokines in allergy

	From	*Actions*
IL-1 TNF-α IL-2	many T-cells	pro-inflammatory: T cell activation; ↑ ICAM-1; ↑ cytokine production T cell proliferation + clonal amplification
IL-3 + IL-5	T cell mast cell	growth + differentiation: stem cells, eosinophils, basophils integrin expression
IL-4	T cell mast cell	co-factor in T cell activation growth and differentiation B cells switch to IgE production
GM-CSF/ G-CSF	fibroblasts epithelium endothelium T cells	growth + differentiation haemopoietic cells activation of mature granulocytes integrin expression
IL-9	T cell	enhances mast cell growth
IL-10	T + B cells	co-factor in mast cell growth inhibits cytokines from Th1 T cells

neutrophils to increase their adhesion to vascular endothelium and hence accumulation of sites of inflammation. Another cytokine, GM-CSF (granulocyte macrophage colony stimulating factor), performs the same function for eosinophils, activates them and can render them corticosteroid resistant. Table 3 shows the cytokines thought to be involved in the allergic response.

Recently, it has been shown that ICAM-1 is the receptor for many rhinoviruses, the major cause of the common cold. Upregulation of ICAM-1 in allergic patients could increase their susceptibility to viral infection. Anecdotal evidence that regular use of inhaled corticosteroids decreases upper respiratory tract infections may have a basis in fact.

The development of anticytokines and cytokine inhibitors should provide a further possible therapeutic option.

CLINICAL EFFECTS

Allergic rhinitis is the commonest immunological disease and the commonest chronic disease of man, affecting 10–15% of the population. It can be seasonal, due to wind-borne pollens, or perennial due to allergens such as the house dust mite and animal dander, or a combination of the two. Occupational allergens, such as flour and ricin (from castor beans), can also cause rhinitis. Inhalant allergens are usually responsible for rhinitis, although, in a small proportion of patients, foods such as cows' milk protein are involved. Interestingly, a proportion of birch pollen-sensitive patients are also allergic to apple, nuts and celery, which show RAST cross-reactivity to birch pollen.

Allergic inhalation results in the degranulation of IgE-sensitized basophils and mast cells, leading to mediator release. There is dilatation of blood vessels with oedema formation and fluid leakage into nasal secretions, together with nerve irritation and glandular secretion. This results in sneeze, itch, rhinorrhoea and congestion.

Augmentation of response

Increased antigen sensitivity in the nose after repeated antigen exposure (priming) has been known since 1967. Increased numbers of mast cells are seen in the nasal mucosa at the end of the grass pollen season compared with the beginning. Allergen challenge to the basal mucosa is followed by an increased sensitivity to histamine lasting up to 10 days. This hyper-reactivity can lead patients to state that they are allergic to smoke or perfume, whereas, in fact, they are simply hyper-reactive having been sensitized earlier by an allergen such as house dust mite.

Chronic problems

Chronic allergen exposure tends to cause obstruction, possibly via a continuing inflammatory response, with less itch and sneeze and with posterior catarrh rather than anterior rhinorrhoea. As such, its underlying allergic nature may not be recognized: the typically 'adenoidal' child is frequently also suffering from undiagnosed perennial allergic rhinitis with swelling throughout the nasal mucosa of the respiratory tract and with enlarged lymphoid tissues, possibly the site of the ongoing IgE response.

Many patients with uncontrolled allergic disease are prone to sinus and middle ear problems. They tend to have symptoms in response to barometric pressure changes and more frequent infections, which tend to involve the middle ear in childhood and the sinuses in adults. Underlying factors are probably poor sinus drainage, apposition of swollen mucosa leading to decreased ciliary function and possibly also decreased ciliary beat frequency secondary to an allergic response.

More generalized effects of nasal inflammation include poor sleep and snoring (with an increased risk of cerebrovascular events), decreased appetite (due to the associated anosmia and mucous drainage into the stomach), impaired social life and occupational problems, e.g. to a singer or public speaker.

DIAGNOSIS

The diagnosis of allergic rhinitis can frequently be made on the patient's history, when particular attention is paid to past and family history of allergy, precipitating factors and the seasonal and/or diurnal nature of symptoms. Continuous allergen exposure frequently goes unrecognized until there has been a gap of at least 2 weeks, such as a holiday, following which the allergen is re-encountered. Symptoms then are usually more marked and include sneezing and rhinorrhoea as well as a recurrence of obstruction. Thus, when a patient says that their cat never causes problems, it is as well to ask whether this is true when the patient returns from holiday.

Skin prick testing

This is a usual adjunct to the history and, when positive, also provides a demonstration for the patient of the swelling which can result in response to allergen exposure. False positive results can occur, and the skin prick test must always be interpreted in the light of the history. It is rarely necessary to take blood for IgE levels (which are normal in 50% of allergic rhinitis patients) or for a radio-allergosorbent test looking for specific IgE. The latter is no more sensitive than skin prick testing and is more expensive. However, it may be necessary for the patient with previous anaphylactic reactions, for those with severe eczema, those who have recently taken antihistamine and for dermatographic patients.

Nasal challenge

Since the IgE response initially occurs locally close to the site of allergen contact, the mast cells and basophils at this site will retain this allergen-specific IgE until they are saturated. Only after this will there be a spill over into the blood with sensitization of cells at other sites such as the skin. This means that it is possible to have a negative skin prick test and yet to give a specific positive allergic response on nasal challenge. Thus nasal challenge with the postulated allergen is the final diagnostic arbiter. The use of objective measurements following challenge increases the incidence of positive responses markedly.

Nasal smears

The demonstration of eosinophils in nasal smears is a good predictor of responsiveness to inhaled corticosteroids. Nasal eosinophilia is seen in allergic rhinitis and in the so-called NARES syndrome, i.e. non-allergic rhinitis with eosinophilia. It is likely that a proportion of NARES patients are, in fact, allergic but undiagnosed, largely because of the excessive reliance placed on skin prick and RAST testing.

TREATMENT

There is limited information available on the natural history of allergic rhinitis and its prognosis without treatment. Complete remission of symptoms occurs in 5–10% of patients, usually in those with mild seasonal disease of short duration. In a further 5–10%, perennial asthma develops. In view of morbidity from the disease itself and from complications, such as sinusitis, eustachian tube dysfunction, dysosmia, sleep disturbance, etc., it seems reasonable to advise treatment.

There are three main principles of treatment of allergic rhinitis: allergen avoidance, pharmacotherapy, and immunotherapy.

Allergen avoidance

This is the first line of treatment and can be curative if complete avoidance is achieved. The efficacy of house dust mite removal has been shown in a group of asthmatic children. Half of these house dust mite-sensitive children had the bedroom dust reduced as much as possible with a subsequent reduction in the number of wheezy days, need for medication and occasions when a low peak flow was recorded. Bronchial hyper-reactivity was also reduced. Meticulous elimination of house dust mite allergen is rewarding in rhinitis, especially in those patients who fail to respond to initial pharmacotherapy. A 40% reduction in symptoms can be achieved by encasing pillows and mattresses in impermeable covers (a water-vapour permeable house dust mite impermeable material which is more comfortable than plastic is now available) together with frequent damp dusting, effective vacuuming and hot washing of bedding.

Ingested allergens are rarely a major cause of rhinitis. Avoidance of food antigens is difficult and should be done on an experimental basis, with complete elimination followed by re-introduction with symptom monitoring throughout. The adequacy of the remaining diet should be assessed by a dietician. The major group with food sensitivity is young children in whom cow's milk protein is the usual cause. It is important to ensure that the treatment is not worse than the initial disease!

Pharmacotherapy

The medications used and their sites of action are shown in Figure 7 and a plan for the treatment of allergic rhinitis is shown in Figure 8. As with asthma, anti-inflammatory therapy is recommended for anything other than mild disease. In general, only corticosteroids are effective against all symptoms, including obstruction, whereas antihistamines provide symptomatic relief of rhinorrhoea, sneeze and itch. Thus they make an effective combination. It is important to use an initial dose of corticosteroids which is sufficient to overcome the nasal inflammation. Betamethasone nose drops used in the head down and forward position are usually more effective than any corticosteroid spray initially. Once symptoms are under control, a spray can usually be used for routine maintenance treatment. The exceptions to this are those patients with nasal polyps or with marked hyposmia, where nose drops taken in the head down and forward position appear more effective at reaching the ethmoid area. In very severely affected or very resistant patients, it may be necessary to start with systemic corticosteroids, either as oral prednisolone or injected adrenocorticotrophic hormone

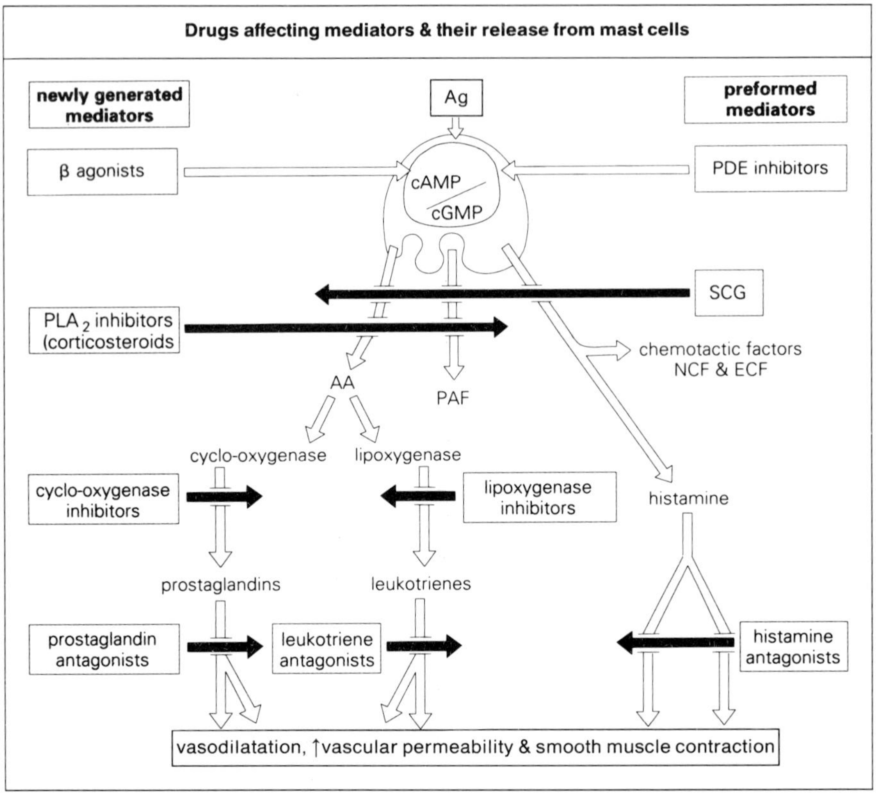

Figure 7 The balance of cyclic AMP and GMP within a mast cell determine its ease of degranulation. *β*-Agonists and phosphodiesterase (PDE) inhibitors increase cyclic AMP and inhibit mediator release; *β*-blockers have the reverse effect and may worsen rhinitis and asthma. Sodium cromoglycate has mast-cell-stabilizing activity, as well as many other actions which are less understood. Corticosteroids probably exert their major effects upon T lymphocytes but can also inhibit breakdown of arachidonic acid to make mediators. Antagonists are under development and testing for various stages of the leukotriene pathway. Aspirin-like compounds inhibit prostaglandin synthetase and cause increased generation of leukotrienes from arachidonic acid. Histamine-receptor blockers are valuable in allergic rhinitis but have little effect in asthma.
Dietary attempts to change the composition of membrane lipids from the E3 to the E2 (less reactive) series by increasing the proportion of polyunsaturated fats have been largely unsuccessful in allergy [Adapted from Brostoff J, Scadding GK, Male D, Roitt IM. Clinical immunology. London: Gower Medical Publishing; 1991, with permission]

(ACTH).

Local sodium cromoglycate (Rynacrom) is unfortunately less effective in the nose than in the lower airways. However, it is a useful first line of treatment in small children, where corticosteroids are relatively contraindicated. It may be necessary, in children, to use a small dose of local corticosteroid at night with Rynacrom throughout the rest of the day. Frequent usage of Rynacrom, at least four times daily, does increase its efficacy, but makes compliance a problem.

Diagnosis of allergic rhinitis
↓
Identification of allergen(s)
↓
Allergen avoidance
↓
Still symptomatic

Mild symptoms	*Watery rhinorrhoea only*	*Moderate symptoms*	*Severe symptoms*	*Very severe symptoms*
Antihistamine as required	Ipratroprium spray	Regular cromoglycate (child) or local corticosteroids (adult). If not controlled, add antihistamine (regular or as required) or local corticosteroid (child)	Betamethasone nose drops plus regular antihistamine ↓ Corticosteroid spray for long-term use with or without regular antihistamine	Short course of oral corticosteroids plus betamethasone drops ↓ If no response, consider immunotherapy

In addition, short courses of *intranasal* decongestants may be needed:
1. at the start of treatment
2. for flying
3. in the 'thick phase' of upper respiratory tract infections

Figure 8 A treatment plan for allergic rhinitis

Table 4 Major immunological changes during immunotherapy. Clinical benefit is not clearly related to any one of these changes, not all of which occur in every patient. Reduced Th2 cell responsiveness may play an important role

– ↑ specific IgG (blocking antibody)
– ↑ IgE over several months; then slow ↓IgE over years abrogation of usual seasonal ↑IgE
– ↑ specific IgG & IgA in nasal secretions
– ↓ mediator release from sensitized cells in some patients
– ↓ lymphocyte proliferation & lymphokine production to immunizing antigen; development of antigen-specific suppressor cells
– Switch of Th2 to Th1 type T cells seen in nasal biopsy

[Adapted from Brostoff J, Scadding GK, Male D, Roitt IM. Clinical immunology. London: Gower Medical Publishing; 1991, with permission]

Some of the new generation of non-sedating antihistamines are claimed to have effects on the late-phase response, with decreased migration of cells, such as the eosinophils, into the tissues. This has not yet been convincingly demonstrated in the nose, although a new intranasal antihistamine, azelastine, does appear to have some effect on nasal blockage.

Immunotherapy

This is the administration by injection of sufficient allergen to atopic individuals to reduce their allergic response following subsequent natural exposure. It began in 1911 when Noon[30] used grass pollen extracts to decrease hay fever symptoms. Hyposensitization appears to reduce the symptoms and the need for medication in 60–90% of rhinitics, although only a small percentage become completely asymptomatic. The mechanism of action is not yet known, but a number of immunological changes have been shown to take place and these are detailed in Table 4.

The occurrence of anaphylactic reactions and death during immunotherapy means that this treatment must be reserved for severely affected individuals who do not respond to conventional therapy. Asthmatics appear to be at particular risk of bad reactions and should probably be excluded. The current regulations in the UK state that immunotherapy must be undertaken only in centres where full cardiorespiratory resuscitation facilities are available and that the patient must be monitored for 2 hours following each injection. In fact, in the past 27 years, twenty-six patients have died from immunotherapy, whereas over 25 000 have died of asthma.

The prospects for safer and more specific immunotherapy in allergic disease are being investigated at the moment and these are dealt with in the final chapter.

Surgery

The place of surgery in uncomplicated allergic rhinitis is limited to structural improvements of the airway (septoplasty, turbinate reduction) to increase the access of local medications. Surgical intervention may well be required in the treatment of chronic sinusitis but should be combined with allergen avoidance and pharmacotherapy for maximum effect. The role of vidian neurectomy (to decrease autonomic input) in the treatment of profuse rhinorrhoea is not established. The production of submucosal fibrosis by cauterization, cryotherapy or laser surgery to the turbinates has not been shown to be of prolonged benefit.

Treatment during pregnancy

Allergen avoidance is the mainstay of treatment and is also sensible from the point of view of the developing child, since early allergen exposure appears to lead to earlier and more severe allergic disease. The fetus of an allergic mother has a 30% chance of being atopic; this increases to about 60% if both parents are allergic.

Pharmacotherapy in pregnancy is difficult and rhinitis symptoms may be severe. Sodium cromoglycate, which is practically non-absorbed, is safe. Of the corticosteroids, betamethasone is best avoided because of systemic absorption; beclomethasone in routine dosage is frequently used. Some antihistamines, e.g. azelastine, can cause fetal malformations; my practice is to give chlorpheniramine at night only when symptoms prevent sleep.

Immunotherapy does not appear to hold any excessive risks in pregnancy as long as systemic reactions are avoided.

Aspirin sensitivity

Some patients suffer from the well-known triad of nasal polyposis, asthma and acute sensitivity to aspirin. Many of these individuals are skin prick test negative and have intrinsic asthma, although skin-prick test-positive aspirin-sensitive patients also occur. The majority of subjects with aspirin sensitivity may be carefully desensitized as in-patients by the oral administration of increasing dosages of aspirin. This may lead to an improvement in the nasal symptoms and the asthma.

The mechanism of aspirin sensitivity is unknown, as is the mechanism of the frequently associated alcohol intolerance. Subjects with aspirin-sensitive asthma and rhinitis are also intolerant of other non-steroidal anti-inflammatory drugs and the capacity of these agents to provoke asthma is related to their potency as inhibitors of the cyclo-oxygenase enzyme. This led to a theory that, following cell degranulation, arachidonic acid, which is normally metabolized by both the cyclo-oxygenase and the lipoxygenase pathways, is forced mainly into the latter resulting in an increased generation of spasmogenic leukotrienes.

This has now been shown to occur: in patients with aspirin-induced rhinitis, the naso-ocular reaction following ingestion of aspirin was associated with increased concentrations of both LTC_4 and histamine in nasal lavage fluid[33]. Following desensitization, the naso-ocular reaction did not occur and concentrations of LTC_4 and histamine did not rise. LTE_4, which is a

Table 5 Low salicylate diet

The very highest levels are in the following, which must be absolutely avoided:
Allspice, aniseed, cayenne, celery powder, cinnamon, curry powder, dill powder, chinese five spices, garam m'sala, mace, mixed dried herbs, mustard, oregano powder, paprika, rosemary powder, sage (dried), tarragon powder, turmeric, thyme (powdered), worcester sauce

High levels are found in the following:

Fruits	*Vegetables*	*Drinks*	*Nuts and seeds*
Berries	Chicory	Rum	Almonds
Dried fruits	Gherkin	Port	Peanuts
Citrus fruits	Endive	Tia Maria	
Figs	Mushrooms (canned)	Tea	
Guava	Olives (canned)	Benedictine	
Kiwi	Radish	Drambuie	
Currants	Watercress		
Pineapple			
Raisins			
Prunes			

The diet can contain up to 200 mg salicylate/day which is equivalent to two thirds of an aspirin tablet. This may be sufficient to cause clinical effects in those with marked salicylate idiosyncrasy. There is some disagreement about the relative content of salicylate in various foodstuffs, but these are generally accepted as containing the highest levels and are worth a trial of avoidance in patients who are still symptomatic despite avoiding all aspirin-containing medication. (Courtesy of Mrs Cherie Ambasma, former Dietician, Middlesex Hospital)

metabolic product of LTC_4, can be shown to be raised in the urine of aspirin-sensitive asthmatics and to rise further following aspirin provocation.

There may also be an increased target organ sensitivity to the leukotrienes in these patients. Leukotriene receptor antagonists decreased the response to aspirin by 43–74% in five of six subjects studied.

The cell source of the mediators is unknown, but, in some patients, mast cells are implicated. In others, platelets may be involved. Aspirin-induced mediator release has been demonstrated by one group to be associated with a platelet abnormality: reduced glutathione peroxidase. The treatment of aspirin sensitivity involves either 'desensitization' followed by regular ingestion, or complete exclusion of aspirin-containing medications and non-steroidal anti-inflammatory drugs. Paracetamol can usually be tolerated except in a small percentage of patients who are also sensitive to this. Up to 200 mg salicylate can be contained in the daily diet; in patients who do not improve, it may be worth enquiring about their intake of salicylate-rich foods (Table 5).

References and further reading

IgE and its receptors

1. Capron A, Dessaint J-P, Capron M, Bazin H. Specific IgE antibodies in immune adherence of normal macrophages to Schistosoma mansoni schistosomules. Nature. 1975;253:474.
2. Capron M, Capron A, Dessaint J-P, et al. Fc receptors for IgE on human and rat eosinophils. J Immunol. 1981;126:2087.
3. Ishizaka K, Ishizaka T, Hornbrook MM. Physicochemical properties of human reaginic antibody. IV. Presence of a unique immunoglobulin as a carrier of reaginic activity. J

Immunol. 1966;97:75.
4. Liu FT, Bolin JW, Ferry EL, et al. Monoclonal dinitrophenol-specific murine IgE antibody preparation, isolation and characterization. J Immunol. 1980;124:2728.
5. Kulczycki A Jr, Vallini VL. Specific binding of non-glycosylated IgE to Fc receptor. Mol Immunol. 1981;18:723.

The genetics of atopy

6. Coca AF, Cooke RA. On the classification of the phenomena of hypersensitiveness. J Immunol VIII. 1923;VIII:163–82.
7. Cookson WOCM, Sharp PA, Faux JA, Hopkin JM. Linkage between immunoglobulin E responses underlying asthma and rhinitis and chromosome 11q. Lancet. 1989;1:1292–4.

Environmental factors

8. Kjellman M. Epidemiology and prevention of allergy. In: Malling H-J, ed. State of the art lectures in allergology. Allergy. 1988;43(Suppl. 8):39–41.
9. Tajafuki S, Suzuki S, Koizumi K et al. Diesel exhaust particulates inoculated by the intranasal route have an adjuvant activity for IgE production of mice. J Allergy Clin Immunol. 1987;79:639–45.
10. Sporik R, Holgate ST, Platts-Mills TAE, Cogswell JJ. Exposure to house dust mite allergen (Der pl) and the development of asthma in childhood – a prospective study. N Engl J Med. 1990;323:502–7.

Control of IgE production

11. Ishizaka K. Regulation of IgE biosynthesis. Hosp Pract. 1989;Sep. 15:51–60.
12. Romagnani S, Ricci M. Present views on the regulation of human IgE synthesis. Allergy Clin Immunol News. 1990;2:192–6.
13. Heusser CH, Brinkmann V, Delespesse G, Kilchherr E, Blaser K, Le Gros G. Current concepts of IgE regulation. Allergy Clin Immunol News. 1991;47–51.
14. Gordon J. CD23 and B cell activation. In: Annual Conference of The British Society for Allergy and Clinical Immunology. Sept. 1991, Book of Abstracts S14.
15. Bradding P, Feather IH, Howarth PH et al. Interleukin 4 is localized to and released by human mast cells. J Exp Med. 1992;176:1381–6.

Mediators

16. Pipkorn U. Mediators and nasal allergy. Clin Exp Allergy. 1989;19:585–9.
17. Featherstone RL, Church MK. Respective roles of mediators in allergic reactions. Allergy Clin Immunol News. 1991;3:81–4.
18. Svensson C, Andersson M, Persson CG, Venge P, Alkner U, Pipkorn U. Albumin, bradykinins and eosinophil cationic protein on the nasal mucosal surface in patients with hay fever during natural allergen exposure. J Allergy Clin Immunol. 1990;85:828–33.
19. Proud D, Reynolds CJ, Lacapra S, Kagey-Sobotka A, Lichtenstein LM, Naclerio RM. Nasal provocation with bradykinin induces symptoms of rhinitis and a sore throat. Am Rev Respir Dis. 1988;137:613–6.

Allergic rhinitis

20. Okuda M. Pathophysiology of allergic rhinitis. Allergy Clin Immunol News. 1989;1:167–76.

21. Enerback L. Mucosal mast cells in the rat and in man. Int Arch Allergy Appl Immunol. 1987;82:249–255.
22. Naclerio RM. Allergic rhinitis. New Engl J Med. 1991;325:860–9.

Late-phase response

23. Gleich GJ. The late phase of the immunoglobulin-E mediated reaction: a link between anaphylaxis and common allergic disease. J Allergy Clin Immunol. 1982;70:160–9.
24. Durham SR. Clinical relevance of late allergic responses. In: Annual Conference of The British Society for Allergy and Clinical Immunology. Sept. 1991, Book of Abstracts S18.
25. Jacobson MR, Varney VA, Sudderick RM, Robinson DS, Mackay IS, Kay AB, Durham SR. Immunohistology of allergen-induced late nasal responses. J Allergy Clin Immunol. 1991;87:305 (Abstract).
26. Kaliner MA. The late-phase reaction and its clinical implications. Hosp Pract. 1987;22: 73–83.

Cytokines

27. Durham SR, Ying S, Varney V, Jacobson MR, Sudderick RM, Mackay IS, Kay AB, Hamid QA. Cytokine messenger RNA expression for IL-3, IL-4, IL-5 and granulocyte/macrophage-colony stimulating factor in the nasal mucosa after local allergen provocation: relationship to tissue eosinophilia. J Immunol. 1992;148:2390–4.
28. Sun Ying D, Robinson S, Varney V, Meng Q, Tsicopoulos A, Moqbel R, Durham SR, Kay AB, Hamid Q. TNF mRNA expression in allergic inflammation. Clin Exp Allergy. 1991;21:745–50.
29. Owen WF. Cytokine regulation of eosinophil inflammatory disease. Allergy Clin Immunol News. 1991;3:85–89.

Diagnosis

30. Navas Romero J, Scadding GK. Nasal eosinophilia in allergic rhinitis; correlation with skin prick tests and nasal challenge. Rhinology. 1992;30:169–75.

Treatment

31. Alexander AG, Barnes NC, Kay AB. Trial of cyclosporin in corticosteroid-dependent chronic severe asthma. Lancet. 1992;339:324–8.

Immunotherapy

32. Noon L. Prophylactic inoculation against hay fever. Lancet. 1911;1:1572.
33. Norman PS. Immunotherapy. In: Ishizaka K, ed. Regulation of the IgE antibody response. Basel: Karger; 1982:318–39. (Progress in Allergy series.)
34. Varney VA, Gaga M, Frew AJ, Aber VR, Kay AB, Durham SR. Usefulness of immunotherapy in patients with severe summer hay fever uncontrolled by anti-allergic drugs. Br Med J. 1991;302:265–9.

Aspirin sensitivity

35. Lee TH (1991) Aspirin-induced asthma. In: Annual Conference of The British Society for Allergy and Clinical Immunology. Sept. 1991, Abstract S20.

7
Food and Allergic Rhinitis

L. J. HAWK

INTRODUCTION

Food problems divide clinically into two categories: immediate and delayed. In the first, the reaction to a food shows a clear time relationship to symptoms which is not difficult to recognize. The difficulty lies in determining the underlying cause. This may be allergic but there are many other possible reasons.

In delayed food reactions there is no obvious time relationship between food ingestion and symptoms. Diagnosis depends on the removal of the food from the diet with an amelioration of symptoms which recur on rechallenge with the food.

ALLERGIC RHINITIS

In a sensitized individual, direct nasal challenge with antigen will cause itching, sneezing, rhinorrhoea and sometimes conjunctivitis within minutes. This early-phase reaction results from the interaction of mast cell membrane-bound antigen-specific IgE and the antigen which stimulates the mast cell to release and to manufacture a cascade of mediators and cytokines. Some mediators, e.g. histamine, are preformed; others, e.g. prostaglandin D_2 (PGD_2), are produced by the cell only after stimulation. Cytokines shown to date to be produced by mast cells include IL-3, IL-4, IL-5 and IL-6 which, individually or in combination, are known to affect basophil activation, IgE synthesis and eosinophil activation.

Some six to twenty-four hours after antigen challenge, a late response may occur. Clinical symptoms may be absent but nasal airflow measurements can be shown to be restricted and a biopsy will demonstrate the influx of cells which include basophils, eosinophils and neutrophils. An interesting finding is that further antigen challenge at this time produces an augmented early response. Such a scenario encourages the view that chronic allergic rhinitis reflects ongoing and recurring antigen challenge.

ACUTE FOOD ALLERGIC PROBLEMS

Food allergies in which specific IgE can be demonstrated tend to alter with age. In infants, the gastrointestinal tract is often targeted. These babies tend to have an atopic family history. The risk to a child of developing an allergic disorder has been shown to double if one parent is atopic and double again if both parents are affected. It has been postulated that sensitization occurs because of a large antigen load crossing an 'extra leaky' gut but recent studies cast doubt on this. As the infants mature, the GI problems resolve and tolerance develops in a proportion, while others proceed to develop asthma, eczema and/or rhinitis. In a recent follow-up study, 43% of food-allergic infants subsequently developed rhinitis. That food-allergic individuals are more likely to be atopic is also substantiated by Fiorini et al.[12] and by Sabah et al.[13] who additionally noted that, in perennial rhinitis, isolated food allergies were rare (6/261), being more commonly found in association with allergies to other environmental elements, e.g. pollen, animal dander etc.

A few foods account for the majority of confirmed food allergic reactions: in adults, nuts, peanuts, fish and shellfish. In children, eggs, milk, peanuts, nuts, fish and soy are the major culprits. The glycoprotein portions of these foods have been implicated as the major allergenic components.

Histamine and histamine releasing factors (HRF)

Ingestion of a food allergen produces an increase in circulating plasma histamine levels. Prolonged ingestion of a food allergen has been shown to lead to an increased production of HRFs by peripheral blood monocytes and basophils in vitro which disappears when the food is eliminated from the diet. Food-allergic patients have a unique form of IgE, called IgE+, which allows HRFs to activate basophils. The induction and prolonged production of HRFs might explain some of the responsiveness to ingested foods noted by rhinitis sufferers.

Crossreacting antibodies

There are demonstrable immunological crossreactions between some inhaled allergens and food allergens (Table 1). For example, the birch antigen shares some features with apple, carrot and potato antigens, and the ragweed antigen with melon and banana antigens. Allergen crossreactions within the legume family, between various fish families and between a variety of nuts, have also been recorded. There is, however, not always a clear clinical relationship, even in individuals in whom a shared antigen epitope has been demonstrated. Dietary advice on 'theoretical' grounds, i.e. to avoid all members of a particular food family because an allergy is demonstrated to

Table 1 Association between respiratory allergies and food hypersensitivities

1. **Complete identity between aeroallergen and food allergen**
   e.g. Occupational garlic dust sensitization → dyspnoea on eating garlic
   Occupational exposure to aerosolized shrimp → anaphylaxis after eating one shrimp
   Occupational exposure to ampicillin dust → positive oral challenge

2. **Partial similarity between aeroallergen and food allergen**
   a. Vegetable
   Sunflower pollen sensitivity → allergy to honey
   Dandelion pollen sensitivity → anaphylaxis with 'bee-pollen' health food

   b. Animal
   Occupational carmine (red dye) sensitivity → asthma and/or gut symptoms on challenge with cochineal and with Campari

   c. Enzyme
   Occupational sensitization to bromelain (protease) → gut symptoms on eating pineapple

3. **Structural similarity between pollens and fruits/vegetables from different sources** (cross-reactive epitopes on RAST)

Ragweed	→	Melon, banana, latex
Birch	→	Nuts, fruit
Grass	→	Tomatoes
Mugwort	→	Celery
Ryegrass	→	What endosperm
Avian antigens	→	Egg

one member, is therefore wrong. An interesting possible mechanism for nasal mucosal sensitization is provided, however.

DIAGNOSTIC TESTS FOR FOOD ALLERGY

Food-specific IgE and IgG can be measured by the radioallergosorbent test (RAST; Figure 1) and IgE can also be assessed with skin prick tests. False positive and false negative results occur with each system. Agreement between the two averages 79%. Neither is therefore sufficient on its own for food allergy diagnosis. This is not entirely surprising as few food allergens have been isolated and test solutions are not highly specific. As the quality of the allergen extract is increased, so might the precision of testing. For example, in Scandinavia, almost 100% of children allergic to codfish, for which the offending allergen has been identified and purified, have positive RAST tests.

For the moment, the diagnosis of the food allergy depends on dietary manipulation. The recommended technique is the double-blind placebo-controlled food challenge (DBPCFC) as described by Bock et al[28]. It is important to recognize the placebo effect of a change in diet and critical to carry out a challenge to confirm the diagnosis. Challenges are not entirely without risk; anaphylactic reactions have been reported.

NON-ALLERGIC ACUTE REACTIONS

Not all acute reactions to food have an allergic basis, though, clinically, allergic and non-allergic reactions may be indistinguishable. Popular opinion

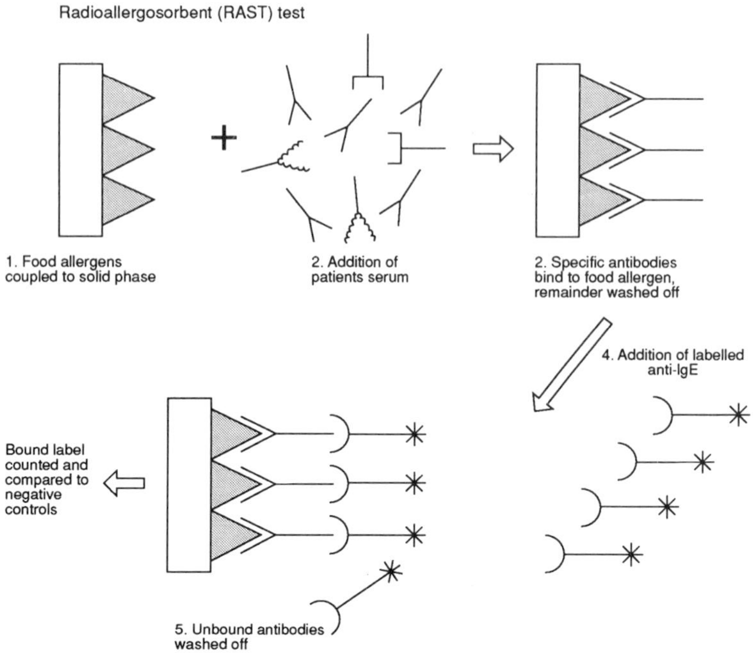

Figure 1 The basis of the RAST test is shown above. There are obvious pitfalls, including the quality of the food allergen, crossreacting antibodies (e.g. grass and wheat) and non-IgE antibodies to food. Only strongly positive reactions (3+, 4+) which correlate with the patient's history are taken into consideration

condemns food additives and colourings yet a study in 1984[31] estimated that symptoms occur in only 0.01–0.26% of the population. Possible mechanisms for acute reactions include:

1. Abnormal intake of biogenic amines, such as histamine and tyramine;
2. Abnormal release of mediators from mast cells other than by IgE triggering;
3. Interference by food or additive with the enzyme or autonomic system.

An example of (3) is gustatory rhinitis described in twelve individuals with acute rhinitis induced by spices and prevented by atropine. Another relevant example is salicylate sensitivity which is discussed in Chapter 6.

DELAYED FOOD REACTIONS

There is little information on the incidence of delayed food effects in rhinitis. Dietary manipulation studies on atopic individuals with asthma or eczema have identified a very small proportion of individuals who benefit clinically from dietary change, the offending food having caused no acute symptoms. A similar result in atopic individuals with chronic rhinitis is likely. It is to be emphasized that these individuals are atopic and that food allergic problems become increasingly likely with increasing degrees of atopy (rhinitis with or without asthma, with or without eczema) and numbers of positive skin tests.

Dietary management is difficult, time consuming and, particularly in the childhood population, potentially hazardous. Alterations to the diet of individuals with no acute food-related symptoms should be confined to the atopic population with chronic rhinitis in whom full therapeutic and environmental measures are failing to control the situation.

References and further reading

Allergic rhinitis

1. Plaut M, Pierce JH, Watson CJ et al. Mast cell lines produce lymphokines in response to cross linkage of Fc RI or to calcium ionophore. Nature. 1989;339:64–7.
2. Wodnal-Filipowicz A, Heusser CH, Moroni C. Production of the haemopoietic growth factors GM-CSF and IL3 by mast cells in response to IgE receptor-mediated activation. Nature. 1989;339:150–2.
3. Iliopoulos O, Proud D, Lichtenstein LM et al. Relationships between early, late and rechallenge responses to nasal challenge. J Allergy Clin Immunol. 1987;790:253–7.
4. Denburgh JA, Dolovich J, Harnish D. Basophil mast cell and eosinophilic growth and differentiation factors in human allergic disease. Clin Exp Allergy. 1989;19:249–55.
5. Naclerio RM, Proud D, Togias AG et al. Inflammatory mediators in late antigen induced rhinitis. N Engl J Med. 1985;312:65–70.
6. Brown M, Peters SP, Adkinson NF et al. Arachidonic acid metabolites during nasal challenge. Arch Otolaryngol Head Neck Surg. 1987;113:178–83.
7. Walden S, Proud D, Bascom R et al. Experimentally induced nasal allergic responses. J Allergy Clin Immunol. 1988;81:940–9.

Acute food allergic problems

8. Jellman K. Atopic disease in 7 year old children. Incidence in relation to family history. Acta Paediatr Scand. 1977;66:465–8.
9. Jenkins HR, Pincott JR, Soothill JF et al. Food allergy: the major cause of infantile colitis. Arch Dis Child. 1984;59:326–9.
10. Heyman M, Grasset E, Ducroc R et al. Antigen absorption by the jejunal epithelium of children with cows' milk allergy. Pediatr Res. 1988;24:1997–202.
11. Bishop JM, Hill DJ, Hoskings CS. Natural history of cows' milk allergy. Clinical outcomes. J Paediatr. 1990;116:862–7.
12. Fiorini G, Rinaldi G, Bigi I et al. Symptoms of respiratory allergies are worse in subjects with coexisting food sensitisation. Clin Exp Allergy. 1990;20:689–92.
13. Sabah A, Drout M, Millet B et al. Perennial rhinitis from food allergy. Allerg Immunol (Paris). 1990;22:51–5.
14. Powell GK, McDonald PJ, Van Sickle GJ et al. Absorption of food protein antigen in infants with food protein induced enterocolitis. Dig Dis Sci. 1989;34:781–8.

Histamine and HRF

15. Sampson HA, Broadbent KR, Bernhisel-Broadbent J. Spontaneous release of histamine from basophils and histamine releasing factors in patients with atopic dermatitis and food hypersensitivity. N Engl J Med. 1989;321:228–32.
16. McDonald SM, Lichtenstein LM, Proud D et al. Studies of IgE dependent histamine releasing factors. Heterogeneity of IgE. J Immunol. 1987;139:506–12.

Crossreacting antibodies

17. Anderson LB, Frefus EM, Logan J et al. Melon and banana sensitivity coincident with ragweed pollinosis. J Allergy. 1970;45:310–9.
18. Dreborg S, Foucard T. Allergy to apple, carrot and potato in children with birch pollen allergy. Allergy. 1983;38:167–72.
19. Barnett D, Bonham B, Howden MEH. Allergenic cross reactions among legume foods – as an in-vitro study. J Allergy Clin Immunol. 1987;79:433–8.
20. De Martino M, Novembre E, Galli I et al. Allergy to different fish species in cod allergic children. In-vivo and in-vitro studies. J Allergy Clin Immunol. 1990;86:909–14.
21. Bernhisel-Broadbent J, Taylor S, Sampson HA. Cross allergenicity in the legume botanical family in children with food hypersensitivity. J Allergy Clin Immunol. 1989;84:701–9.

Diagnostic tests for food allergy

22. Eriksson NE. Total IgE influences the relationship between skin test and RAST. Ann Allergy. 1989;63:65–9.
23. Johansson SGO, Yman L. In-vitro assays for immunoglobulin E. Methodology indications and interpretation. Clin Rev Allergy. 1988;6:93–139.
24. Guerin B, Watson RD. Skin tests. Clin Rev Allergy. 1988;6:211–27.
25. Bahna SL. Diagnostic test for food allergy. Clin Rev Allergy. 1988;6:259–83.
26. Aas K, Lundkvist V. The radio-allergosorbent test with a purified allergen for codfish. Clin Allergy. 1973;3:255.
27. Hill DJ, Duke AM, Hosking CS et al. Clinical manifestations of cow's milk allergy in childhood. II. The diagnostic value of skin tests and RAST. Clin Allergy. 1988;18:481–90.
28. Bock SA, Sampson HA, Atkins FM et al. Double blind, placebo controlled food challenge (DBPCFC) as an office procedure: a manual. J Allergy Clin Immunol. 1988;82:986–97.
29. David TJ. Hazards of challenge tests in atopic dermatitis. Allergy. 1989;9(Suppl.):101–7.
30. Metcalf DD, Sampson HA. Workshop on experimental methodology for clinical studies of adverse reactions to foods and food additives. J Allergy Clin Immunol. 1990;86:421–2.

Non-allergic acute reactions

31. Ortolani C, Pastorelo E, Luraghi MT et al. Diagnosis of intolerance to food additives. Ann Allergy. 1984;53:587.
32. Raphael G, Raphael MH, Kaliner M. Gustatory rhinitis. J Allergy Clin Immunol. 1989;83:110–5.
33. Young E, Patel S, Stonehak M et al. The prevalence of reaction to food additives in a survey population. J R Coll Physicians. 1987;21:241–7.

Delayed food reactions

34. Ogle KA, Bullock JD. Children with allergic rhinitis and/or bronchial asthma treated with elimination diet: A five year follow-up. Ann Allergy. 1980;44:275–8.
35. Burks AW, Mallory SB, Williams LW et al. Atopic dermatitis: clinical relevance of food hypersensitivity reactions. J Paediatr. 1988;113:447–51.
36. Robertson DA, Ayres RC, Smith CL et al. Adverse consequences arising from misdiagnosis of food allergy. Br Med J. 1988;297:719–20.
37. Atherton DJ, Sewell M, Soothill JF et al. A double-blind controlled crossover trial of an antigen avoidance diet in atopic eczema. Lancet. 1978;1:401–3.

8
Wegener's Disease

V. J. LUND

This relatively rare condition, though bearing Wegener's name after an article on rhinogenic granulomatosis in 1939[1], was probably first described by Klinger in 1931[2]. The true incidence of the condition is difficult to establish though it is certainly more common than originally supposed. Up to 1967, only 138 unequivocal cases had been recorded[3] but a greater awareness of the condition combined with the recognition of a wider clinical spectrum has expanded the numbers[4,5].

In a recent study from Leicester[6], the incidence of Wegener's granulomatosis increased nearly four-fold in 1987–89 compared with 1980–86, suggesting increased diagnostic awareness among physicians since the introduction of tests for antineutrophil cytoplasmic antibodies (ANCA). Later cases had less-severe renal disease and improved renal outcome on treatment.

Age/sex

The patients are usually previously healthy individuals of young or middle-age though the age at presentation to the Institute of Laryngology and Otology has varied between 15 and 64 years, and the disease has also been reported in children[7]. Indeed, it has been suggested that the pattern of disease manifestation is different in younger patients[8]. There does not appear to be any sexual predilection.

Site

The condition is characterized by:

1. Necrotizing granulomas with vasculitis of the upper and lower respiratory tracts,
2. Systemic small vessel vasculitis, and
3. Focal necrotizing glomerulitis[9].

Table 1 Clinical features of Wegener's granulomatosis: incidence of system involvement (per cent)

System	*Wolff et al* 1974[12]	*Kornblut et al* 1980[13]	*Lawson et al* 1982[14]	*Nicklasson and Strangeland* 1982[15]	*McDonald and Deremee* 1983[16]	*D'Cruz et al* 1989[17]
	Authors					
Nose and sinuses	95	89	90	95	80	100
Ears	38	36	35	38	19	
Lungs	100	100	95	100	56	77
Kidneys	81	85	85	85	42	27
CNS	24	15		20	11	
Joints	57	48		52		73
Eyes	43	55	60	49	22	73
Skin	48	40		44	14	
Heart	29	17		23		

As originally described, it constituted a rapidly progressive systemic disease which proved fatal within a few months. However, it is now recognized that more limited forms of the disease can present with less accelerated clinical deterioration. Thus, the upper respiratory tract and lungs can be affected alone or in combination and, having received therapy, patients may not manifest renal involvement though subclinical focal glomerulitis may be present[10]. Such pathological change in the kidneys alone is too non-specific to be recognized as a single disease entity and patients rarely, if ever, present with renal failure in the absence of systemic disease[11].

Whilst some form of respiratory tract involvement may predominate, the condition is systemic and can affect any organ. The frequency with which this occurs will depend upon the specific interests of the clinician and the stage of presentation. Table 1 shows the frequency of system involvement in a number of published series, emanating from respiratory, ENT, ophthalmic and rheumatology departments[12–17].

Aetiology

This remains essentially unknown. Certain similarities with tuberculosis initially suggested a bacterial cause[18] but no causative organism has ever been found. The possibility of an autoimmune or hypersensitivity reaction to drugs or tissue breakdown products has also been suggested[19,20]. Shillitoe et al. found a depression of certain immunological reactions and concluded that the cell-mediated response might be deficient[21]. The deposition of immune complexes is responsible for vasculitis in many conditions[22–24] and the presence of such circulating immune complexes has been reported in Wegener's disease in a proportion of cases. Travers[25] reported their presence in two thirds of cases whilst Shillitoe et al.[21] found them in one seventh, though Friedmann and Osborn[26] observed that most of these patients had previously received chemotherapy. Howell and Epstein[27] found that they were only present during the acute phase of the disease, disappearing during therapeutically induced remission.

It has been proposed that following deposition of such complexes in the vessel wall, inflammation and leukocyte destruction leads to platelet aggregation and fibrin deposition producing further vascular obstruction and necrosis. This behaviour has been observed in ultrastructural studies of pulmonary Wegener's disease[28] and appears to be suppressed by cytotoxic agents, such as cyclophosphamide.

However, more recent studies by Weiss and Crissman[29] failed to demonstrate any evidence for an immune complex pathogenesis and McDonald and DeRemee[16] reported that, whilst occasional immunofluorescence studies of renal biopsies have shown scattered deposition of IgG, IgA and C3, these are more usually absent.

Abnormal serum immunoglobulin levels have been reported in Wegener's disease with elevation of IgA[30], IgE[31] and IgD[32] in certain individuals though they are, again, the exception rather than the rule. Raised concentrations of C-reactive protein have also been described[3]. However, it has been suggested that the findings of increased C-reactive protein and immune complexes reflect infection rather than disease activity[33,34] which would explain the discrepancy in the various reports.

Antineutrophil cytoplasmic antibodies (ANCA)

These antibodies were first reported in 1982 in patients with a febrile illness and glomerulonephritis, thought to be due to a viral infection[35]. However, their association with Wegener's granulomatosis was first clearly defined by Van der Woude et al.[33], who used an indirect immunofluorescence technique to identify antibodies binding in a granular pattern to cytoplasm of normal neutrophils and monocytes (ANCA). These findings were readily reproduced by other groups, and the assay was found to be highly specific and sensitive (around 95%) in patients with active generalized disease[36]. However, in disease localized to the respiratory tract, only about 60% of cases are positive.

It soon became apparent that ANCA were also detectable in microscopic polyarteritis (MP) and certain other forms of vasculitis[36]. In 1988, Falk and Jennette[37] described a different pattern of ANCA binding in patients with rapidly progressive glomerulonephritis (RPGN). Staining was concentrated around the nucleus, and these antibodies were described as perinuclear or P-ANCA, as opposed to cytoplasmic or C-ANCA. In general, patients with Wegener's granulomatosis have C-ANCA, whereas those with MP or RPGN may show either pattern (Figure 1).

The antigenic targets of ANCA have been largely defined over the last two years. Most C-ANCA recognize a 29-kDa serine proteinase in neutrophil primary granules[38–40]. This has now been identified as proteinase-3, and a cDNA clone encoding it has been isolated[41]. However, it seems that a minority of C-ANCA do not recognize proteinase-3, and binding to cationic antimicrobial protein (CAP) 57, another neutrophil granule protein, has been reported[42]. Most P-ANCA recognize myeloperoxidase (MPO), which is also present in the primary granules. The perinuclear staining pattern is therefore

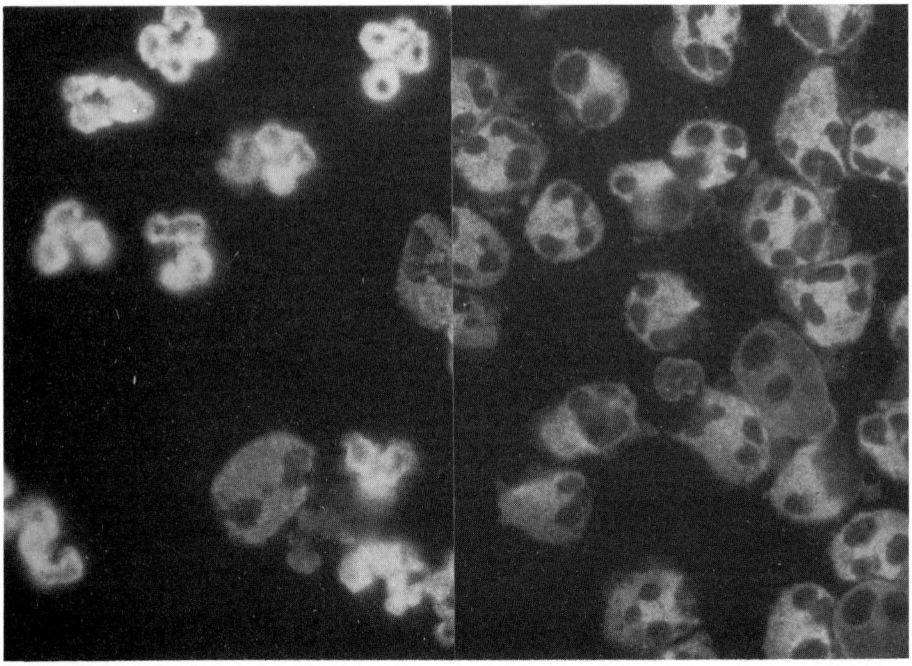

Figure 1 Immunofluorescence study of C-ANCA (*left*) and P-ANCA (*right*) ×360. [Courtesy of Dr J Cambridge, Department of Rheumatology, University College and Middlesex Hospital, London]

artefactual, and thought to result from release of MPO from granules by ethanol fixation[37]. Rarely, P-ANCA appear to recognize elastase or lactoferrin. The development of solid-phase immunoassays using purified MPO, proteinase-3, and other candidate autoantigens, should soon resolve the question of specificity of ANCA in vasculitic disorders.

Although the pathogenicity of ANCA is not proven, there is mounting evidence for their role in disease. ANCA are more readily detected in patients with active Wegener's granulomatosis[33] and titres of ANCA have been found to correlate with disease activity[43,44]. Cohen-Tervaert et al.[45] showed that a four-fold rise in titre of ANCA predicted clinical relapse, and went on to perform a trial of treatment in response to rising titres. Patients showing a four-fold rise in titre were randomized to receive immunosuppressive drugs or to be observed until there was clinical evidence of disease. The control group showed a higher incidence of relapse whereas the treated group showed no relapse[46]. However, it has been widely reported that ANCA can be present without overt disease, and the case for treating patients on serological grounds alone remains controversial.

Finally, there is more direct evidence for the pathogenetic role of ANCA from in vitro experiments. Incubation of C- and P-ANCA, or their $F(ab)_2$ fragments, with normal neutrophils (primed with TNF) leads to degranulation and to a respiratory burst[47]. There is also preliminary evidence that ANCA can stimulate primed neutrophils to cause endothelial cell injury[48].

In addition to ANCA, several groups have now reported antiendothelial cell antibodies in Wegener's granulomatosis[49,50]. These occur only in a proportion of patients, and are non-specific, also occurring in systemic lupus erythematosus and other connective tissue diseases. Their significance is unclear at present, and they could represent a response to endothelial injury.

Histology

The condition is characterized in the lungs by two types of lesion:

1. Areas of destructive necrosis in the parenchyma, resembling caseation and surrounded by an inflammatory reaction of lymphocytes, plasma cells, eosinophils and polymorphs. Giant cells of the foreign body and Langhan's type are found in the exudate.
2. Vasculitis of small arteries and veins.

In the nose, these features are often absent and only a non-specific chronic inflammatory reaction is seen. In the kidneys, a focal necrotizing glomerulonephritis occurs which, again, is not specific to Wegener's disease.

Evidence of repair and fibrosis proceeding simultaneously with destruction can be seen and, though the presence of epithelioid necrotizing granulomas is not pathognomonic, it provides important corroborative data to clinical findings.

Clinical features (Table 1)

The majority of patients present with a short history of progressive malaise, pyrexia and weight loss, feeling disproportionately unwell compared to clinical findings which are often non-specific and trivial. The patient may complain of nasal obstruction and crusting due to a chronic rhinosinusitis, sometimes associated with a secondary infection, which is frequently *Staphylococcus aureus*. Examination of the nasal cavity shows changes on the septum and inferior turbinate similar to atrophic rhinitis or sarcoid. There may be erosion of the septum and saddling of the bridge which can sometimes be coincident with nasal surgery. About one quarter of patients with nasal symptoms develop external nasal deformity (Figure 2).

Other ENT symptoms include hoarseness and stridor secondary to subglottic stenosis and tracheal involvement. Although mucosal lesions of the mouth and pharynx can occur, they are rarely extensive and midline destruction of the hard palate should suggest other pathology. Patients may also develop otorrhoea due to an otitis externa or acute otitis media[15]. A more chronic serous otitis media may produce deafness but this can also be sensorineural in nature as part of a specific neuritis. Similarly, vertigo[51] can occur.

Pulmonary involvement produces a cough, which, as cavitation progresses, may be associated with haemoptysis. Progressive fibrosis leads ultimately to diminished respiratory reserve and dyspnoea. Pleuritic pain is frequently

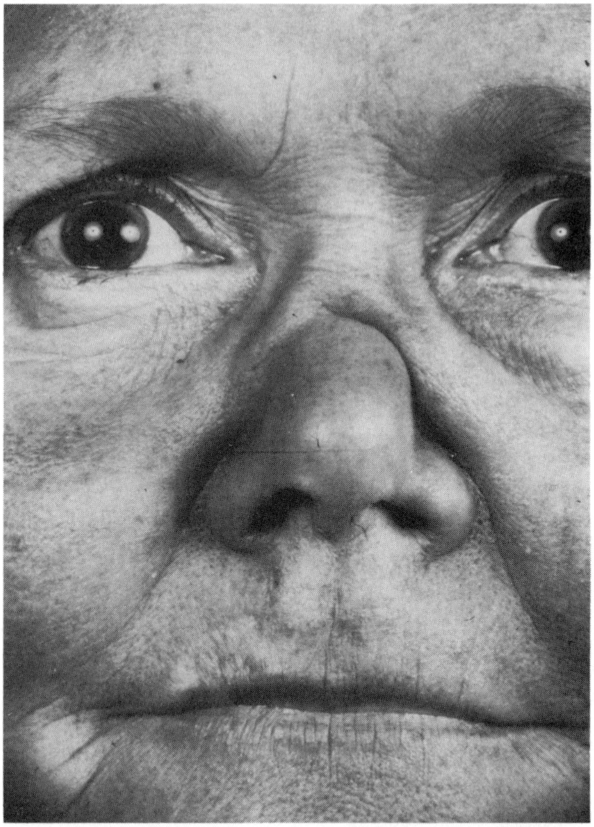

Figure 2 Saddle deformity of nasal bridge in Wegener's granulomatosis

encountered, though evidence of hilar lymphadenopathy should raise the possibility of other conditions.

In the orbit, corneoscleral ulceration, keratitis and conjunctivitis can occur. The nasolacrimal duct may be obstructed with fibrous tissue at either end and infiltration of periglobal tissues can produce a type of pseudotumour ultimately composed of firm fibrous tissue resulting in proptosis. Specific involvement of individual nerves can produce ophthalmoplegia and blindness, sometimes presenting as an acute superior orbital fissure syndrome.

Such mononeuritis is not uncommon, manifesting itself in up to 25% of patients[52]. Cranial nerve palsies are particularly obvious. Muscle involvement per se is unusual but can occur secondarily to vasculitis or neuritis. In the heart, valvulitis or pericarditis can occur; in the joints, synovitis; and a variety of skin lesions, including purpura, are found in up to half of patients.

A wide variety of oral lesions has been described, the most common of which is a distinctive hyperplastic gingivitis originating in the area of the interdental papillae. The gingiva are usually described as granular and, if extensive, gingivitis may cause tooth mobility or loss[53]. Once a tooth is lost, the socket fails to heal which may be the first sign of this disease[54,55]. Extensive ulcerative stomatitis has also been reported and, in most cases, the prognosis for patients presenting initially with disease in the oral cavity is poor[53].

Renal involvement marks a fulmination of the disease with progressive renal failure and ultimately death from a combination of uraemia and infection.

It is impossible to generalize as the clinical course of each patient is unique and the manifestations of the disease protean. The need for rapid recognition of the condition cannot be overemphasized if rapid clinical deterioration is to be averted and renal involvement avoided.

Investigations

These include full blood count, erythrocyte sedimentation rate (ESR), serum urea and creatinine with urinalysis for casts and red cells. A creatinine clearance or other clearance studies, such as chromium-51 edetic acid, are needed as an initial base-line. Immunoglobulin and autoantibody studies may be done for interest and differential diagnosis.

Of these tests, the ESR has provided the most convenient and accurate indication of disease activity. Whilst not specific to Wegener's granulomatosis, it correlates well with clinical activity and therapeutic response, and therefore offers a useful measure of the clinical situation, particularly in the out-patient clinic. Thus, medication can be titrated against ESR to maintain it within normal limits[56,57].

Tissue biopsy may be helpful though, taken alone, rarely diagnostic. It is a combination of the clinical features and a markedly raised ESR which more accurately indicate the condition.

As noted earlier, ANCA is positive in 95% of patients with generalized active disease but in only 60% of patients with disease localized to the respiratory tract. A four-fold rise in ANCA titre predicts clinical relapse and patients in whom C-ANCA persists despite treatment are more likely to relapse in the long term than those who become seronegative.

Previously, the time required to obtain a preliminary assessment on a sample was 2 days with indirect immunofluorescence and 4.5 hours with radioimmunoassay[36]. Immunofluorescence for C-ANCA has now decreased in time to 2 hours but requires considerable experience for accurate interpretation. ANCA is of particular use in equivocal cases at the more benign end of the spectrum and in determining when and in whom to decrease medication.

Radiology

In Wegener's granulomatosis, plain X-rays of the sinuses reveal only minimal bone destruction in 25% of patients with mild generalized mucosal thickening. CT and MRI are, therefore, of little value unless there is marked orbital involvement when active granulations can be expected to produce a strong

Table 2 Differential diagnosis of nasal granulomas

Non-specific	*Specific*
Wegener's granulomatosis	Syphilis
Sarcoid	Tuberculosis
Midline granuloma	Yaws
Polymorphic reticulosis	Leprosy
Lymphoma	Rhinoscleroma
Pyogenic granuloma	Rhinosporidiosis
Churg–Strauss syndrome	Mucormycosis
SLE	Aspergillosis
	Histoplasmosis
	Blastomycosis
	Sporotrichosis
	Actinomycosis
	Moniliasis
	Cryptococcosis
	Leishmaniasis

Table 3 The spectrum of vasculitic disease

Vessel size	*With granulomata*	*Without granulomata*
Small	Wegener's granulomatosis (WG)	Microscopic polyarteritis (MP) (idiopathic focal necrotizing glomerulonephritis = focal form) (FNGN or RPGN)
Medium	Churg–Strauss syndrome (+asthma + eosinophilia)	Polyarteritis nodosa (PAN)
Large		Giant cell arteritis* Takayasu's arteritis*

*Sometimes occur with granulomata

signal on T2-weighted sequences whereas residual fibrous disease produces a low signal on all sequences[58].

The chest X-ray shows progressive cavitation followed by fibrosis, though, as mentioned previously, hilar lymphadenopathy is not a feature of Wegener's granuloma.

Differential diagnosis

The many conditions from which Wegener's granuloma must be distinguished have been listed by Batsakis[9] (Table 2). The position of Wegener's granulomatosis in the spectrum of primary vasculitides is shown in Table 3.

Treatment

The most effective treatment appears to be a combination of high-dose prednisolone (80 mg/day initially) and a cytotoxic agent, such as azathioprine (200 mg/day) or cyclophosphamide (2 mg/kg). The possibility of haemorrhagic cystitis with cyclophosphamide has been the main reason for our favouring azathioprine which is effective with few associated complications, although both drugs can potentially cause bone marrow hypoplasia, decreased resistance to infection and hepatotoxicity. Other centres favour induction therapy with oral prednisolone and cyclophosphamide, with additional plasma exchange in fulminant disease. After 2–3 months, azathioprine is substituted for cyclophosphamide for maintenance therapy.

Once in remission, dosage, particularly of the steroid, may be reduced but it is important not to do so precipitously and most patients require a baseline maintenance dose of 10 mg/day or less once long-term therapy has effectively ablated adrenal function. Drugs are only tapered and discontinued after a disease-free period of at least one year. Patients with persistently or recurrently positive C-ANCA should probably be maintained on therapy.

The nose can be managed with alkaline douching and topical preparations, such as glucose and glycerine drops or betamethasone sodium phosphate. The temptation to operate on saddle deformities should be resisted and the most which should be attempted, albeit during clinical quiescence, is a silastic implant.

The laser has been used with limited success in the subglottis but tracheostomy may be needed in severe cases. Orbital decompression has also been performed on a number of cases but, again, the fibrous nature of the condition precludes any dramatic improvement.

Established renal failure has been managed with dialysis and even transplantation but the disease process can be expected to involve the new kidney.

The finding of potentially specific autoantibodies opens up the possibility of identification and synthesis of antigenic components which might be used in immunoadsorptive therapy in the future[59].

Natural history

Although the speed of progression may vary, without treatment, all patients are dead within 2 years from a combination of renal failure and infection. Rapid implementation of treatment can arrest progress and even reverse pulmonary and renal damage, producing a variable period of remission though, thereafter, the patient walks a tightrope between exacerbations of the disease and the side-effects of the long-term steroid and cytotoxic therapy, from which he may ultimately succumb. The best prognosis obviously results from early diagnosis before systemic involvement occurs. Once remission is produced, the clinician should be cautioned against injudicious reduction in medication as his anxiety to avoid the therapeutic complications may precipitate catastrophic clinical deterioration from which a remission cannot be achieved.

Acknowledgements

Grateful thanks are due to Dr C.D. Pusey for his advice and to Dr J. Cambridge for Figure 1.

References

1. Wegener F. Uber eine eigenartige rhinogene Granulomatose mit besonderer Beteilgung des Arteriensystems und der Nieren. Beitr Pathol. 1939;102:36–68.
2. Klinger H. Grenzformen der Periarteritis nodosa. Frankf Z Pathol. 1931;42:455–80.
3. Editorial. Br Med J. 1971;3:446.
4. Carrington CB, Liebow AA. Limited forms of angiitis and granulomatosis of Wegener's type. Am J Med. 1966;41:497–527.
5. Cassan SM, Coles DT, Harrison EG. The concept of limited forms of Wegener's granulomatosis. Am J Med. 1970;49:366–79.
6. Andrews M, Edmunds M, Campbell A, Walls J, Feehally J. Systemic vasculitis in the 1980s. Is there an increasing incidence of Wegener's granulomatosis and microscopic polyarteritis? J R Coll Phys London. 1990;24:284–8.
7. Allen JC, France TD. Pseudotumour as the presenting sign of Wegener's granulomatosis in a child. J Pediatr Ophthalmol. 1977;14:158–9.
8. Halstead LA, Karmody CS, Wolff SM. Presentation of Wegener's granulomatosis in young patients. Otolaryngol Head Neck Surg. 1986;94:368–71.
9. Batsakis JG. Wegener's granulomatosis and midline (nonhealing) 'granuloma'. Head Neck Surg. 1979;1:213–22.
10. Fauci AS, Johnson RE, Wolff SM. Radiation therapy of midline granuloma. Ann Intern Med. 1976;84:140–7.
11. Fauci AS, Wolff SM. Wegener's granulomatosis and related disease. Disease-a-Month. 1977;23:5–56.
12. Wolff SM, Fauci AS, Horn RG. Wegener's granulomatosis. Ann Intern Med. 1974;81:513–25.
13. Kornblut AD, Wolff SM, DeFries HO, Fauci AS. Wegener's granulomatosis. Laryngoscope. 1990;90:1453–65.
14. Lawson VG, Reid AJ, Cardella CJ, DeVeber GA. Wegener's granulomatosis and the respiratory system. J Otolaryngol. 1982;11:60–4.
15. Nicklasson B, Strangeland N. Wegener's granulomatosis presenting as otitis media. J Laryngol Otol. 1982;96:277–80.
16. MacDonald TJ, DeRemee RA. Wegener's granulomatosis. Largyngoscope. 1983;93:220–31.
17. D'Cruz DP, Baguley E, Asherson RA, Hughes GRV. Ear, nose and throat symptoms in subacute Wegener's granulomatosis. Br Med J. 1989;299:419–22.
18. Mills CP. Malignant granuloma of the nose and paranasal sinuses. J Laryngol Otol. 1958;72:849–87.
19. Walton EW. Giant cell granuloma of the respiratory tract (Wegener's granulomatosis). Br Med J. 1958;2:265–70.
20. Blatt IM, Seltzer HS, Rubin P, Furstenberg AC, Maxwell JH, Schull WJ. Fatal granulomatosis of the respiratory tract. Archiv Otolaryngol. 1959;70:707–57.
21. Shillitoe EJ, Lehner T, Lessof MH, Harrison DFN. Immunological features of Wegener's granulomatosis. Lancet. 1974;1:281–4.
22. Schroeter AL, Copeman PWM, Jordan RE, Sams MW, Winkelmann RK. Immunofluorescence of cutaneous vasculitis associated with systemic disease. Archiv Dermatol. 1971;104: 254–9.
23. Parish WE. Cutaneous vasculitis: antigen–antibody complexes and prolonged fibrinolysis. Proc R Soc Med. 1972;65:276–8.
24. Sams MV, Thorne EG, Small P, Mass MF, McIntosh RM, Stanford RE. Leucocytoclastic vasculitis. Archiv Dermatol. 1976;112:219–26.
25. Travers RL. Polyarteritis and related disorders. Br J Hosp Med. 1979;22:38–45.
26. Friedmann I, Osborn DA. Pathology of granulomas and neoplasms of the nose and paranasal sinuses. Edinburgh, London: Churchill Livingstone; 1982.
27. Howell SB, Epstein WV. Circulating immunoglobulin complexes in Wegener's granulomatosis. Am J Med. 1976;60:259–68.
28. Donald KJ, Edwards RL, McEvoy DS. An ultrastructural study of the pathogenesis of tissue injury in limited Wegener's granulomatosis. Pathology. 1976;8:161–9.
29. Weiss MA, Crissman JD. Renal biopsy findings in Wegener's granulomatosis: segmental necrotizing-glomerulonephritis with glomerular thrombosis. Hum Pathol. 1984;15:943–56.
30. Fauci AS, Haynes BF, Katz P. The spectrum of vasculitis. Ann Intern Med. 1978;89:

660–76.
31. Conn DL. Raised serum immunoglobulin E in Wegener's granulomatosis. Ann Rheum Dis. 1976;35:377–9.
32. Koornneef L, Melief CJM, Peterse HL, Wilmink JM. Wegener's granulomatosis of the orbit. Orbit. 1983;2:1–10.
33. Van der Woude FJ, Rasmussen N, Lobatto S, Wik A, Permin H, Van E's, LA, Van der Giessen M, Van der Hem GK, The TH. Autoantibodies against neutrophils and monocytes: tool for diagnosis and marker of disease activity in Wegener's granulomatosis. Lancet. 1985;1:425–9.
34. Pinching AJ, Rees AJ, Pussell BA, Lockwood CM, Mitchison RS, Peters DK. Relapses in Wegener's granulomatosis, the role of infection. Br Med J. 1980;281:836–8.
35. Davies DJ, Moran JE, Niall JF, Ryan GB. Segmental necrotising glomerulonephritis with antineutrophil antibody: possible arbovirus aetiology? Br Med J. 1982;285:606.
36. Savage CO, Winearls CG, Jones S, Marshall PD, Lockwood CM. Prospective study of radioimmunoassay for antibodies against neutrophil cytoplasm in diagnosis of systemic vasculitis. Lancet. 1987;1:1389–93.
37. Falk RJ, Jennette JC. Anti-neutrophil antibodies with specificity for myeloperoxidase in patients with systemic vasculitis and idiopathic necrotising and crescentic nephritis. N Engl J Med. 1988;318:1651–7.
38. Goldschmeding R et al. Wegener's granulomatosis autoantibodies identify a novel diisopropylfluorophosphate-binding protein in the lysosymes of normal human neutrophils. J Clin Invest. 1989;84:1577–87.
39. Ludemann J, Utrecht B, Gross WL. Anti-neutrophil cytoplasm antibodies in Wegener's granulomatosis recognize an elastolytic enzyme. J Exp Med. 1990;171:357–62.
40. Niles JL, McCluskey RT, Ahmad MF, Arnaout MA. Wegener's granulomatosis autoantigen is a novel neutrophil serine proteinase. Blood. 1989;74(6):1888–93.
41. Campanelli D et al. Cloning of cDNA for proteinase 3: a serine protease, antibiotic and autoantigen from human neutrophils. J Exp Med. 1990;172:1709–15.
42. Falk RJ, Terrell RS, Charles LA, Jennette JC. Anti-neutrophil cytoplasmic autoantibodies induce neutrophils to degranulate and produce oxygen radicals in vitro. Proc Natl Acad Sci USA. 1990;87:4115–9.
43. Nolle B, Specks U, Ludemann J, Rohrbach MS, DeRemee RA, Gross WL. Anticytoplasmic autoantibodies: their immunodiagnostic value in Wegener's granulomatosis. Ann Intern Med. 1989;111:28–40.
44. Specks U, Wheatley CL, McDonald TJ, Rohrbach MS, DeRemee RA. Anticytoplasmic autoantibodies in the diagnosis and follow-up of Wegener's granulomatosis. Mayo Clin Proc. 1989;64:28–36.
45. Cohen-Tervaert JW et al. Association between active Wegener's granulomatosis and anticytoplasmic antibodies. Arch Intern Med. 1989;149:2461–5.
46. Cohen Tervaert JW et al. Prevention of relapses in Wegener's granulomatosis by treatment based on antineutrophil cytoplasmic antibody titre. Lancet. 1990;336:709–11.
47. Falk RJ. ANCA-associated renal disease. Kidney Int. 1990;38:998–1010.
48. Savage COS, Pottinger BE, Gaskin G, Pusey CD, Pearson JD. Autoantibodies developed to myeloperoxidase and proteinase 3 in systemic vasculitis stimulate neutrophil cytotoxicity towards cultured endothelial cells. Am J Pathol. 1992;141:335–42.
49. Brasile L, Kremer JM, Clarke CL, Cerilli J. Identification of an antibody to vascular endothelial cell-specific antigens in patients with systemic vasculitis. Am J Med. 1989;87: 74–86.
50. Ferraro G, Pusey CD. Systemic vasculitis. Oxford Textbook of Clinical Nephrology. OUP; 1992.
51. Bennett RW, Staker LV. Wegener's granulomatosis presenting as vertigo. West J Med. 1987;146:359–61.
52. Anderson JM, Jamieson DG, Jefferson JM. Non-healing granuloma and the nervous system. Q J Med. 1975;44:309–23.
53. Hanlers JP, Waterman J, Abrahams AM. Oral features of Wegener's granulomatosis. Arch Otolaryngol. 1985;111:267–70.
54. Israelson H, Binnie WH, Hurt WC. The hyperplastic gingivitis of Wegener's granulomatosis. J Periodontol. 1981;52:81–7.

55. Scott J, Finch LD. Wegener's granulomatosis presenting as gingivitis. Oral Surg. 1972;34:920–33.
56. Harrison DFN. Non-healing granulomata of the upper respiratory tract. Br Med J. 1974;4:205–9.
57. Lund VJ, Howard DJ. Wegener's granulomatosis. Br Med J. 1988;297:556.
58. Lloyd GAS. Diagnostic Imaging of the Nose and Paranasal Sinuses. London, Berlin: Springer Verlag; 1988:73–7.
59. Lockwood CM, Bakes D, Jones S, Whitaker KB, Moss DW, Savage CO. Association of alkaline phosphatase with an autoantigen recognised by circulating anti-neutrophil antibodies in systemic vasculitis. Lancet. 1987:1:716–9.

9
Sarcoidosis

V. J. LUND

Scadding and Mitchell[1] recommended the following definition in 1985:

> "Sarcoidosis is a disease characterized by the formation in all of several affected organs or tissues of epithelioid-cell tubercles, without caseation though fibrinoid necrosis may be present at the centres of a few, proceeding either to resolution or to conversion into hyaline fibrous tissue."

It is a condition of particular interest to the otorhinolaryngologist as, although it is uncommon, it is a cause of florid nasal symptoms, especially mucopurulent catarrh, and patients may present in a general ENT clinic with this as the first manifestation of the disease.

Besnier, in 1889[2], first described cutaneous lesions of the face and upper extremities which he named 'lupus pernio'. Hutchinson described similar findings which he termed 'Mortimer's malady' after the patient concerned[3]. Boeck, in 1899[4], was the first to recognize the generalized nature of the disease which he called 'multiple benign sarcoid' and, in 1905[5], he noted that 4 out of 9 cases had nasal lesions which preceded those in the skin, whilst, in two other patients, the relationship was coincident. In 1908, Kreibach and Kraus[6] described a case of sarcoid affecting the skin of the nose and forehead with nasal symptoms due to thickening of the mucosa, though this was not examined histologically.

Laryngeal involvement was first described by Ulrich in 1918[7] who noted epiglottic and aryepiglottic changes. Subsequently there have been many reports of changes in the upper respiratory tract but relatively few studies of the incidence of these changes in unselected series of cases of sarcoid presenting in other ways. Thus the situation has been confused by reports in the literature from two separate groups of the medical profession, the chest physicians and the ENT surgeons, implying two populations of patients: those with primary florid upper respiratory tract manifestations of sarcoid and those with generalized disease who may have upper respiratory tract involvement.

Table 1 Upper respiratory tract involvement in sarcoidosis

Author	*Total no. patients*	*Upper respiratory tract involvement**				
		Total no.	*Nose*	*Mouth/pharynx*	*Larynx*	*Other*
Barmwater (1936)[9]	42	13	—	—	—	—
Gravesen (1942)[10]	112	39	37	14	6	—
Reisner (1944)[11]	35	4	2	—	2	—
Robinson and Pound (1950)[12]	30	6	6	—	—	—
Lindsay and Perlman (1951)[13]	50	9	2	2	5	—
James (1956)[14]	150	1	—	—	1	—
Weiss (1960)[15]	345	4	4	—	—	—
Kampfer (1964)[16]	277	11	9	1	1	—
McKelvie et al (1968)[17]	14	14	11	—	5	—
Neville et al (1976)[18]	100	6	6	—	—	—
Selroos and Niemisto (1977)[19]	192	14	14	—	—	—
James et al. (1982)[20]	818	53	51	—	8	10
McCaffrey and MacDonald (1983)[21]	2319	23	23	—	—	—
Wilson et al (1988)[8]	750	27	27	—	5	—

*More than one site may be affected

INCIDENCE

In a series of 750 patients with generalized sarcoidosis, 27 patients (3.6%) were found to have nasal manifestations of the disease[8], which is similar to the findings of other workers[8–21] (Table 1). It is, however, readily apparent that nasal manifestations are almost always part of multisystem sarcoid which may have been present for some years (1–20 years, average 4.4 years). Similarly, the larynx is rarely, if ever, affected alone and is almost always affected in association with nasal involvement[15].

AGE/SEX

Generally the condition affects young adults, between the third and fifth decades. Women are affected twice as often as men, and this female preponderance may be higher in those with upper respiratory tract manifestations.

Adult coloured people living in rural areas of south-east United States, West Indians and Scandinavians appear to be more susceptible than other racial groups. A 12:1 ratio of black to Caucasian patients has been found in the United States[22,23].

SITE

Sarcoidosis is a multisystem disease, most frequently affecting the lungs and lymph nodes. In the upper respiratory tract, the inferior turbinate and the

Table 2 Incidence of sarcoid in other organs of patients with nasal sarcoid

Lung	66%
Skin	56%
Peripheral lymph nodes	30%
Lupus pernio	26%
Eyes	22%
Bone	19%
Larynx	19%
Lacrimal glands	15%
Conjunctiva	11%
Uveitis	11%
Brain	11%
Joint	11%
Spleen	4%

adjacent part of the nasal septum are most commonly affected with extension into the nasal bones and overlying skin. The maxillary and occasionally ethmoid sinuses can also be involved.

The larynx is affected in 3–5% of cases[17,24] where it is predominantly the supraglottis which suffers rather than the glottis or subglottis though neither area is immune. The process begins with the posterior and lateral aspects of the epiglottis, spreading to involve aryepiglottic folds, false cords and ventricle. This pattern is probably related to the distribution of lymphoid tissue and takes the form of granularity and oedema, occasionally polypoid masses and later fibrosis. The trachea may occasionally be affected, usually by direct extension from the larynx[9].

The nasopharynx, hypopharynx and soft palate are less frequently affected. Enlargement of lymphoid tissue can result in serous otitis media[25] and adenoidal infiltration has led to the diagnosis of sarcoid in some children[26]. Similarly, histological infiltration of the tonsil has been reported but is an incidental finding in most cases[10,15,27].

The incidence with which other systems were found to be affected in a group of patients with nasal sarcoid is shown in Table 2.

IMMUNOLOGICAL ASPECTS AND AETIOLOGY

It has been known for some time that Type IV delayed hypersensitivity reactions are depressed in patients with active sarcoid[28]. This is evidenced by diminished skin test reactions to tuberculin or purified protein derivatives and can also be demonstrated in vitro. This depressed response was first noted by Boeck[29] and subsequently confirmed in larger studies though its capacity to change in response to disease activity is variable. There is generalized depression of Type IV hypersensitivity to other skin antigens, such as *Candida*, *Trichophyton* and mumps but this should not be interpreted as a depression of cell-mediated immunity as there is no increased susceptibility to viral or fungal infections[30]. In approximately half of such patients, the tuberculin reaction could be made positive by a concomitant injection of cortisone[31,32] which suggests that this is a paradoxical response.

However, Type I hypersensitivity appears normal and humoral antibody responses are unaffected or increased. Similarly, total plasma protein levels are increased, in particular γ-globulin, first reported in 1935[33], a response thought to be more pronounced in those of African descent than in Caucasians. Individual immunoglobulin class elevation is variable with IgG, A, M and even E affected[34–36].

Immunohistology demonstrates IgG, A, M and D in lymph nodes and biopsies of other tissues, such as skin, lung and blood vessels[37]. There appears to be an increase in circulating immune complexes, associated with recent acute onset of the condition, especially when erythema nodosum and bilateral hilar lymphadenopathy are present[34,38,39]. Levels of C3 can rise with long-standing disease.

In active sarcoid levels of circulating lymphocytes are decreased[40], with T cells being most affected[41], of which 10–20% are atypical. If stimulated with an irritant, such as pokeweed mitogen, the number of T cells also decreases compared with controls and the proportion of suppressor T cells increases, whilst helper T cells fall[42]. In sarcoid, peripheral blood monocytes seem to have a suppressor effect on the lymphocytes and additional serum factors have been described inhibiting cellular processes concerned in immune responses[43–47].

Broncho-alveolar lavage (BAL)

One method which has been widely employed to obtain representative cells for study is broncho-alveolar lavage[48]. The cells obtained from normal individuals are predominantly macrophages and a few lymphocytes. In sarcoidosis, an excess number of lymphocytes can be retrieved from the lower respiratory tract. These are predominantly T lymphocytes of the helper–inducer phenotype (CD4+)[49], which also express activation markers: IL-2R (the interleukin-2 receptor)[50], class II major histocompatibility complex (MHC) markers[51] and VLA-1 (a late activation marker)[52]. (In the peripheral blood of sarcoid patients, the reverse phenomenon is seen with a depletion of CD4+ T cells.) The lung T cells are spontaneously replicating and secreting various cytokines, including interleukin-2 (IL-2)[53], interferon-γ[54], monocyte chemotactic factor and macrophage migration inhibition factor[55].

Lavage fluid from sarcoid patients also contains increased numbers of macrophages, which also show signs of activation. There is increased density of MHC class II expression at the cell surface[56]. Levels of DP and DQ in particular correlate with lymphocyte numbers and the degree of lymphocyte activation in lavage fluid. DQ levels also correlate with the decrease in pulmonary function, suggesting that DQ may be particularly relevant to clinical disease[57]. This enhanced class II expression is consistent with the observation that sarcoid alveolar macrophages are capable of enhanced antigen presentation to autologous lymphocytes compared with those from control subjects[58,59].

These macrophages show the phenotype of newly recruited cells. A proportion, which increases with pulmonary disease severity as assessed by X-ray, shows an unusual phenotype[60]: RFD1 +, RFD7 +. This subpopulation is glass adherent, expresses strong lysozymal enzyme activity and suppresses mixed lymphocyte reactivity when co-cultured with allogeneic lymphocytes[61].

The relationship between T lymphocytes and macrophages in BAL has been recently studied[62]. In cytospin preparations, T lymphocytes were often seen closely adherent to macrophages. Corticosteroid treatment decreased the T4/T8 ratio in BAL, but increased the numbers of macrophage/T8 (suppressor cell) interactions.

Sarcoid alveolar macrophages can spontaneously release IL-1[63] and, on stimulation, release enhanced quantities of tumour necrosis factor (TNF-α) and reactive oxygen intermediates (ROIs)[64]. They also show increased angiotensin convertase activity (ACE) in active disease (vide infra). Recent data have also emphasized the role of 1,24-dihydroxy vitamin D3 (1,25,$(OH)_2D3$-calcitriol)[65,66]. Under the influence of interferon-γ, macrophages acquire 1,25-hydroxy vitamin D3, α_1-hydroxylase activity. This accounts for the hypercalcaemia and hypercalcuria seen in sarcoidosis and occasionally in tuberculosis. Calcitriol promotes monocyte differentiation and macrophage fusion to form granulomas. It also enhances various macrophage functions, including killing of mycobacteria. It inhibits T cell production of IL-2 and interferon-γ. Macrophages are also known to synthesize and secrete factors which cause fibroblasts to grow and divide[67].

IMMUNOHISTOLOGY

Lung tissue obtained by transbronchial biopsy shows the same cell composition as the BAL, but also reveals spatial organization. The granuloma contains a central core of epithelioid cells together with CD4+ T cells. CD8+ T cells are present around the periphery and occur only rarely in the centre. Mature tissue macrophages are also peripherally distributed, together with a few CD4+ T cells[68].

PATHOGENESIS

Figure 1 shows the current concept of the pathogenesis of sarcoidosis.

Current data are consistent with sarcoidosis being an antigen-driven process rather than a non-specific accumulation of inflammatory cells. There is a bias in the T cell receptor (TCR) variable region gene expression: large cells from a subgroup of patients show an increase in the numbers of cells expressing the β chain variable region, Vβ8[69]. Analysis of the Vβ8+ cDNA clones produced from mRNA extracted from these large cell populations reveals a significant homology in gene sequence in the hypervariable regions of these clones, suggesting preferential T cell selection or replication. A different subgroup of patients shows expanded numbers of T cells expressing the $\gamma\delta$ receptor[70]. Studies of the constant region of the β chain showed a

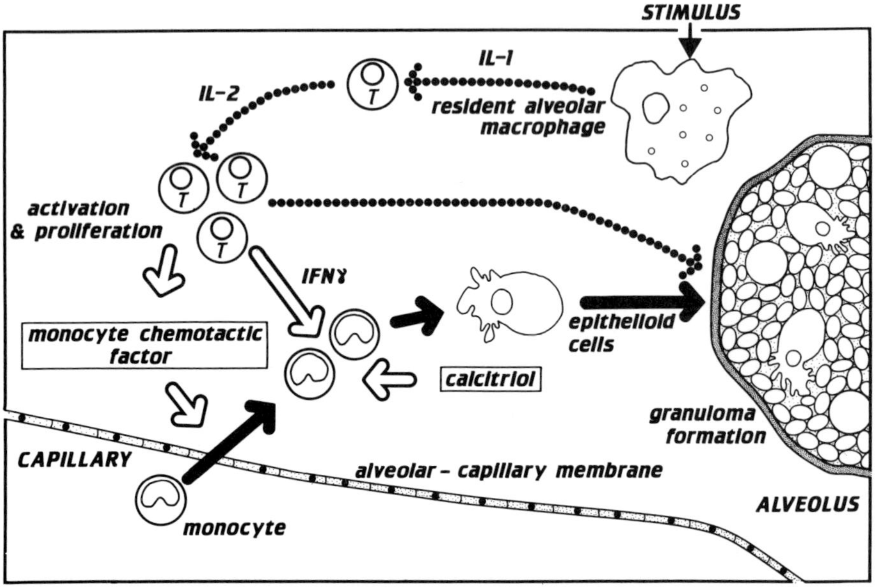

Figure 1 Current concepts of the pathogenesis of sarcoidosis. The initial event is stimulation of an antigen presenting cell, probably an alveolar macrophage. Subsequently there is an IL-1, IL-2 driven T lymphocyte proliferation. Monocytes are attracted from the blood by monocyte chemotactic factor (IL-8) and held at the site of reaction by macrophage migration inhibition factor. Monocyte activation by IFN-γ occurs and this stimulates calcitriol production, which, in turn, causes macrophage fusion to epithelioid cells and granuloma formation

preferential bias of Cβ1 over Cβ2 in the lung T lymphocytes of sarcoid patients compared with sarcoid blood, normal blood and normal lung. Again, a subgroup showed a very exaggerated Cβ1 usage of more than 3 standard deviations above the mean[71].

These studies suggest not only that sarcoid is the result of antigen triggering, but that the antigen (or epitope) may differ in different groups of patients. The relationship of sarcoidosis to tuberculosis and the possibility of atypical mycobacteria as initiating organisms has been reviewed[72]. Mycobacterial DNA (or RNA) has recently been demonstrated in material from similar proportions of patients with diagnoses of mycobacterial tuberculosis and sarcoidosis[73] leading to further discussion[74].

Persistence of the granuloma can be ascribed to

1. Persistence of antigen,
2. Failure of suppressor regulating mechanism,
3. Abnormalities in the regulation of cytokine networks,

or to a combination of these factors.

Models of antigen persistence, such as *Schistosoma mansoni* egg granulomata, involve a chronic stage with suppressor cell populations and factors. Poulter[61] has suggested that the mantle zone of the granuloma may represent a delayed hypersensitivity reaction to the inner contents. Interferon-γ injected

Table 3 Incidence of symptoms in patients with nasal sarcoidosis

Nasal stuffiness and obstruction	88%
Crusting	63%
Blood-stained discharge	37%
Purulent discharge	30%
Facial pain	22%
Mucoid discharge	15%
Anosmia	4%

into foreign body granulomas results in their resolution, indicating that active immune mechanisms may be needed for granuloma removal. In those individuals where sarcoid granulomas fibrose instead of regressing, it is possible that a defect in immune function is occurring, possibly related to the presence of suppressive RFG1+, RFD7+ macrophages in the mantle zone. The enhancement of skin delayed hypersensitivity by corticosteroids, long noted in sarcoid patients, is of interest in this context[31,32]. Further studies of immunohistology and molecular biology should lead to a resolution of the puzzle of sarcoidosis within the next decade.

HISTOLOGY[75]

The tubercles are composed of groups of epithelioid cells with no caseation. The epithelioid cells may be derived from macrophages or monocytes. The tubercles remain discrete, even if closely packed, and minute amounts of central necrosis are occasionally present as are multinucleated giant cells, often of the Langhans variety, but sometimes resembling the foreign body type. A number of crystalline or calcified inclusions are sometimes found in older lesions, such as asteroid inclusions or Schaumann bodies. The latter consist of concentrically arranged lamellated membranes, often enclosing mitochondria and other organelles, and are rich in mucopolysaccharides, phospholipids and lipoproteins. They are relatively infrequent in upper respiratory tract lesions.

However, in all cases, the histological picture is not pathognomonic and the diagnosis of sarcoid requires additional supporting clinical evidence.

CLINICAL FEATURES

In the upper respiratory tract, the nasal symptoms may be quite pronounced (Table 3). They consist of nasal stuffiness and obstruction, crusting and mucopurulent postnasal drip, which is often bloodstained, and, occasionally, anosmia. Facial pain may be present. These symptoms are present from initial presentation with the disease in the majority but can develop as a later problem after 1–9 years.

On examination, the nasal mucosa may show the classical appearances of tiny firm yellow nodules. These may spread into plaques and, occasionally, large polyploid granulomatous masses are present. However, sometimes,

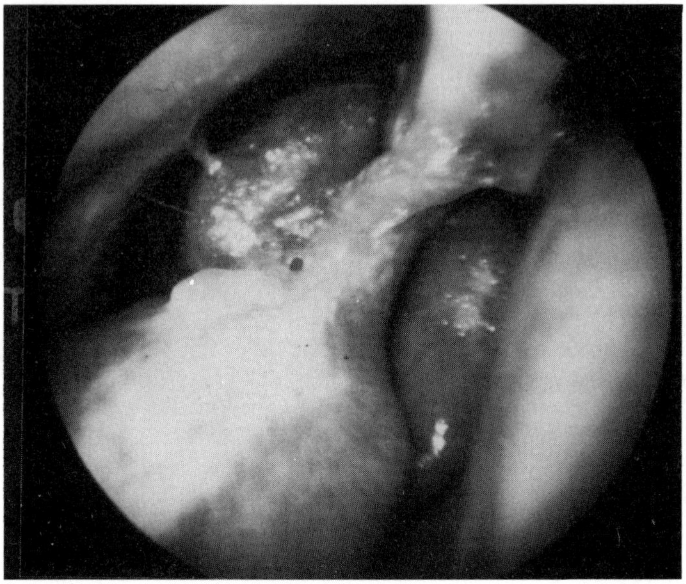

Figure 2 Intranasal photograph of a septal perforation

simple hypertrophy of the mucosa with crusting is seen and this may be excoriated with slight spotting of blood.

Septal perforations (Figure 2) are occasionally seen, sometimes following septal surgery. There may be marked external deformity of the nose, which may take the form of collapse of the bridge (Figure 3) associated with the septal perforation or infiltration and destruction of the cartilage and bone (Figure 4). The nose may be generally swollen without evidence of skin involvement and this swelling can be very marked. If there is skin involvement, this may originate from the vestibule, spreading towards the upper lip or through the nasal bones onto the bridge, often with subcutaneous nodules or erythema nodosum (Figure 5). Furthermore, classical lupus pernio is seen in nearly a quarter of these patients.

In the larynx, fusion of nodules and subsequent fibrosis in the supraglottis produce changes in the voice and more extensive involvement of the glottis and/or subglottis can lead to stridor and dyspnoea. Central neurological manifestations may include vocal cord palsy and hoarseness and, whilst it is probable that anosmia may sometimes result from the nasal problems themselves, more frequently it can be due to actual involvement of the olfactory nerves and their connections. Autopsy findings suggest that olfactory damage is present in 1.4% of cases but is frequently overlooked clinically[76]. Other cranial nerves may be affected, e.g. facial and vestibulocochlear, and patients may develop diabetes insipidus and a basal meningitis.

Reference has already been made to conductive deafness due to serous otitis media and, though sarcoid infiltration of the palate and tonsils is usually symptomless, occasionally sleep apnoea and sore throats can occur.

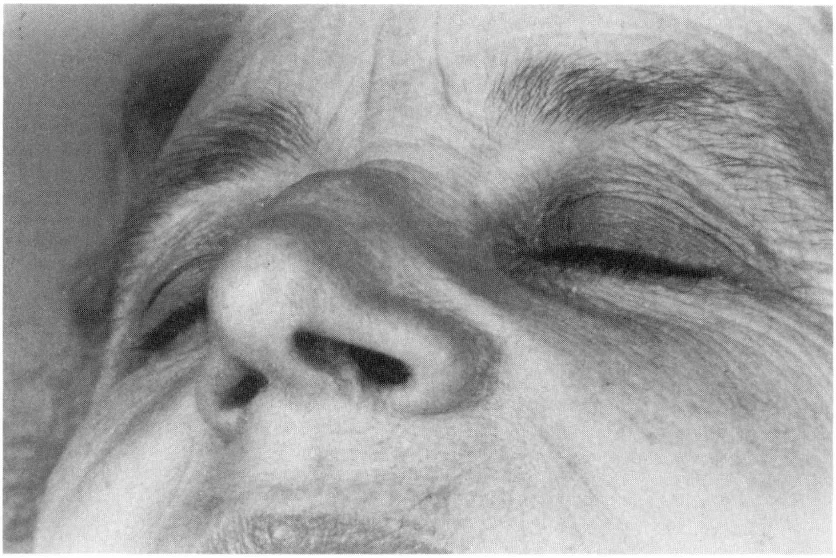

Figure 3 Clinical photograph showing collapse of the nasal bridge in sarcoidosis

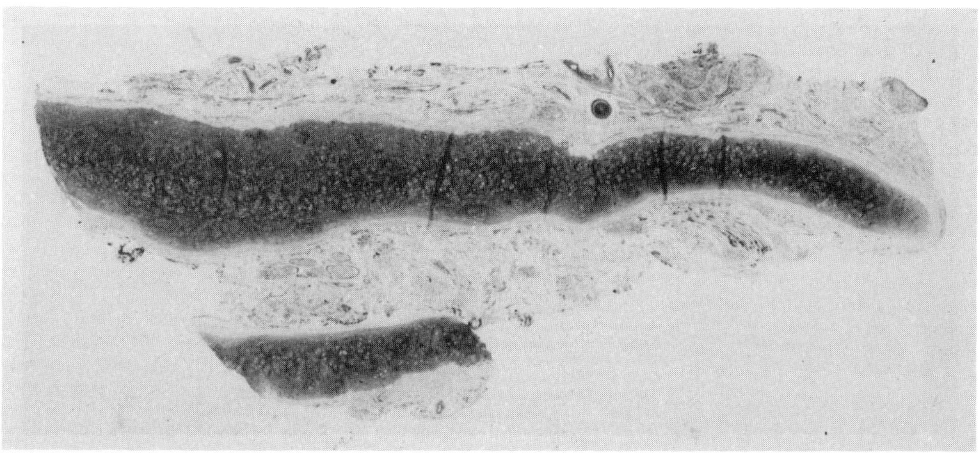

Figure 4 Photomicrograph of coronal section through nasal septum demonstrating early erosion of cartilage (× 15, PAS)

Uveoparotid fever, first described by Heerfordt in 1909[77], may also come to the attention of the ENT surgeon with its clinical features of fever, parotid enlargement, uveal tract disease and a bilateral and transient facial nerve palsy[78].

The clinical effects of sarcoid on the other systems of the body have been extensively documented[1].

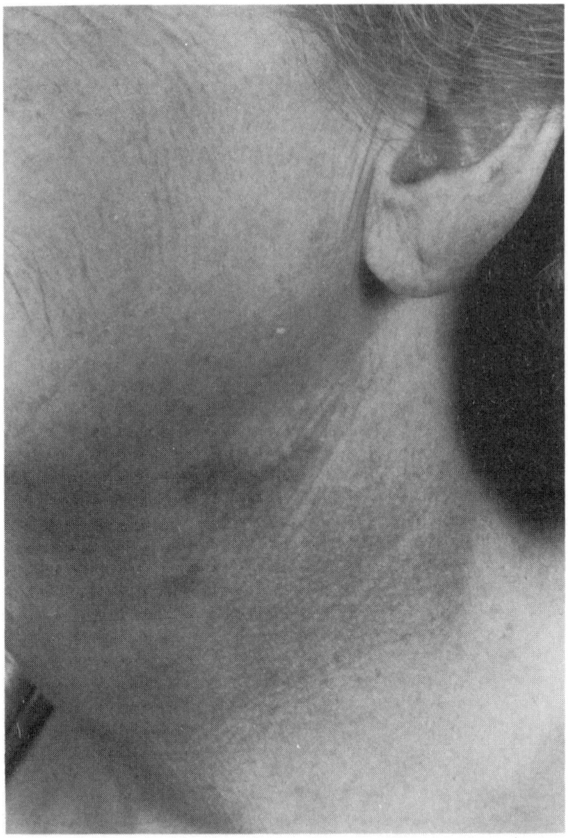

Figure 5 Clinical photograph showing typical patch of violaceous erythema nodosa on the skin of the neck

Table 4 Incidence of positive results of investigations in patients with nasal sarcoid

Kveim test	86%
Serum angiotensin converting enzyme	77%
Sinus X-rays	68%
Sedimentation rate	22%
Full blood count	5%
Serum calcium	5%

INVESTIGATIONS (Table 4)

The majority of patients have a positive Kveim test and raised serum angiotensin converting enzyme [ACE] at some stage during the course of the disease though the ACE is rarely persistently elevated.

ESR, serum globulin, and serum and urinary calcium levels are sometimes elevated and a full blood count may show mild anaemia, leucopenia, thrombocytopenia and eosinophilia.

Kveim test

In 1941, Kveim[79] described a reaction to an intradermal injection of sarcoid tissue suspension which produced a slowly developing nodule with histology consistent with sarcoid in individuals suffering from the condition. This response is dependent upon the evolution of the disease and is not pathognomonic, occurring in other granulomatous conditions, such as Crohn's disease, tuberculosis, leprosy and brucellosis. Furthermore, it is inhibited by administration of oral steroids and is open to considerable observer error in the interpretation of subsequent histology, though accuracy of 80–85% has been claimed[21]. Thus, it is advisable to avoid terms like 'positive' and 'negative' in favour of a description of the histological findings which may be used to corroborate the clinical features.

It is important to use a test solution which is known to be potent and selective; human spleen is most commonly used. The reaction begins to develop within two weeks and the biopsy is taken at 4–6 weeks when the epithelioid cell follicles are well formed.

Attempts to demonstrate an immunological basis for the Kveim reaction have given negative or equivocal results, though it is thought that it detects some form of altered reactivity.

Serum angiotensin converting enzyme

Angiotensin converting enzyme (ACE) is found in macrophages, epithelioid and giant cells of the granulomas and increases in active disease proportional to its extent and activity. However, it is also increased in other conditions, such as Gaucher's disease, tuberculosis, leprosy and primary biliary cirrhosis, so, again, it is a contributory test rather than diagnostic.

^{67}Gallium scanning

This has also been used to detect areas of active sarcoid but also demonstrates malignancy and other granulomas.

Biopsy

Biopsy of potentially affected tissue, such as lymph nodes, liver, skin and lung, may demonstrate histology compatible with a diagnosis of sarcoid.

As nasal mucosa is readily accessible, it would be an attractive site for diagnostic biopsy. However, random biopsy of macroscopically normal mucosa in patients with proven sarcoid[8] was found to be negative in 92%. Conversely, if the nasal mucosa looks abnormal, biopsy is almost always positive and shows the typical appearances of a non-caseating epithelioid granulomatous process.

Biopsy of maxillary sinus mucosa in the presence of abnormal X-ray appearances is also positive in a high proportion of cases, but, unless there is obvious macroscopic involvement in the upper respiratory tract, random biopsy produces a low yield and is not a useful screening test.

Radiology

Sinus X-rays in patients with nasal symptoms are often abnormal, showing varying degrees of mucosal thickening, polypoid masses and opacification. Bone destruction can sometimes be seen[80,81]. Similarly, X-rays of the nasal bones may show rarefication, a wide-meshed trabecular pattern, disappearance of suture lines and even punctate osteolysis in 15–26% of cases[15].

The chest X-ray demonstrates abnormalities in the majority of cases. Initially, 50% show some abnormality and this may increase to 90% during the course of the disease. A ground-glass appearance of the lung fields is frequently found, though large confluent infiltrations may also be seen in addition to the commonest finding of bilateral hilar lymphadenopathy. X-ray evidence of pulmonary disease is not always present and, in 33% of a series of patients with nasal sarcoid, the chest X-ray was normal[8].

Differential diagnosis – see Chapter 8, Table 2, page 130.

TREATMENT

Medical

In the nasal cavity, symptomatic relief can be obtained from alkaline nasal douches, glucose and glycerine drops and the application of topical steroids, such as betamethasone drops, in the 'head down and forwards' position.

Local depot steroid injections in the upper respiratory tract have been advocated[17] but it seems that systemic steroids at doses of 30–60 mg/day are the most effective medication, both for generalized disease and also to control nasal symptoms. On this regimen, two thirds of patients remain stable or improve. It is, however, rarely possible to completely withdraw this medication without relapse though the dosage may be decreased with the addition of topical steroids. Though the mucosa may improve in appearance, it hardly ever returns to normal.

Surgical

It is probably safe to debulk large inferior turbinates and polypoid masses but other surgical procedures, particularly on the septum, are to be avoided as they are associated with a significant incidence of perforation and nasal collapse[18,82].

Spontaneous regression of the disease has been observed but may be associated with fibrosis and structural distortion. It is obviously important to be sure that the disease is completely burnt out before contemplating any surgical reconstruction.

As sarcoid can present in the upper respiratory tract in a variety of forms, one should always consider it when confronted by a patient complaining of mucopurulent catarrh or an unexplained septal perforation, or even requesting rhinoplasty, and not allow one's enthusiasm for surgery to override a consideration of the aetiology of the deformity.

Acknowledgements

I would like to thank Dr G.K. Scadding for her considerable contribution and advice on the immunological aspects of sarcoid.

REFERENCES

1. Scadding JG, Mitchell DN. Sarcoidosis. 2nd Ed. London: Chapman and Hall; 1985.
2. Besnier E. Lupus pernio de la face. Ann Dermatol Syphiligr. 1889;10:333–6.
3. Hutchinson J. Cases of Mortimer's malady. Arch Surg Lond. 1898;9:307–14.
4. Boeck C. Multiple benign sarcoid of the skin. J Cutan Dis. 1899;17:543–53.
5. Boeck C. Forgestzte untersuchugen uber des multiple benigne Sarkoid. Arch Dermatol Syph Wien. 1905;73:301–32.
6. Kreibach K, Kraus A. Beitrage zur Kenntnis des Boeckschen benignen Miliarlupoid. Arch Dermatol Syph Wien. 1908;92:173–204.
7. Ulrich K. Die Schleimhautveranderungen der oberen Luftwege beim 'Boeckschen Sarkoid' und ihre Stellung zum lupus pernio. Arch Laryngol Rhinol Berl. 1918;31:506–34.
8. Wilson R, Lund V, Sweatman M, Mackay IS, Mitchell DN. Upper respiratory tract involvement in sarcoidosis and its management. Eur Respir J. 1988;1:269–72.
9. Barmwater K. Uber Boeck's Sarkoid auf den Schleimnauten. Hals-Nas u Ohrenartz. 1936;27:259–64.
10. Gravesen PB. Lymphogranulomatosis benigna. Odense. 1942.
11. Reisner D. Boeck's sarcoid and systemic sarcoidosis: a study of 35 cases. Am Rev Tuber. 1944;49:289–307.
12. Robinson B, Pound AW. Sarcoidosis: a survey with report of 30 cases. Med J Aust. 1950;2:568–82.
13. Lindsay JR, Perlman HB. Sarcoidosis of the upper respiratory tract. Ann Otol Rhinol Laryngol. 1951;69:549–66.
14. James DG. Diagnosis and treatment of sarcoidosis. Br Med J. 1956;2:900.
15. Weiss JA. Sarcoidosis in otolaryngology: report of 11 cases. Laryngoscope. 1960;70: 1351–98.
16. Kampfer R. Über extrapulmonale Organmanifestationen des Morbus Boeck unter besonderer Berucksichtigung der Schleimhaut der oberen Luftwege. Prax Pneumol. 1964;18:204–17.
17. McKelvie P, Goesson C, Pokhrel RP, Jackson P. Sarcoidosis of the upper air passages. Br J Dis Chest. 1968;62:200–5.
18. Neville E, Mills RGS, Jash DG. Sarcoidosis of the upper respiratory tract and its association with lupus pernio. Thorax. 1976;31:660–4.
19. Selroos O, Niemisto M. Sarcoidosis of the nose. Scand J Respir Dis. 1977;58:57–62.
20. James DG, Barter S, Jash D, MacKinnon DM, Carstairs IS. Sarcoidosis of the upper respiratory tract (SURT). J Laryngol Otol. 1982;96:711–8.
21. McCaffrey TV, MacDonald TJ. Sarcoidosis of the nose and paranasal sinuses. Laryngoscope. 1983;93:1281–4.
22. Cummings MM, Dunner E, Schmidt RH, Barnwell HB. Concepts of epidemiology of sarcoidosis: Preliminary report of 1,194 cases reviewed with particular reference to geographic ecology. Postgrad Med. 1956;19:437–46.

23. Creston JE, Dibble PA. Nasal sarcoidosis. Arch Otolaryngol. 1961;74:210–8.
24. Devine KD. Sarcoidosis and sarcoidosis of the larynx. Laryngoscope. 1965;75:533–69.
25. Fishman SM, Canalis RF. Nasopharyngeal sarcoidosis. Ear, Nose Throat. 1979;58:4–9.
26. Wilson R, Sweatman M, Mackay IS, Mitchell DN. Adenoidal tissue as an aid to the diagnosis of sarcoidosis in childhood. Thorax. 1986;41:66–7.
27. Schaumann J. Etude sur le lupus pernio et ses rapports avec les sarcoides et la tuberculose. Ann Dermatol Syphiligr. 1917;6:357–73.
28. Scadding JG. Insensitivity to tuberculin in pulmonary tuberculosis. Tubercle. 1956;37: 371–80.
29. Boeck C. Nochmals zur klinik und zur Stellung des 'beningen Miliarlupods'. Arch Dermatol Syph Wien. 1916;121:707–41.
30. Friou GJ. Delayed cutaneous hypersensitivity in sarcoidosis. J Clin Invest. 1952;31:630–5.
31. Gross NJ. The paradoxical skin response in sarcoidosis: a hypothesis. Am Rev Respir Dis. 1973;107:798–801.
32. Pyke DA, Scadding JG. Effect of cortisone upon skin sensitivity to tuberculin in sarcoidosis. Br Med J. 1952;2:1126–8.
33. Salvesen HA. The sarcoid of Boeck, a disease of importance to internal medicine. Acta Med Scand. 1935;86:127–51.
34. Norberg R. Studies in sarcoidosis. IV. Serum immunoglobulin levels. Acta Med Scand. 1967;175:497–504.
35. Celikoglu S, Vieira LODB, Siltzbach LE. Serum immunoglobulin levels in sarcoidosis. In Levinsky L, Macholda F, eds. 5th International Conference on Sarcoidosis. University Karlova, Prague; 1971:168–70.
36. Bergmann KC, Zaumsell J, Lachmann B. Quantitative IgE – Bestimmung bei sarkoidose. Z Erkr Atmungsorgane. 1973;37:351–2.
37. Wanstrup J, Elling P. Immunochemistry of sarcoidosis. Acta Pathol Microbiol Scand. 1968;73:37–48.
38. Hedfors E, Norberg R. Evidence of circulating immune complexes in sarcoidosis. Clin Exp Immunol. 1974;16:493–6.
39. Saint-Remy J-MR, Mitchell DN, Cole PJ. Variation in immunoglobulin levels and circulating immune complexes in sarcoidosis. Am Rev Respir Dis. 1983;127:23–7.
40. Hoffbrand BI. Occurrence and significance of lymphopenia in sarcoidosis. Am Rev Respir Dis. 1968;98:107–10.
41. Hedfors E. Activation of peripheral T-cells of sarcoidosis patients and healthy controls. Clin Exp Immunol. 1974;18:379–90.
42. Katz P, Haynes BF, Fauci A. Alteration of T lymphocyte subpopulations in sarcoidosis. Clin Immunol Immunopathol. 1978;10:350–4.
43. Mangi RJ, Dwyer JM, Kantor FS. The effect of plasma upon lymphocyte response in vitro – demonstration of a humoral inhibitor in patients with sarcoidosis. Clin Exp Immunol. 1974;18:519–28.
44. Maderazo EG, Ward PA, Wjronick CL, Kubik J, DeGraff AC. Leukotactic dysfunction in sarcoidosis. Ann Intern Med. 1976;84:414–9.
45. Campbell PB. Defective monocyte leukotaxis in sarcoidosis. Am Rev Respir Dis. 1977;116:251–9.
46. Williams JD, Smith MD, Davies BH. Interaction of immune complexes and T-suppressor cells in sarcoidosis. Thorax. 1982;37:602–6.
47. Davies J, Nellen M, Goodwin JF. Reversible pulmonary hypertension in sarcoidosis. Postgrad Med J. 1982;58:282–5.
48. Hunninghake GW, Gadek JW, Kawanami O, Ferrans VJ, Crystal RG. Inflammatory and immune processes in the human lung in health and disease: evaluation by bronchoalveolar lavage. Am J Pathol. 1979;97:149–206.
49. Hunninghake GW, Crystal RG. Pulmonary sarcoidosis. N Engl J Med. 1981;305:429–34.
50. Semenzaid G, Agostini C, Trentin L et al. Evidence of cells bearing interleukin-2 receptor at sites of disease activity in sarcoid patients. Clin Exp Immunol. 1984;57:331–7.
51. Costabel U, Bross KJ, Ruhle KH et al. Ia-like antigens on T cells and their subpopulations in pulmonary sarcoidosis and in hypersensitivity penumonitis. Analysis of bronchoalveolar and blood lymphocytes. Am Rev Respir Dis. 1985;131:337–42.
52. Saltini C, Hemler ME, Crystal RG. T lymphocytes compartmentalised on the epithelial

surface of the lower respiratory tract express the very late activation complex VLA-1. Clin Immunol Immunopathol. 1988;46:221–33.
53. Pinkston P, Bitterman PB, Crystal RG. Spontaneous release of IL-2 by lung T lymphocytes in active pulmonary sarcoidosis. N Engl J Med. 1983;308:793–800.
54. Robinson BWS, McLemore TL, Crystal RG. Gamma interferon is spontaneously released by alveolar macrophages and lung T lymphocytes in patients with pulmonary sarcoidosis. J Clin Invest. 1985;75:1488–95.
55. Hunninghake GW, Gadek JW, Young RC et al. Maintenance of granuloma formation in pulmonary sarcoidosis by T lymphocytes within the lung. N Engl J Med. 1980;302:594–8.
56. Campbell DA, du Bois RM, Butcher RG, Poulter LW. The density of HLA-DR antigen expression on alveolar macrophages is increased in pulmonary sarcoidosis. Clin Exp Immunol. 1986;65:165–71.
57. Haslam PL, Parker DJ, Townsend PJ. Increases in HLA-DQ, DP, DR and transferrin receptors on alveolar macrophages in sarcoidosis and allergic alveolitis compared with fibrosing alveolitis. Chest. 1990;97:651–61.
58. Venet A, Hanle AJ, Saltini C et al. enhanced alveolar macrophage-mediated antigen-induced T lymphocyte proliferation in sarcoidosis. J Clin Invest. 1985;75:293–301.
59. Lem VM, Lipscomb MF, Weissler JC et al. Bronchoalveolar cells from sarcoid patients demonstrate enhanced antigen presentation. J Immunol. 1985;135:1766–71.
60. Ainslie GM, Poulter LW, du Bois RM. Relation between immunocytological features of bronchoalveolar lavage fluid and clinical indices in sarcoidosis. Thorax. 1989;44:501–9.
61. Poulter LW. Immune aspects of sarcoidosis. Postgrad Med J. 1988;64:536–43.
62. Van Maarseveen TCMT, Mullink H, Stam J, De Groot J. Macrophage-T suppressor cell interference in the lungs of steroid-treated sarcoidosis patients. Am Rev Respir Dis. 1991;143:839–43.
63. Hunninghake GW. Release of interleukin-1 by alveolar macrophages of patients with active pulmonary sarcoidosis. Am Rev Respir Dis. 1984;129:569–72.
64. Bachwich PR, Lynch JP III, Larrick J et al. Tumour necrosis factor production by human sarcoid alveolar macrophages. Am J Pathol. 1986;125:421–5.
65. Kunkel SL, Chensue SW, Streiter RM et al. Cellular and molecular aspects of granulomatous inflammation. Am J Respir Cell Mol Biol. 1989;1:439–47.
66. Kelley J. Cytokines of the lung. Am Rev Respir Dis. 1990;141:765–88.
67. Rennard SI, Hunninghake GW, Bitterman PB, Crystal RG. Production of fibronectin by the human alevolar macrophage: mechanism for the recruitment of fibroblasts to sites of tissue injury in interstitial lung diseases. Proc Natl Acad Sci USA. 1981;78:7147–51.
68. Du Bois RM. Recent advances in the immunology of interstitial lung diseases. Clin Exp Allergy. 1991;21:9–16.
69. Moller DR, Konishi K, Kirby M et al. Bias toward use of a specific T cell receptor B-chain variable region in a subgroup of individuals with sarcoidosis. J Clin Invest. 1988;82: 1183–91.
70. Balbi B, Moller DR, Kirby M et al. Increased numbers of T lymphocytes with positive antigen receptors in a subgroup of individuals with pulmonary sarcoidosis. J Clin Invest. 1990;85:1353–61.
71. Tamura N, Moller DR, Balbi B, Crystal RG. Preferential usage of the T-cell antigen receptor B-chain constant region CB1 element by lung T-lymphocytes of patients with pulmonary sarcoidosis. Am Rev Respir Dis. 1991;143:635–9.
72. Lyons DJ, Fielding JF. What's in a relationship? Sarcoidosis and tuberculosis. Irish Med J. 1990;83:76–9.
73. Fidler HM, Rook GA, Johnson N McI, McFadden J. Mycobacterium tuberculosis DNA in tissue affected by sarcoidosis. Br Med J. 1993;306:346–9.
74. Letters. Br J Med. 1993;306:1269–71.
75. Friedman I, Osborn DA. Pathology of granulomas and neoplasms of the nose and paranasal sinuses. London: Churchill Livingstone; 1982.
76. Delaney P, Henkin R, Manz H, Satterley RA, Bauer H. Olfactory sarcoidosis. Arch Otolaryngol. 1977;103:717–24.
77. Heerfordt CF. Uber eine 'Febris uveo-parotidea subchronica'. Graefes Arch Ophthalmol. 1909;70:254–73.
78. Thompson WC. Uveoparotitis. Arch Intern Med. 1937;59:646–59.

79. Kveim A. En ny og specifikk kutan-reaksjon ved Boecks sarcoid. Nord Med. 1941;9: 169–72.
80. Bordley JE, Proctor DF. Destructive lesion in paranasal sinuses associated with Boeck's sarcoid. Arch Otolaryngol. 1942;36:740–2.
81. Dodd GD, Jing B-S. Radiology of the nose, paranasal sinuses and nasopharynx. Baltimore: Williams and Wilkins; 1977.
82. Hammond BL, Kataria YP. Nasal sarcoidosis with perforation. J Otolaryngol. 1980;9: 31–4.

10
Nasal Polyps

A. B. DRAKE-LEE

INTRODUCTION

Breathing has been closely linked with the spirit of man since antiquity: the word inspiration is an obvious example. The importance of nasal function was recognized early and the ancient Indian culture had an elementary knowledge of rhinology. They were the first to describe nasal polyps but the word polyp was first used by Hippocrates (poly pous means many footed or feet) and accurately describes the condition that occurs in the ethmoid sinuses.

Originally, the term was applied to any polypoidal lesion in the nose with no reference to any pathological classification. During the nineteenth century, histological classification improved the understanding of diseases and, in the nose, neoplasms were differentiated from simple nasal polyps which were considered inflammatory in nature. Today, the term is most commonly used to describe simple benign nasal polyps which are bilateral and arise from the ethmoid sinuses. It must be remembered that polyps are neither a diagnosis nor a disease but the end result of inflammation in the sinuses and, in some cases, the respiratory tract in general.

GENERAL CONSIDERATIONS

Simple nasal polyps are usually found in both sides of the nose but may occur unilaterally. However, when unilateral, polyps must be removed and examined histologically to exclude neoplasia.

Polyps are the linings of the ethmoid sinuses that prolapse into the nose. They appear as pale masses, unless traumatized when they can become reddened. The turbinates can also undergo polypoidal changes. Antrochoanal polyps, which arise from the maxillary sinus and usually descend into the post-nasal space where they are visible with a mirror, are a different entity.

If the patient has had an intransal antrostomy, this polypoidal mucosal can enter the nasal cavity.

Polyps have a constant histological character and so are usually considered as a single entity. However, the nose is only capable of acting in a number of ways and so the same histological picture may be produced by a number of different aetiologies. The histological features will be described in detail later. The aim is to exclude the rare known causes from the majority of patients who have no obvious underlying cause.

Although, for reasons that become apparent later, most polyps are considered either due to allergy or infection, these premises are incorrect. Polyps are, in general, a disease of adults.

AETIOLOGY

Age

Polyps may arise in children, but most children have enlarged inferior turbinates that are mistaken for polyps. The age of onset is important. The ethmoid sinuses are not well enough developed before the age of 2 years for polyp formation to occur. If polyps are encountered before 2 years of age, a defect of the anterior cranial fossa should be suspected and a CT of the cranium, sinuses and nose performed. Diagnosis by biopsy of neural tissue is contraindicated!

If polyps are seen after 2 years, they may be a presenting manifestation of cystic fibrosis[1]. Polyps usually arise in established cases and, in some, may be particularly recurrent. They may cause expansion of the floor of the anterior cranial fossa before the symphyses unit and result in hypertelorism as the child grows.

Benign simple polyps present in adulthood and they are rare before 20 years. Initial presentation occurs equally in each decade up to 60; after this, they are encountered more rarely. They also become less troublesome as the patient ages.

Incidence

The true incidence of polyps is difficult to determine. It would appear that between 20 and 100 per 1000 of the adult population have nasal polyps at sometime in their lives. This would fit in with the general incidence of nasal disease in the UK. Allergic rhinitis occurs in about 10% of the population and non-allergic rhinitis occurs in a further 5%. A proportion of the latter have nasal polyps.

The number of patients with some degree of late-onset asthma is about 1% and about one third of these patients have nasal polyps; about one third of patients with nasal polyps have some evidence of bronchospasm.

Sex

A strong male predominance is found both in children with cystic fibrosis and adults who have nasal polyps. Figures vary from series to series but the ratio is between 2 and 4 to 1. This is not found in patients who have asthma in addition to polyps, where the incidence is equal[2], suggesting that this is a different group of patients.

Racial groups

All racial groups have nasal polyps and, as yet, there are no comparable studies between the 4 major groups. Most of the research work has been published on people of European extraction and confirmed by workers in Japan.

Animal studies

Polyps are virtually confined to man, occuring very rarely in other primates, usually chimpanzees. Cats occasionally have Eustachian polyps and cows can have granulation polyps of the nasal septum but this is confined to cows of European extraction living in Australia! The difference in development of the ethmoturbinal system in other animals may account for the species differences. This means that there are no animal models in which to study the disease processes and so work must be performed on human tissue.

CYSTIC FIBROSIS AND NASAL POLYPS

Polyps occur in 8% of cases with cystic fibrosis[3] and they are associated with the respiratory rather than the gastrointestinal manifestations of the disease[4]. This may help to explain the lack of increase in polyps in children now alive because of control of gastrointestinal symptoms in the first year of life and the better survival of those presenting with meconium ileus.

The genetic abnormality of this autosomal recessive condition lies on the seventh chromosome in three quarters of the patients. The disease results in colonization of the lower respiratory tract by both *Pseudomonas* and staphylococci. The sinuses do not appear to act as a reservoir for infection for the chest disease[5].

Polyps become less of a problem as the child ages. The disease is not associated with an increased incidence of allergy to dust and pollens although the serum IgE to *Aspergillus* spp. does appear to be raised in polyp patients in adulthood. The immunological changes in cystic fibrosis are not yet well worked out.

OTHER INTRINSIC RESPIRATORY ABNORMALITIES

While the deficit in cystic fibrosis is in the function of the exocrine glands, other abnormalities in the respiratory mucosa may result in polyp formation.

Immotile cilial syndrome (Kartagener's syndrome) can result in polyps eventually because of stasis of mucus, as can hyperviscous mucus seen in Young's syndrome. These two are very rare causes of polyps in adults and often follow a long period of respiratory illness in childhood which should alert the clinician.

ASTHMA AND NASAL POLYPS

Asthma and other respiratory diseases

The association between nasal polyps and other diseases, particularly asthma has been widely documented. Maloney and Collins[6] reviewed the literature and stated that between 20 and 40% of patients with polyps had some degree of bronchospasm. The association is with late-onset asthma and the aetiology here is open to debate. Although IgE-mediated allergy is not common, mast cell reactions would appear to have some place in the initiation of the symptoms.

The incidence of childhood asthma among polyp patients is the same as in the general population. The number of children with asthma is rising and around 5% of the population have some evidence of asthma during childhood. The incidence of childhood asthma in cases of nasal polyps is 3.5%[2]. While the aetiology of adult-onset asthma is extensively debated, cases developing asthma during childhood have a strong allergic bias.

As mentioned earlier, the sex ratio of patients with nasal polyps and asthma is different from that found with polyps alone, suggesting disease heterogeneity.

Aspirin hypersensitivity

There is a well-recognized triad of asthma, aspirin hypersensitivity and nasal polyps, occurring in up to 8% of patients who present with nasal polyps[7]. The mechanism is uncertain but it is not an allergic reaction and both prostaglandins[8] and leukotrienes have been implicated in the production of the oedema. This is presumably mediated via mast cell degranulation[9].

In conclusion, respiratory diseases, such as asthma, cystic fibrosis, immotile cilial syndrome and Young syndrome, which result in an unstable respiratory mucosa, may result in the development of nasal polyps.

ALLERGY

Allergy has been considered to predispose to polyp formation for some considerable time but it is the result of a loose association of features. Histologically, over 90% of polyps show tissue eosinophilia, over 20% of polyp patients have asthma and many of the patients have a prodromal period of rhinitis with blockage, running and sneezing. The term 'allergy' has been used in a number of ways but is now defined as a Type 1

Table 1 The incidence of allergic and respiratory diseases in patients with nasal polyps

	Polyp patients	*Normal population*
Allergic diseases		
Hayfever	10%	10%
Childhood asthma	5%	5%
Eczema	11%	3%
Penicillin allergy	7%	<15%
Positive skin tests	25%	20–25%
Non-allergic diseases		
Late-onset asthma	>25%	3%
Aspirin intolerance	8%	0.1%

The figures for the controls are gathered from a number of different studies which are referenced in Drake-Lee, Lowe, Swantson, Grace. Clinical profile and recurrence of nasal polyps. J Laryngol Otol. 1984;98:783–93.

hypersensitivity reaction caused by a known allergen reacting with an allergen-specific immunoglobulin (most commonly IgE) which is situated on a mast cell. Certain clinical conditions are known to be mediated by these reactions, e.g. seasonal allergic rhinitis and perennial rhinitis caused by dust-mite sensitivity. Several authors have felt that allergic diseases are no more common in polyp patients than in the normal population[2,10].

Table 1 shows the incidence of allergic diseases in polyp patients compared with literature controls. Hay fever, childhood asthma, penicillin hypersensitivity (which may be mediated by IgE) and multiple positive skin tests are no more common than expected. The presence of allergy would appear to be coincidental and the presence of an allergic disease in patients is not associated with a more severe recurrence pattern.

THE ROLE OF BACTERIA IN THE PATHOGENESIS OF POLYPS

There is considerable debate on the place of bacteria in the pathogenesis of nasal polyps, with some authors drawing different conclusions although using the same data. Part of the problem comes from terminology and part from understanding the role of bacteria, as this role may range from frank infection through to bacteria acting as allergens. The normal nose harbours bacteria which may become pathological given the right conditions (Table 2).

Sinusitis

Virtually every patient with nasal polyps has some degree of radiological change in the sinuses which is not confined to the ethmoids alone. Unfortunately, sinusitis does not necessarily mean infected sinuses. At least 2 types are recognized: true infective sinusitis and hyperplasia.

Purulent sinusitis results from infection, usually by bacteria, and may become chronic. Inflammation responds to appropriate treatment with

Table 2 Comparison of bacterial cultures from the nose and paranasal sinuses

	Normal nose		*Maxillary sinuses*		
	Anterior	*Posterior*	*Acute*	*Polyposis*	*Nasal polyp tissue*
Staphylococcus aureus	30%	10%	4%	—	12%
Streptococci (all)	—	15%	30%	10%	25%
Gram −ve	1%	10%	10%	—	10%
Haemophilus influenzae	—	40%	20%	10%	—
Anaerobes	—	—	6%	—	5%

These figures are presented as percentages for comparison. Figures are derived as follows: the normal nose – Reference 38; acute axillary sinusitis – aggregated figures; chronic sinus disease in patients with nasal polyps – Reference 39; polyp homogenates – Reference 11

antimicrobial chemotherapy and surgical treatment if necessary. The incidence of chronic sinusitis has decreased dramatically over the last 50 years; nasal polyps have not become any less frequent.

Hyperplastic sinusitis is associated with mucus hypersecretion and when the ostium of a sinus is blocked, then secretions remain in the sinus. These may then become colonized and bacterial sinusitis ensues.

Nasal polyp homogenates have been cultured for organisms and 24 out of the 40 grew aerobic bacteria; Gram-negative cultures were obtained in 6 cases whereas 14 were completely sterile[11]. Streptococci were cultured most frequently and were more common in asthmatics and patients on inhaled steroids. If the polyps showed a polymorph infiltration, then bacteria were more likely to be cultured. Cultures were completely negative for mycobacteria, mycoplasmata and viruses.

The presence of bacterial specific IgE in nasal polyp oedema fluid has been investigated by Calenoff and his co-workers[12]. They stated that 59 of the 61 patients had bacterial specific IgE in the polyp oedema and the most commonly raised immunoglobulin was to *Proteus*. They defined a positive result on the basis of a count 150% above background noise. It would appear from their studies that the activity was lost on incubation of sera at 56°C. They gave no information on the anti-IgE used and some of the commercial anti-IgEs have had purity and specificity problems. The results appear to be inconclusive.

Nasal polyp tissue has been challenged with bacteria to release histamine[13] and a wide and variable amount of histamine was released with anti-IgE. The study concluded that, although there was some response to challenge with streptococcal and staphylococcal extracts, bacterial allergy was only a possibility.

A further indirect argument against a direct bacterial role is the dramatic response of about half the cases to glucocorticosteroids. If the process were primarily infective, an exacerbation of the condition should occur, and, even in those cases who do not respond, there is no exacerbation of symptoms. No studies have shown that nasal polyps respond dramatically to antibiotics which should eradicate organisms and remove the source of allergens.

HISTOLOGY

The histological features of polyp tissue, sinus mucosa and the lining of the bronchi from patients dying in status asthmaticus are the same. Respiratory epithelium lies on a thickened basement membrane which covers a grossly oedematous submucosa. The oedematous nature of the stroma has been well demonstrated histologically by Taylor[14]. If there has been repeated trauma to the polyp, the epithelium may undergo squamous metaplasia.

The submucosa contains few vessels, mainly capillaries. The cellular infiltrate is mainly composed of plasma cells, small lymphocytes and macrophages, and the most striking feature, which is present in over 90% of polyps, is eosinophilia. This varies within and between polyps. Their part in the pathogenesis of polyps remains unclear. Sensitized eosinophils are believed to be important in the initiation of mucosal oedema in patients with aspirin hypersensitivity[15].

There is little nervous tissue. Some of the cells may show atypia in the stroma[16].

LOCAL NASAL ALLERGY

It is possible that, even though the patients are no more allergic as a group, a local allergy occurs in the nasal cavity that is not manifest systemically. If this were the case, a local allergic reaction should occur in the nose. Evidence for such a reaction would be found by looking at mast cell morphology, the presence and the generation of mast cell mediators, the local production of IgE and at allergen challenge studies.

Mast cells

Although there is extensive debate on the subgrouping of mast cells in animals, there do not appear to be any obvious distinct subgroups in man, more a spectrum of cells which have metachromatic granules under light microscopy and electron-dense granules ultrastructurally. Ultrastructural studies have shown that mast cells in polyps are degranulated[17,18]. The degranulation could give rise to eosinophilia and the presence of inflammatory mediators would account for the oedema.

Polyp oedema

The polyp oedema is easy to collect and has been studied several times, the first of which was by Berdal[19]. Serum may also be collected and levels of compounds compared in both samples from the same patient. The fluid is mainly oedema since all the plasma proteins may be demonstrated in smaller amounts than in serum. All the immunoglobulins are present but IgA and IgE are produced locally in greater amounts than can be accounted for by diffusion alone.

IgE levels

Levels of IgE in polyp oedema have been shown to be higher than the corresponding levels in serum in several studies[20–22]. Although some authors feel that this may be related to the presence of an allergic response, others feel that the production is purely a function of local plasma cells because elevated levels of IgE may be found in nasal secretions in non-atopics[23]. Polyps are capable of local production and this has been demonstrated by comparing the levels of IgE with those of either albumin or macroglobulin which are produced elsewhere. Serum values for these compounds are usually below those in polyp oedema.

Allergen-specific IgE

Since house dust mite and grass pollen are the two most common causes of allergic rhinitis and produce the most frequent positive skin tests in these patients, activity against these allergens has been sought in the polyp oedema fluid. Raised levels of allergen-specific IgE may be found rarely. Elevated levels are less common than positive skin tests. Local IgE may be elevated when the serum RAST is negative, suggesting local production of allergen-specific IgE in the nasal mucosa.

Cell-bound IgE

Difficulty in determining the purity of some of the earlier commercial anti-IgEs means that some of the earlier studies which looked at the presence of cell-bound IgE are open to criticism. It is important to demonstrate the distribution of local plasma cells as some mast cells have little surface IgE but have cytoplasmic staining[24]. Mast cells stain metachromatically but the intensity of the stained granules may disguise the IgE which is stained brown by a peroxidase–antiperoxidase method. Using a dilute toluidine blue, which stains all nuclei a light blue and mast cell granules metachromatically a light purple, it is possible to combine both techniques[24]. A few IgE-producing plasma cells may be found in all polyps. Some polyps have far fewer mast cells than others but they may be found in all polyps. Approximately half the mast cells have an intense staining for IgE, whereas the other cells appear to have very little IgE on their surface. There is no obvious subgrouping into those patients who are atopic and those who are not.

Vasoactive compounds and mediators

Histamine, the prostaglandins and the leukotrienes mediate inflammation. Some of the mediators, namely histamine, prostaglandin D_2 and the leukotrienes C_4 and D_4 appear to be derived from mast cell reactions whereas others are less specific. Histamine is preformed and stored in the granules and arachidonic acid is metabolized in the cell wall by two pathways to produce the other compounds. Histamine is easy to measure and a number of assays are available to do this. A small but variable amount of histamine is found in nasal secretions[25]. Levels are far higher in polyp fluids with values several hundred times those of serum on average[22]. Since histamine is preformed and detoxified locally by the tissue histaminases, as well as being metabolized in the lungs and the liver, these levels suggest that local mechanisms are overcome and the circulation is inadequate to transport the excess away.

Arachidonic acid metabolites are not easy to quantify since they are relatively unstable and may be generated by trauma. The results from the four main studies which looked at these compounds[26–29] are difficult to interpret because there is little work on normal levels in nasal tissues and two of the studies induced the generation of metabolites by challenge. It appears that the levels of thromboxanes are elevated and that challenge will produce 5-, 12- and 15-hydroxyeicosatetraenoic acid (HETE), the most elevated being 15-HETE. There is some suggestion that levels are higher in patients with aspirin sensitivity but whether this is due to a more severe inflammation is not clear. Leukotrienes C_4 and D_4 may be demonstrated in polyp oedema fluid (see above). Prostaglandins E_2, F_2 and 6-keto are also present in the oedema.

Allergen challenge to polyp tissue

Bacterial challenge has been discussed already. The first report of pollen allergen challenge to nasal polyp tissues was by Kaliner and his colleagues in 1973[30]. They used a heterogeneous collection of tissue, including that taken from children with cystic fibrosis, and either challenged allergic tissue or passively sensitized non-allergic tissue with pollen extract and demonstrated that it was possible to release histamine. Challenge to non-sensitized tissue with mixed grass pollen and house dust mite extracts has shown that it is possible to release tissue histamine. Polyp tissue is less reactive than peripheral blood and, even then, only releases histamine rarely on direct challenge, suggesting that allergic reactions are not common.

CYTOKINES AND MICROENVIRONMENTAL DIFFERENTIATION

Cytokines are proteins produced by cells. They act locally, either on the same cell type (autocrine function) or, more frequently, on other cell types. The elevation of certain cytokines, such as GM-CSF (granulocyte macrophage colony stimulating factor) in polyp tissue has been described. This could explain eosinophil accumulation in polyps. Nasal polyp epithelial cells and fibroblasts are capable of stimulating eosinophil and basophil differentiation in blood from atopic individuals. Mononuclear cell colonies derived from polyp tissue show many eosinophil/basophil precursors; polyp fibroblasts show increased growth in vitro. In addition, an elevation of epithelial growth factor receptor has been demonstrated immunohistologically, as has insulin-like growth factor, a neuropeptide. Using this information, a scheme for polyp formation is shown in Figure 1.

Similar tissue-driven responses probably occur in asthma, in which eosinophil and basophil progenitors are also chronically increased. Anatomical factors could account for the localization of polyps. Local inflammatory reactions occur throughout the nose but the anatomical development of the ethmoids facilitates persistent oedema since the blood supply is far less well developed in the sinuses. The process is dynamic so polyps may vary in size.

SYMPTOMS AND SIGNS

Symptoms

All patients, without exception, have nasal obstruction to some degree. This is frequently bilateral although it is not always equal in severity. Sneezing and anterior rhinorrhoea are present in about half the patients and are often found together. Loss of sense of smell and taste occurs in three quarters of the cases. This is usually partial and is the most difficult symptom to treat. The grossly congested mucosa may produce excess mucus that results in a post-nasal drip which may become green if infected. The eosinophilia may colour the mucus a yellow-green. Pain around the face is present occasionally but patients complain more frequently about pressure in the nose and face. Epistaxis is uncommon and suggests malignancy in unilateral polyps but may occur if the patient tries to blow his nose with excessive force.

Signs

Patients talk with a hyponasal voice and are often asked if they have a cold. If the polyps are severe, they can prolapse out of the nose but are usually seen inside the nares where they appear as semitranslucent masses in the nasal cavity (Figure 2). If they are injected or the examiner cannot determine whether the structure is a polyp then it can be probed lightly. Polyps are relatively insensitive because they have a poor nerve supply.

If polyps are present before the facial bones fuse, as in children with cystic fibrosis, the resulting pressure in the ethmoids will force the sutures apart in the growing skull and produce hypertelorism. Polyps rarely produce bone erosion but it may be seen following surgery or if the patient develops a mucocoele. The latter is very rare in polyp patients and usually arises sometime after surgery.

Figure 1 Opposite. (a) A scheme for the development of nasal polyps. Insulin-like growth factor stimulates the growth and cytokine production of local nasal tissues, leading to local accumulation of granulocyte progenitors. In the presence of T lymphocytes and further cytokines IL-3 and IL-5 produced by them, the final stages of differentiation occur, producing eosinophils, basophils and possibly mucosal mast cells. Polyp oedema results from degranulation reactions involving these cells. (b) Nasal polyp epithelium stained for granulocyte macrophage colony stimulating factor (GM-CSF). Courtesy of Dr Robin Poston, Guy's Hospital. (c) Nasal polyp epithelium stained for epithelial growth factor (EGF). Courtesy of Mr Ian Bottrill, Royal National Throat, Nose & Ear Hospital.

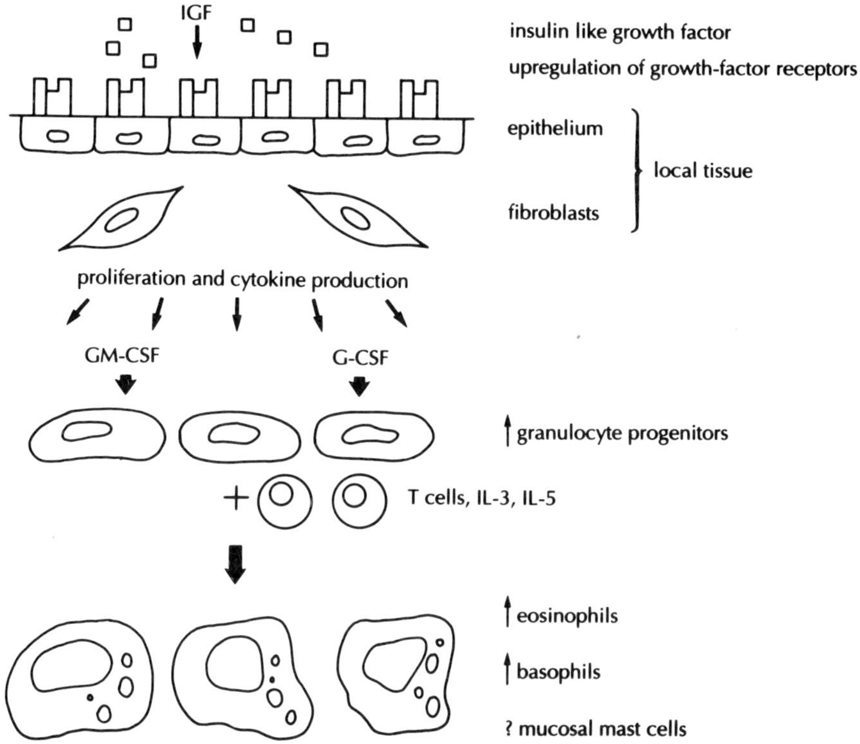
IGF
insulin like growth factor
upregulation of growth-factor receptors
epithelium
fibroblasts
local tissue
proliferation and cytokine production
GM-CSF
G-CSF
granulocyte progenitors
T cells, IL-3, IL-5
eosinophils
basophils
? mucosal mast cells

(a)

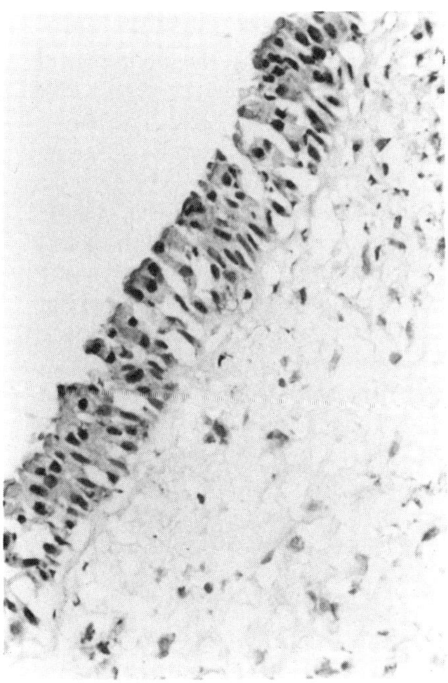

(b)

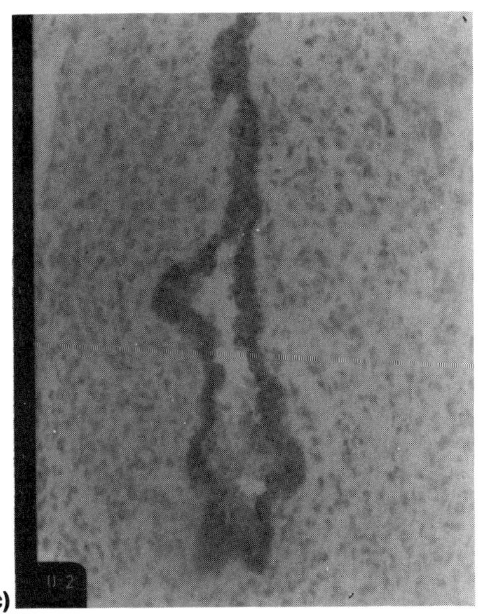

(c)

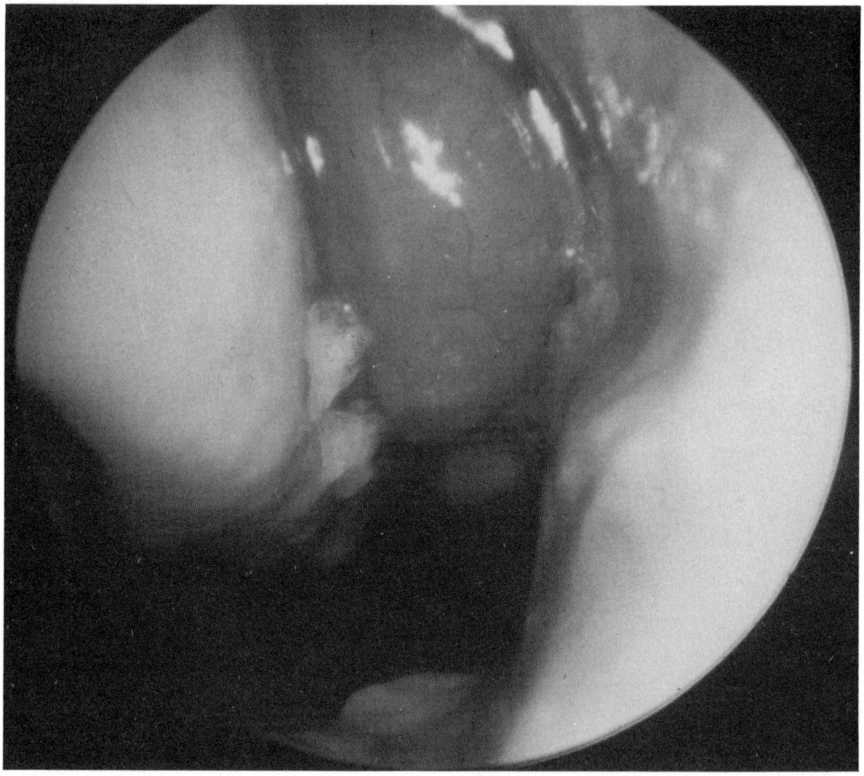

Figure 2 Polyps in the nasal cavity can be seen as pale structures which are next to the inferior turbinate and lateral to the nasal septum

Investigation

There are no diagnostic investigations. Plain radiographs of the sinuses demonstrate mucosal disease in the sinuses to some degree in virtually every patient whereas the sinuses are usually clear or there are only very minor changes in patients with perennial allergy. Surgeons who use the nasendoscope for resecting polyps, advocate computerized scanning prior to surgery to define the normal anatomy and the extent of the disease.

If any unusual cause for nasal polyps, such as immotile cilial syndrome, cystic fibrosis or immune deficiency, is suspected, the relevant investigations should be undertaken. Except in research centres, no allergic work up is required unless the patient has a coexisting allergic condition.

TREATMENT

Unfortunately, much of the earlier work on the treatment of nasal polyps was anecdotal, particularly the efficacy of surgery in preventing recurrence and its effect on the lower airway. Some authors felt that surgery caused asthma. Polyps and asthma are both manifestations of the same pathology in the respiratory mucosa and, if surgery does have any effect, then it tends to improve the asthma[6]. Since the nose resumes its normal physiological function, i.e. warms and humidifies the inspired air, the reconstitution of nasal breathing prevents cold air inducing bronchospasm in hyper-reactive individuals.

Although most physicians consider that if the polyps are no longer present then the condition is controlled, patients expect to be symptom free, and many are not relieved of their loss of sense of smell and taste. Similarly, the post-nasal drip and attacks of running and sneezing may not be controlled. It is important to counsel the patients on the limitations of treatment.

Initial medical treatment

As mentioned previously, about half the cases respond to corticosteroids. Although polyps regress when corticosteroids are given orally and oral corticosteroids are as effective as surgery[31], because of the risk of side-effects, they are usually given intranasally. It is worth trying intranasal corticosteroids on all patients since they will help to avoid surgery in up to half of the patients. Betamethasone drops, two each side twice a day with retention, should be tried or an aqueous spray, such as beclomethasone or flunisolide two puffs each side twice a day[32,33].

If medical treatment is to work, then it must be given in a way which will ensure contact for a reasonable length of time. Nose drops may be given in either the head down and forward position (praying to Mecca) or lying prone with the head dependent and the patient should stay in the position for at least a minute, preferably longer. Betamethasone is absorbed systemically; whether its effect is due to this or the position in which it is applied has yet to be evaluated. Cushing's syndrome has been described following betamethasone abuse[34].

Sprays are easier to use and probably have a better compliance. Unfortunately, despite requests, betamethasone has yet to be produced as a spray. Although it is felt that the position of a nasal spray is important, as long as the spray ends up on the ciliary epithelium, ciliary action will transport the spray posteriorly and cover the nasal lining. Medical treatment should be given for a trial period of a month. If the polyps do not respond, they may be removed surgically.

Surgical treatment

There are many different views on the best surgical treatment for nasal polyps. The attitude to surgery is coloured by those patients with severe recurrence. The majority of patients who have occasional recurrences every ten or so years may be treated very effectively by simple polypectomy (Figure 3).

Unfortunately, no trials have ever been performed on patients who have

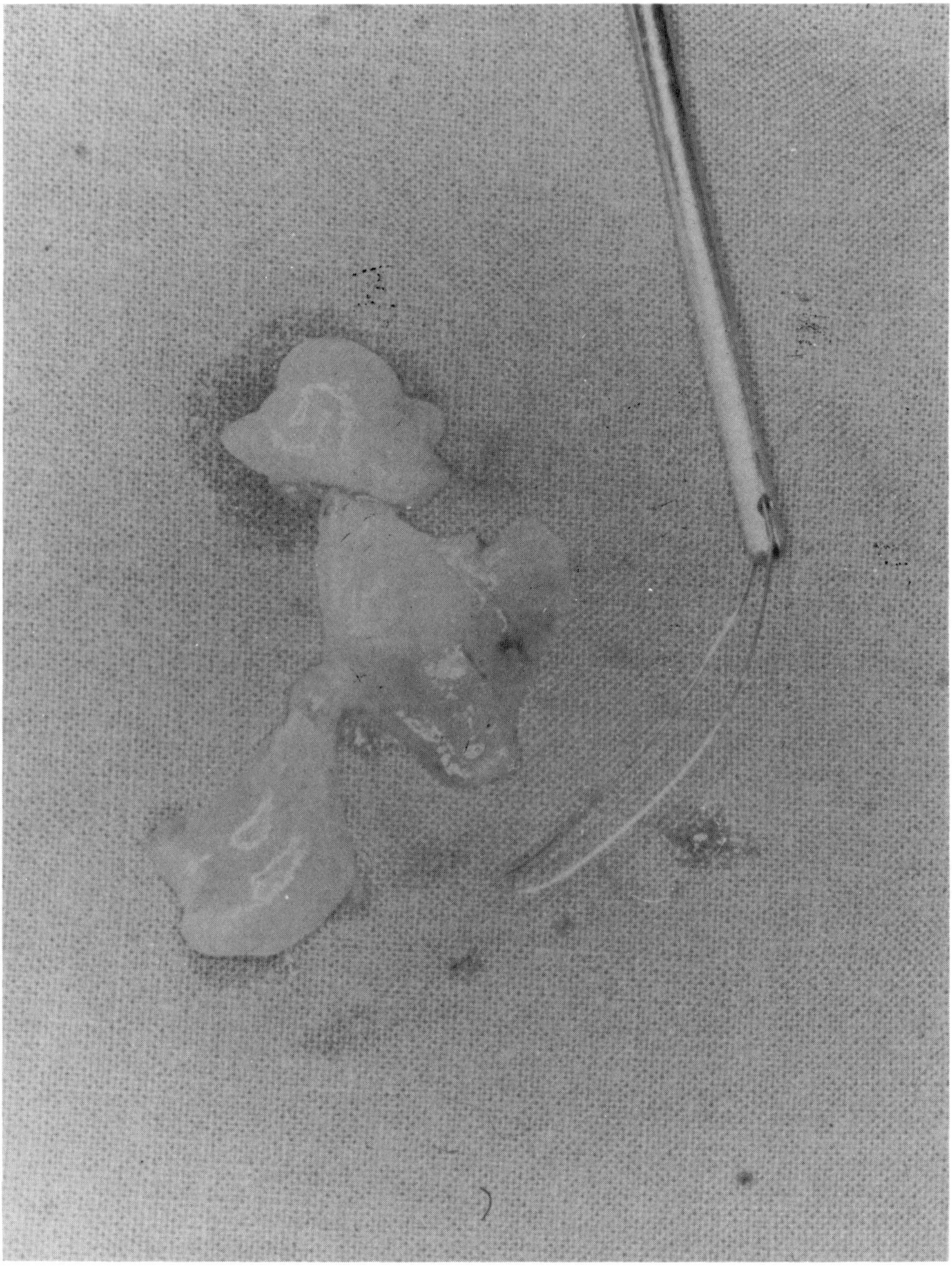

Figure 3 Avulsed nasal polyp which shows the polyp and the ethmoid sinus tag with a waist between the two

radical surgery to all the sinuses despite the enthusiasm of some authors[35]. The current 'flavour of the month' is functional endoscopic nasal surgery; as yet, no trials have demonstrated that it is better at controlling recurrence but it does have a considerably increased risk of complications.

Recurrence

This is not a complication of surgery but a problem in the management of some cases of nasal polyps and it is severe in about 5% of patients. There is no way a surgeon can know beforehand which cases will recur but an earlier age of onset is associated with more severe recurrence, as is the presence of asthma, both alone and with aspirin hypersensitivity. These last two suggest a more aggressive respiratory mucosal disease. Allergy is associated with neither nasal polyps nor more severe recurrence.

Postoperative therapy

The place of postoperative corticosteroids has yet to be determined but evidence suggests that long-term postoperative treatment reduces the severity of recurrence[36,37] although not all patients require therapy. Patients who present for the first time and those with several years between recurrences do not necessarily require treatment. Those who have rhinitis should be treated to control the symptoms. Both beclomethasone and flunisolide or other fluorinated corticosteroid nasal sprays may be used. Oral corticosteroids, such as prednisolone, may be required to control nasal symptoms in those patients where neither surgery nor inhaled corticosteroids prevent severe recurrences.

Diets

Since there is a link between aspirin and the natural salicylates and tartrazine dyes, it is worth trying patients on a diet free from those compounds. It is difficult to perform controlled trials but about half the patients with aspirin hypersensitivity who try this diet say that they feel better and have fewer nasal symptoms. Wheat flour hypersensitivity may produce nasal symptoms and so exclusion diets may be tried. This should be undertaken only with the help of a dietician.

CONCLUSION

Polyps are a multifactorial disease which affects the nasal lining and sinus mucosa and, in about a third of patients, they are associated with asthma and are prone to recurrence. Polyps may occur in other respiratory diseases, such as cystic fibrosis, immotile cilial syndrome and immune deficiencies. Allergy does not predispose to polyp formation but mast cell reactions appear to be important. This may explain why corticosteroids are effective in controlling some cases and helping to prevent recurrence in some others. Polyp formation in the sinuses is due to three factors: the balance between the inflammatory response and the local homeostatic mechanisms; the relatively poor blood supply of the sinuses; and the complex anatomy of the ethmoids which aggravates the existing oedema. Half the cases regress on inhaled corticosteroids and do not require surgery primarily. Simple polypectomy is the treatment of choice in those cases requiring surgery and this can be followed by inhaled corticosteroids in more severe cases and in those with symptoms of rhinitis.

REFERENCES

1. Lurie H. Cystic fibrosis of the pancreas and the nasal mucosa. Ann Otol Rhinol Laryngol. 1959;68:478.
2. Drake-Lee A, Lowe D, Swanston A, Grace A. Clinical profile and recurrence of nasal polyps. J Laryngol Otol. 1984;98:783–93.
3. Schwachman H, Kulcyzchi I, Mueller H, Flake C. Nasal polyposis in patients with cystic fibrosis. Paediatrics. 1962;30:389–401.
4. Drake-Lee A, Pitcher Wilmott R. The clinical and laboratory correlates of nasal polyps in cystic fibrosis. Int J Paediatr Otolaryngol. 1982;4:209–14.
5. Drake-Lee A, Morgan D. Nasal polyps and sinusitis in children with cystic fibrosis. J Laryngol Otol. 1989;103:753–5.
6. Maloney J, Collins J. Nasal polyps, nasal polypectomy, asthma and aspirin sensitivity. J Laryngol Otol. 1977;91:837–46.
7. Samter M, Lederer F. Nasal polyps: their relationship to allergy, particularly bronchial asthma. Med Clin N Am. 1958;42:175–97.
8. Sczeklik A, Gryglewski R, Czerniawske-Mysik G. Relationship of inhibition of prostaglandin biosynthesis by analgesics to asthma attacks in aspirin sensitive patients. Br Med J. 1975;1:67–9.
9. Pearson D, Suarez-Mendez V. Abnormal platelet hydrogen peroxidase metabolism in aspirin sensitivity. Clin Exp Allergy. 1990;20:157–63.
10. Settipane G, Chafee F. Nasal polyps in asthma and rhinitis. J Allergy Clin Immunol. 1977;58:17–21.
11. Dunnette S, Hall M, Washington J, Kern E, McDonald T, Facer G, Gleich G. J Allergy Clin Immunol. 1986;78:102–8.
12. Calenoff E, Guilford T, Green J, Engelhard C. Bacterial specific IgE in patients with nasal polyps. Arch Otolaryngol. 1983;109:372–5.
13. Baenkler H, Schaubschlager W, Behnsen H. Antigen induced histamine release from the mucosa in nasal polyposis. Clin Otolaryngol. 1983;8:227–30.
14. Taylor M. Histochemical studies on nasal polyps. J Laryngol Otol. 1963;77:326–41.
15. Sasaki Y, Nakahara H. Granule core loss in eosinophils from a patient with aspirin induced asthma: an electron microscope study. Ann Allergy. 1989;63:306–8.
16. Freedman I, Osbourne D. Miscellaneous granulomas and nasal polyps. Chapter 2. In: Pathology of granulomas and neoplasms of the nose and paranasal sinuses. Edinburgh: Churchill Livingstone; 1982:28–35.
17. Cauna N, Hindover K, Manzethi G, Swanson E. Fine structure of nasal polyps. Ann Otol Rhinol Laryngol. 1972;81:41–58.
18. Drake-Lee A, Barker T, Thurley K. Nasal polyps. II. Fine structure of mast cells. J Laryngol Otol. 1984;98:783–93.
19. Berdal P. Serological examination of nasal polyp fluid. Acta Otolaryngol. 1954;Suppl. 115.
20. Donovan R, Johansson S, Bannich H, Soothill J. Immunoglobulins in nasal polyp fluid. Int Arch Allergy Appl Immunol. 1970;37:154–66.
21. Chandra R, Abrol B. Immunopathology of nasal polypi. J Laryngol Otol. 1974;88: 1019–24.

22. Drake-Lee A, McLaughlin P. Clinical symptoms, free histamine and IgE in patients with nasal polyps. Int Arch Allergy Appl Immunol. 1982;69:268–71.
23. Mygind N, Weeke B, Ullman S. Quantitative determination of immunoglobulins in nasal secretions. Int Arch Allergy Appl Immunol. 1975;49:99–107.
24. Drake-Lee A, Barker T. Free and cell bound IgE in nasal polyps. J Laryngol Otol. 1984;98:795–801.
25. Eggleston P, Owen Hendley J, Gwaltney J. Histamine in nasal secretions. Int Arch Allergy Appl Immunol. 1978;57:193–200.
26. Salari H, Borgeat P, Steffenrud S, Richard J, Bedard P, Hebert J, Pelletier G. Immunological and non-immunological release of leukotrienes and histamine from human nasal polyps. Clin Exp Immunol. 1986;63:711–7.
27. Nigam S, Kunkel G, Herold D, Baumer F, Jusuf L. Nasal polyps and their content of arachidonic acid metabolites. N Engl Reg Allergy Proc. 1986;7:109–12.
28. Smith D, Gerrard J, White J. Comparison of arachidonic acid metabolites in nasal polyps and eosinophils. Int Arch Allergy Appl Immunol. 1987;82:83–8.
29. Jung T, Juhn S, Hwang D, Stewart R. Prostaglandins, leukotrienes and other arachidonic acid metabolites in nasal polyps and nasal mucosa. Laryngoscope. 1987;97:184–9.
30. Kaliner M, Wasserman S, Austen K. Immunologic release of chemical mediators from human nasal polyps. N Engl J Med. 1973;289:277–81.
31. Lildholdt T, Forgstrup J, Kortholm B, Ulsoe C. Surgical versus medical management of nasal polyps. Acta Otolaryngol (Stockholm). 1988;105:140–3.
32. Charlton R, MacKay I, Wilson R, Cole P. Double blind placebo controlled trial of beclomethasone nose drops for nasal polyps. Br Med J. 1985;2:788–9.
33. Dingsor G, Kramer J, Olshot R, Sonderstrom J. Flunisolide nasal spray 0.025% in the prophylactic treatment of nasal polyposis after polypectomy. Rhinology. 1985;23:49–53.
34. Stevens D. Cushing's syndrome due to the abuse of betamethasone nasal drops. J Laryngol Otol. 1988;102:219–21.
35. Hughes R. The role of radical surgery in the treatment of nasal polyps. J Laryngol Otol. 1973;87:117–122.
36. Mygind N, Pedersen C, Prytz S, Sorensen H. Treatment of nasal polyps with intranasal beclomethasone diproprionate aerosol. Clin Allergy. 1975;5:159–64.
37. Deuschl L, Dretner B. Nasal polyps treated by beclomethasone nasal aerosol. Rhinology. 1977;15:17–23.
38. Gwaltney J, Hayden F. The nose and infection. Chapter 16. In: Proctor D, Anderson I, eds. Upper airway physiology and the atmospheric environment. Amsterdam: Elsevier; 1982: 399–422.
39. Dawes P, Bates G, Watson D, Lewis D, Lowe D, Drake-Lee A. The role of bacterial infection of the maxillary sinus in nasal polyps. Clin Otolaryngol. 1989;14:447–50.

11
Inner Ear Disorders

G. B. BROOKES

INTRODUCTION

The impact of immunological processes in inner ear disturbances has only become apparent relatively recently. Although there is already an abundance of contemporary experimental and clinical evidence demonstrating the many diverse ways in which these processes may affect cochleovestibular function, many fundamental questions remain unanswered. The umbrella term autoimmune (AI) inner ear disease has perhaps rather loosely been applied to all such disorders.

The concept was first postulated by Lehnhardt in 1958[1], on the basis of clinical observation in cases of recurrent bilateral sudden sensorineural hearing loss. McCabe[2], however, was the first to bring autoimmune inner ear disease to the attention of otologists in 1979. It is now becoming generally accepted as an uncommon, quite well-defined, but poorly understood entity. The term may well embrace several different clinical syndromes, which could explain why both cell-mediated and humoral-mediated pathways appear to be involved in the pathogenesis. It may occur as a primary autoimmune disorder confined to the inner ear, or may appear as an occasional local manifestation of a major systemic disease due to an underlying immune system defect (Table 1). Most attention in this chapter will be devoted to the primary inner ear disorders of progressive sensorineural hearing loss with vestibular failure, Meniere's disease, delayed endolymphatic hydrops and the sensorineural hearing loss associated with chronic suppurative otitis media. Although considered separately, it is possible that these disorders represent different parts of the same spectrum of cochleovestibular pathology.

APPLIED ANATOMY AND PHYSIOLOGY

The inner ear is encased in very hard bone, the otic capsule, and consists of two main parts: the auditory organ (cochlea) and the vestibular organ

Table 1 Autoimmune inner ear disease

(1)	Localized
(2)	Systemic
	(a) Systemic lupus erythematosus
	(b) Vasculitis Hypersensitivity vasculitis Polyarteritis nodosa Wegener's granulomatosis Temporal arteritis Cogan's syndrome Behçet's disease
	(c) Relapsing polychondritis
	(d) Polymyositis and dermatomyositis
	(e) Immunodeficiency diseases T-cell deficiency B-cell deficiency Disorders of phagocytosis Complement system disorders

After Hughes et al., 1986[80]

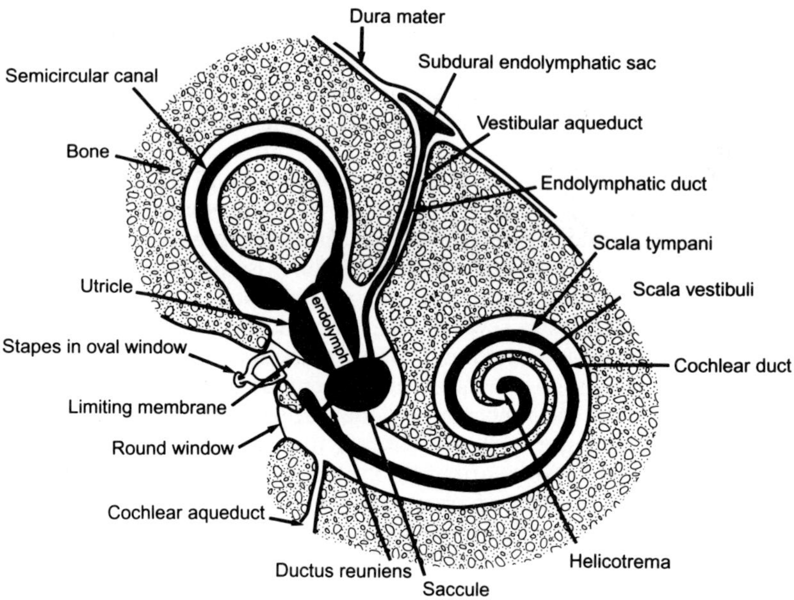

Figure 1 Schematic diagram of the inner ear fluid system. (After Reference 82)

(labyrinth). These sensory organs contain the receptors which efficiently transform mechanical stimulation into electrical impulses for neuronal transmission to the auditory cortex (Figure 1).

The cochlea is divided into two fluid-filled compartments by membranes.

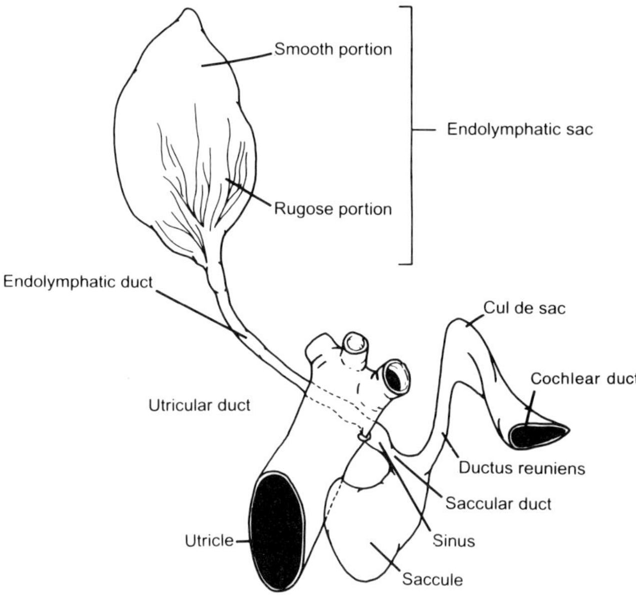

Figure 2 Schematic diagram of the endolymphatic duct system. (After Reference 5)

The organ of Corti is located centrally on the basilar membrane, contains inner and outer cochlear hair cells and is filled with endolymph. The endolymph fluid in the cochlea and endolymphatic duct contains a high concentration of potassium (120 mEq/L), low sodium (13 mEq/L) and a high electrical potential relative to the hair cells which is maintained by active metabolic processes. This endolymphatic space is connected to a blind extradural sac, the endolymphatic sac, via the vestibular aqueduct (Figure 2). The endolymphatic sac is divided into an intraosseous rugose part, with extensive rugae and villi, and an intradural smooth part. In humans, many of the epithelial cells lining the endolymphatic sac have numerous mitochondria and microvilli, whilst others have a well-developed Golgi apparatus, engorged rough endoplasmic reticulum and lysosomal granules. These cellular features reflect metabolic activity and absorptive properties. The subepithelial connective tissue of the sac contains a very rich capillary network and lymphatics. There are also fibrils which appear to communicate directly with the perilymphatic spaces of the inner ear. The cells in the endolymphatic sac lumen are mainly macrophages, whilst lymphocytes are also occasionally seen[3]. An osmophilic substance is also present which contributes to the very high protein concentration in the sac. This concentration is some forty times greater than in the endolymphatic duct. It has been suggested that the proteinaceous material acts as an osmotic pump and draws endolymph from the cochlear duct and vestibule.

In contrast, the scala vestibuli and scala tympani are perilymphatic spaces which communicate with the cerebrospinal fluid (CSF) through the cochlear aqueduct. As a result, perilymph is biochemically similar to CSF, and contains a high sodium (150 mEq/L), and low potassium (6 mEq/L) concentration. Approximately 25% of the perilymph comes from the CSF via the cochlear aqueduct, whilst the remaining 75% is derived locally as an ultrafiltrate from vessels in the perilymphatic space. The stria vascularis, with its extensive capillary network, and spiral ligament form the lateral wall of the cochlear duct. The marginal cells of the stria are morphologically similar to renal tubule cells and are probably involved in fluid and ion transport. It is believed that the stria vascularis generates the unique high positive endocochlear potential. Experiments suggest that most endolymph is produced by the stria vascularis, and is very largely absorbed by the endolymphatic sac. Interestingly, contemporary studies have shown that the endolymph of the endolymphatic sac is similar in composition to perilymph[4]. The vestibular organs are composed of the utricle and saccule, which can be considered gravity receptors, and the semicircular canals and cristae, which are sensitive to rotational stimuli. Some parts of the walls of the utricle and cristaie contain dark cells which exhibit morphological similarities to the marginal cells of the stria vascularis, and are believed to be involved in the production and maintenance of endolymph in these labyrinthine structures.

Inner ear disorders may be caused by factors which impair the local blood supply, thereby reducing perfusion of the capillary networks of the stria vascularis and/or endolymphatic sac with a consequent adverse effect on the metabolic activity in these regions. Alternatively, there may be a disturbance of the cochleovestibular endolymph fluid balance, a pathophysiological condition known to be associated with Meniere's disease and found in other specific otological conditions producing a similar clinical syndrome. The third pathogenetic possibility is a direct primary effect on the sensory hair cells in both the cochlea and labyrinth. In addition, it is quite possible that these three mechanisms may be inter-related and co-exist in certain inner ear disorders.

INNER EAR IMMUNOLOGY

One's initial impression from histopathological examination of inner ear tissues is that it does not appear to have the essential cellular constituents which are necessary to generate immune responses. Thus there are no obvious local collections of lymphoid tissue, no plasma cells in the lamina propria, and, in addition, a lymphatic drainage system for the membranous labyrinth cannot be demonstrated. Nonetheless, there is now substantial evidence that the inner ear does indeed possess its own functioning host immune defence system. Lim and Silver first suggested in 1974[5] that the endolymphatic sac might be primarily involved in these processes on the basis of light and electron microscopic investigations. The subsequent findings of Rask-Anderson and Stahle[3] offered strong support to their hypothesis. These workers demonstrated interaction between macrophages and lymphocytes within the endolymphatic sac lumen, and speculated that these cells were probably the first line of defence when foreign material gained access to the inner ear. They also described the presence of a rich network of lymphatic capillaries and venules surrounding the sac and duct in guinea pigs. Rask-Anderson and Stahle concluded from these studies that the endolymphatic sac could well be the main site in the inner ear for antigen processing activity, and could best be considered as analogous to a functioning lymph node. The hypothesis of an inner ear immune defence system primarily located in the endolymphatic sac was subsequently supported by the studies of Arnold, Altermatt and Gebbers[6], who observed free and tissue-bound IgA and IgG immunoglobulins restricted to the endolymphatic sac region in human ears.

Because the inner ear tissues are surrounded with the specialized endolymph and perilymph fluids, early attention focused on their possible role in the defence of the inner ear against invading organisms or antigens. IgG is the main immunoglobulin in CSF. This is derived from serum across the blood–brain barrier but may also be produced locally in certain diseases of the central nervous system. Several groups have measured immunoglobulins in the inner ear fluids. As in CSF, IgG is the main immunoglobulin in human and animal perilymph, and is also present in endolymph. Smaller amounts of IgA and IgM are also found[7–9]. The transfer of antibody to perilymph is much greater than to CSF. This suggests that, in the normal ear, most perilymph immunoglobulins are derived locally as a filtrate from the blood across a selective blood–brain barrier, or that the inner ear can concentrate antibody in a selective manner. In fact, both processes are known to occur. In addition, Arnold and Altermatt[10] showed that epithelial cells lining the endolymphatic sac lumen stain with antibody to secretory component (SC). SC is essential for transepithelial transport of secretory immunoglobulins, such as IgA and IgM, and indicates that humoral mediated mucosal immune processes protect the inner ear as well.

EXPERIMENTAL IMMUNE STUDIES

The introduction by Lehnhardt of the concept of inner ear autoimmunity in the late 1950s[1] provided the impetus for many animal studies. These have enabled models of the immunopathological effects on the inner ear to be documented. Beickert[11] immunized guinea-pigs to inner ear antigen and produced lesions in the cochlea. Soon after, Terrayama and Sasaki[12] replicated these results in a similar study, though they were not able to confirm the presence of anticochlear antibodies or inflammatory infiltration around local blood vessels due to technical limitations at this time. Yoo et al.[13,14] reported the induction of sensorineural hearing loss and endolymphatic hydrops in rats and guinea-pigs by stimulating autoimmunity to inner ear collagen. After sensitization with type II collagen, a booster dose was given before sacrifice. Histological examination showed ganglion cell degeneration, angiopathy, and degeneration of the organ of Corti as well as hydrops. Pathological changes in the endolymphatic sac were not seen, and further immunohistochemical studies showed that type II collagen was localized in the endolymphatic duct. More recently, Harris et al.[15] described an animal model of autoimmune inner ear dysfunction following exposure to heterologous cochlear tissue. Guinea-pigs already previously immunized

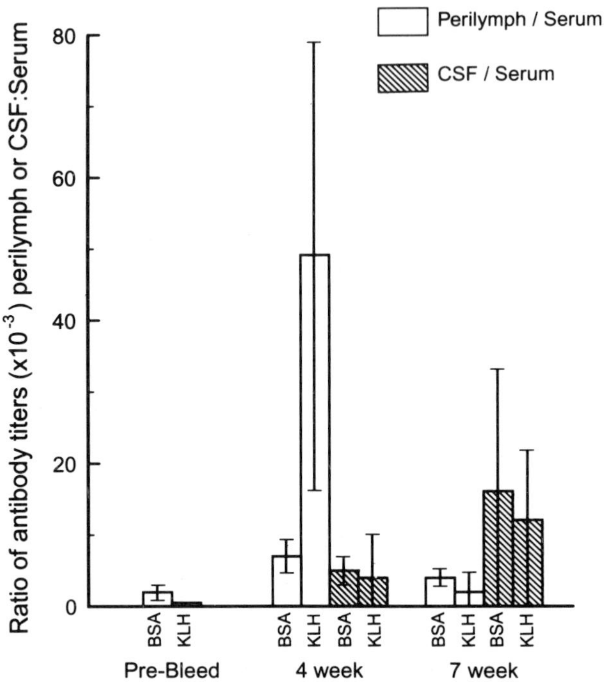

Figure 3 Primary inner ear KLH immunization in BSA-sensitized animals, Perilymph/serum and CSF/serum antibody ratios for KLH and BSA. (After Reference 17)

with fresh bovine cochlear antigen developed significant hearing impairment after further antigen administration compared with a control group. Anti-cochlear antibodies were detected in all animals in the experimental group, whilst one third of the 38 ears tested had marked hearing loss. Some animals only displayed unilateral changes, whereas others had varying degrees of bilateral inner ear damage. The authors pointed out the similarity of their findings with the clinical features of the syndrome of autoimmune sensorineural hearing loss in humans as described by McCabe[16].

Harris[9,17] conducted critically important studies which established how the normal inner ear immune defence mechanisms operated. He demontrated that the inner ear reacted to antigenic challenge by mounting both a primary and secondary immune response. Thus, direct sensitization of the perilymphatic compartment with the antigen keyhole limpet haemocyanin (KLH) in non-sensitized guinea-pigs resulted in a low local perilymph antibody production and systemic immune response. However, when the animals had been initially immunized systemically with bovine serum albumin (BSA), the introduction of KLH into perilymph produced an eight-fold increase in the perilymph/serum KLH antibody ratio after 4 weeks, which was not mirrored by similar changes in the CSF (Figure 3). Seven weeks after antigen challenge to the inner ear the perilymph/serum KLH antibody ratio was found to decline towards pre-immunization values.

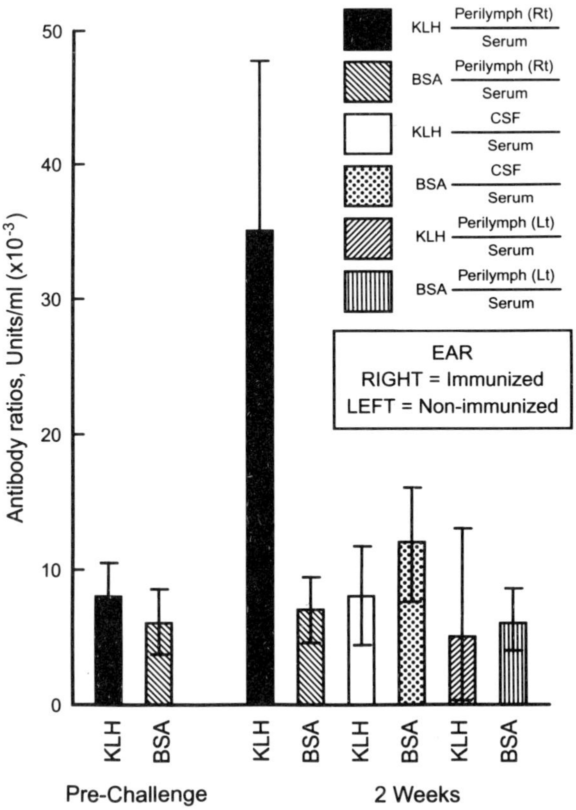

Figure 4 Secondary inner ear immune response. Effect of KLH inner ear inoculation in animals systemically sensitized to KLH and BSA. Antibody ratios are significantly increased for perilymph–serum anti-KLH ratio only on the side of the injection. (After Reference 17)

The secondary immune response occurring in animals previously sensitized to both KLH and BSA, is shown in Figure 4. As expected, anti-KLH antibodies persist in both perilymph and serum following primary sensitization (pre-challenge). Two weeks after KLH inner ear challenge, a significant increase in the anti-KLH perilymph level was seen in the immunized animals. However, antibody titres in the non-immunized ear and CSF did not change. Further experiments showed that these phenomena were due to a local inner ear response and not due to increased vascular permeability or to a CSF antibody response. A limited infiltration of plasma cells and lymphocytes under the basilar membrane of the basal turn of the cochlea was invariably present histologically in animals exhibiting a primary inner ear immune response, though both sensory and neural elements of the membranous labyrinth were preserved. Subsequently, Tomiyama and Harris[18] confirmed that an intact endolymphatic sac was a prerequisite for these responses. They showed that experimental destruction of the endolymphatic duct resulted in a reduced perilymph antibody response to KLH antigen challenge. In addition, although increased infiltration of plasma cells and lymphocytes occurred in previously immunized animals in the cochlear and perisaccular connective tissues, hardly any chronic inflammatory cells were seen when the endolymphatic duct was obliterated.

The secondary inner ear immune response following antigenic challenge of presensitized animals is an amplification of the primary responses. Histologically, an even greater infiltration of plasma cells and lymphocytes occurred throughout the cochlea, endolymphatic sac lumen and perisaccular tissues. Perivascular cuffing was widespread and involved the posterior spiral modiolar veins. Woolf and Harris[19] conducted electrophysiological auditory measurements in animals exhibiting a secondary immune response and showed a progressive reduction in cochlear function. Microscopic features included degeneration of spiral ganglion cells and partial or complete loss of the organ of Corti, with an extensive cellular infiltration throughout the cochlea. These various results have affirmed the central role which the endolymphatic sac plays in antigen processing and immune stimulation within the inner ear in addition to its absorptive function. Systemic immunity develops following the locally generated response when sensitized lymphocytes reach regional lymph nodes. Antigens may also leak directly out of the endolymphatic sac into the general circulation. Cells are then recruited to sites where antigens have been deposited in the cochlea via venules surrounding the endolymphatic sac and duct via the posterior spiral modiolar veins. A diagrammatic simplification of the afferent and efferent limbs of the inner ear immune response proposed by Harris and his colleagues is shown in Figures 5 and 6. The inner ear undoubtedly fulfils a protective role by neutralizing infective organisms within the cochlea. Thus, Harris et al.[20] demonstrated that protection of the guinea-pig from cytomegalovirus labyrinthitis was correlated with the perilymph antibody titre generated by prior immunization. Quite clearly though, secondary immune responses, as elsewhere, can have a marked deleterious effect, whilst, in some instances, virulent organisms may overwhelm the normal defence mechanisms.

AUTOIMMUNE INNER EAR DISEASE

Pathophysiology

Several specific types of immune response are currently recognized, and any of these may, individually or in combination, contribute to the development of autoimmune inner ear disease and cause adverse effects on inner ear function. The most useful classification of tissue-damaging hypersensitivity reactions between antigen and antibody is still that devised by Gell and Coombs[21]. They distinguished three types of initiating mechanisms involving humoral antibodies and a further type involving cell-mediated antibodies associated with delayed hypersensitivity reactions.

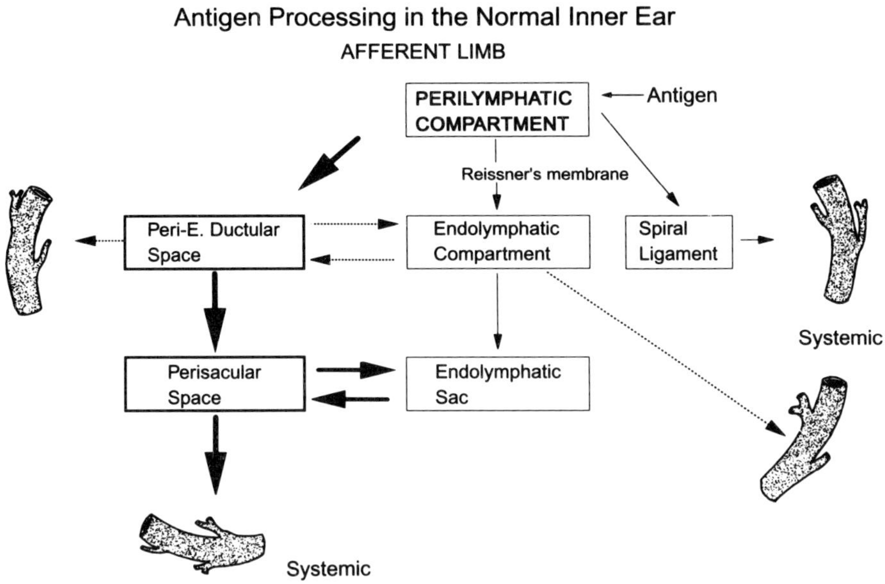

Figure 5 Proposed afferent limb (antigen processing) of inner ear immune response. Large arrows depict principal pathways; small arrows less important pathways. (After Reference 15)

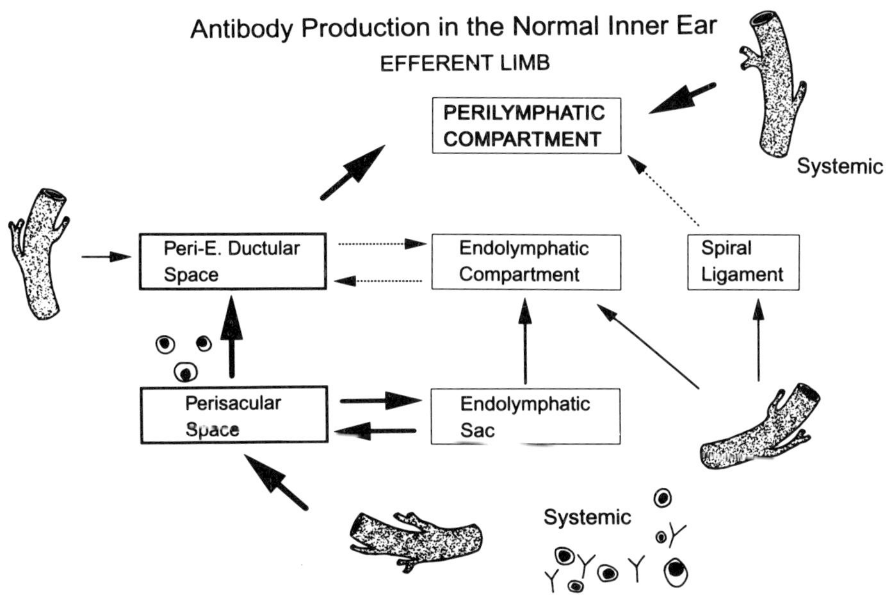

Figure 6 Proposed efferent limb of inner ear immune response. (After Reference 15)

Type I

The Type I reaction (anaphylactic) occurs as a result of free antigen interacting with cell-bound IgE antibody in the tissues. Enzyme activation quickly causes the release of vasoactive substances from mast cells or basophils which increase capillary permeability, alter vascular tone and stimulate smooth muscle contraction. Many allergic reactions take place locally, where the antibody is bound, and do not necessarily induce a generalized anaphylactic response. Allergies, particularly those associated with foods or chemicals, are believed to cause cochleovestibular disturbances[22]. Eliminating the offending antigen from the diet in conjunction with appropriate antiallergic drug therapy may reverse a long-standing sensorineural loss[23,24]. The author has managed a few patients with Meniere's syndrome and intolerance to dairy products in whom dietary management proved efficacious, but, generally, allergies do not appear to have a major impact in the pathogenesis of inner ear disorders.

Type II

This reaction (cytotoxic) occurs when free circulating antibody interacts with fixed antigen which already forms part of a cell surface or tissue membrane. Invariably, this results in membrane change and, in the case of a cell, lysis and cell death. These processes involve complement fixation and activation. Immunofluorescent studies conducted by Arnold and Gebbers[25] suggest that this mechanism is important in a number of immune-mediated inner ear disorders, on occasions in combination with delayed cell-mediated activity.

Type III

When both antigen and antibody are freely circulating, the resulting circulating immune complexes are still, on occasions, able to provoke a tissue response. Immune complexes are usually rapidly and harmlessly removed from the circulation by the phagocytic cells of the reticuloendothelial system. They can, however, become harmful if they are deposited in body tissues, when complement activation enhances local inflammatory processes and cell damage. Immune complex reactions may be related to autoimmunity, or may occur in response to exogenous antigens such as micro-organisms and drugs. Recognized clinical disorders relevant to otology which are probably mediated by immune complexes include systemic lupus erythematosis, polymyositis, and the various vasculitides. These are considered later.

The tissues involved depend on the size and specificity of the complexes. Biologically active complexes are of intermediate size and are poorly cleared from the circulation. They may become arrested on the endothelial lining of small blood vessels or in other tissues. There are specific receptors in some sites for the immune complexes or their breakdown products, and hence certain tissues may become preferentially involved to cause isolated organ or system disorders. Immune complex and complement activation in a vessel

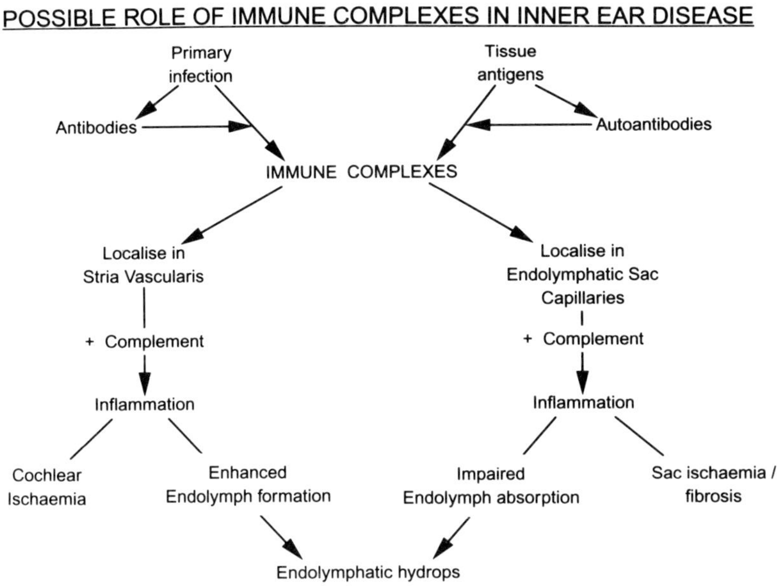

Figure 7 Theoretical mechanism to explain possible primary causative role of circulating immune complexes in the pathogenesis of inner ear disease

wall leads to a local inflammatory reaction, increased vascular permeability and permanent vessel damage. The stria vascularis vessels may be a possible location for immune complex deposition, whilst the capillaries of the endolymphatic sac are another (Figure 7). The cochlear capillaries are non-fenestrated[26] and differ from the capillaries of the endolymphatic sac which are fenestrated[27] and arise from the external carotid system. The endolymphatic sac capillaries almost certainly have a filtration function and interference by antigen–antibody complexes may lead to inner ear fluid imbalance and secondary hydrops.

Syphilis is one specific disease in which the associated cochleovestibular features are believed to have an immunological basis, most probably due to immune complex deposition. Free circulating complexes have been identified in the serum of humans[28,29] and animals[30]. Engel and Diezel[29] found elevated circulating immune complexes (CICs) in 41% of a series of 51 patients with early syphilis, and were able to prove that complexed antibodies were specifically antitreponemal. Moreover, the complexes only decreased to levels within the normal range in about half of the cases following treatment. This indicates the persistence of viable organisms after treatment, and corroborates earlier reports of residual spirochaetes in various sites such as lymph nodes, aqueous humour and cerebrospinal fluid. The author has suggested previously[31] that a persisting low-grade syphilitic infection, causing continuous antigenic stimulation, may lead to continuous and excessive CIC production with secondary pathological changes, including inner ear involvement.

The precise role of immune complexes in the pathogenesis of sensorineural hearing loss remains to be defined. The association was reported by Kanzaki and Ouchi[32] and Stephens et al.[33] and subsequently reviewed by this author[31]. Although circulating complexes may effect a final common pathophysiological pathway in a variety of cochleovestibular disorders, it is also possible that they are merely secondary epiphenomena resulting from local tissue damage.

Type IV

Cell-mediated delayed hypersensitivity reactions occur as a result of preliminary sensitization of T lymphocytes in the recirculating pool of immunologically competent cells. These subsequently become arrested and interact at the site of local concentration of antigen-liberating chemotactic factors leading to infiltration of macrophages which cause tissue damage. Some tissue antigens are functionally sequestrated from the blood and reticuloendothelial system and do not produce an antibody response. However, a cell-mediated response may be induced following tissue damage, when the release of previously 'hidden' antigens results in a secondary immune response in similar tissues. Sympathetic ophthalmia is a well-known example of this type of disorder, when an immune-mediated ocular inflammation and progressive visual impairment follows a penetrating injury or surgery to the contralateral eye. Harris et al.[34] postulated the likelihood of an analogous otological disorder which they termed 'sympathetic cochleolabyrinthitis'. They found a very small but consistent incidence of unexplained sensorineural hearing loss following previous translabyrinthine acoustic tumour surgery to the contralateral ear. As in sympathetic ophthalmia[35], humoral antibodies causing immediate Type II cytotoxic reactions can probably also occur. In other situations, an infective condition of the middle or inner ear may prime a cell-mediated otological immune response (vide infra). Although the aetiology of autoimmunity is unknown, it has been suggested that involved tissues are either of ectodermal or endodermal origin and are recognized as 'foreign' by the immune system, which is mesodermal. The entire labyrinth is ectodermal in origin, and, according to this theory, is therefore a potential site for autoimmune activity.

Clinical features

McCabe described 18 patients seen over a 10-year period who presented with a similar clinical course and showed a uniform response to treatment[16]. The main features consisted of progressive sensorineural hearing loss, often of sudden onset, fluctuant and bilateral, with associated aural pressure or fullness and variable tinnitus. Vestibular symptoms were frequently mild and transient but uncommonly acute and severe, whilst caloric tests showed reduced responses. Very occasionally, disruption of soft tissue of the middle and external ear with facial paralysis was present. It was a disorder of young people in their 30s and 40s and, characteristically, the deafness progressed

Table 2 Presenting diagnosis in 52 patients with autoimmune inner ear disease

Diagnosis	*No.*	*Unilateral*	*Bilateral*
Meniere's syndrome	27	8	19
Sensorineural hearing loss	15	2	13
Cogan's syndrome	7	1	6
Dandy syndrome	3	—	3

After Hughes et al., 1987[38]

rapidly over weeks to months. On long-term follow up, just under 20% went on to develop autoimmune diseases in other organ systems[16]. The lymphocyte inhibition test, in which the patient's own lymphocytes are challenged against inner ear antigen, was positive in about 25%. Treatment with steroids and cyclophosphamide either produced sustained hearing improvement or stabilization. The validity of the clinical concept of autoimmune deafness has been supported by others[36,37], although soft-tissue destruction and facial paralysis has only rarely been encountered.

Investigations

Unfortunately, there are no absolute diagnostic laboratory criteria, and, often, only a beneficial response to treatment has enabled a 'therapeutic' diagnosis to be made. Cell-mediated immunity may be assessed by the antigen-specific lymphocyte transformation test[36] and immunofluorescence, as well as the lymphocyte migration inhibition test. However, a negative result does not necessarily exclude the diagnosis. The levels of serum immunoglobulins are probably of little relevance. Antigen-non-specific tests include assays of circulating immune complexes and complement, which may indicate enhanced immune activity, perhaps due to an immune complex disorder if the levels are persistently elevated. A raised erythrocyte sedimentation rate may reflect systemic disease activity. Additional tests may be carried out to screen for rheumatoid factor and anti-DNA autoantibodies to various non-otological tissues, but these investigations are certainly less specific and their relevance uncertain.

Hughes and his colleagues have now treated more than 100 patients with a presumptive diagnosis of autoimmune inner ear disease[38,39] and have long-term follow up in 47 cases. Table 2 lists the presenting diagnosis in the first 52 patients. Symptoms indistinguishable from Meniere's syndrome were present in more than half the cases, whilst several cases of Dandy syndrome, or idiopathic bilateral labyrinthine failure, were seen. Although so-called 'antigen-specific' tests were used, Hughes acknowledges that these rely on crude inner ear preparations from tissues removed during translabyrinthine surgery, so that the precise antigens are not, in fact, known. Moreover, most of the inner ear tissue would normally be expected to consist of vestibular neuroepithelium, as the cochlear duct is not routinely removed in these procedures.

Arnold and his colleagues[40] enjoyed less success with their own lymphocyte transformation test, and therefore elected to search for cross-reacting antibodies against inner ear structures using immunohistochemical methods with sections from healthy human temporal bones. They studied patients with bilateral inner ear disease of unknown aetiology and found antibodies against inner ear structures in more than half the cases. Antibodies bound preferentially to the cells of the stria vascularis in more than 75%, whilst organ of Corti antibodies were found in less than 10%. Just over 40% of 12 Meniere's disease patients had antibodies exclusively to the stria vascularis. Arnold et al. conclude that their researches only justify the designation 'disease with autoimmune markers', as histopathological evidence of lymphocytic, plasma cell or macrophage infiltration in the temporal bones of patients with Meniere's disease or progressive sensorineural hearing loss is still lacking. Furthermore, because the inner ear is able to produce those antibodies that are required locally via the endolymphatic sac, it may well not be possible to identify them in the circulation. This might explain why conventional clinical serum immunological parameters are negative in patients with presumed isolated autoimmune inner ear disease. In addition, the active stage of the disease may well be long past by the time temporal bone material becomes available for examination.

Harris and Sharp[41] also found limitations in the lymphocyte transformation assay, and, accordingly, used the more specific Western blot technique to study inner ear reactivity. In this technique, both cochlear and vestibular bovine membranous inner ear tissue were processed to form an antigen preparation which could then be electrophoresed onto a polyacrylamide gel for incubation with diluted test sera. The sera of animals in their guinea-pig model of experimental autoimmune sensorineural hearing loss, produced following immunizations with bovine inner ear tissue, all contained specific antibodies to inner ear antigens by this technique[42]. Subsequently, patients with rapidly progressive sensorineural hearing loss have been investigated by a similar blot assay. Thirty-five per cent showed autoantibodies to an antigen of 68 000 molecular weight, similar to those in the sensitized animals. Two-dimensional gel electrophoresis confirmed that both animals and patients reacted to identical components of inner ear antigen.

Western blot techniques are complex and time consuming. They can be considered as a 'molecular dissection' and are probably more suited to research studies. The author has therefore preferred the application of a more straightforward screening test using an enzyme-linked immunoabsorbent assay (ELISA). This assay only requires very small amounts of antigen, perhaps less than one tenth of that required for Western blotting. The inner ear tissues have been dissected from frozen human temporal bones into five individual parts thus allowing more specific localization of antibodies. The test is relatively rapid, and a hundred samples can be screened at a time, as opposed to the single assay technique in Western blot studies. Our preliminary results are highly promising though more normative data are required for standardization. Other workers have also reported successful applications with their own ELISA laboratory technique[43].

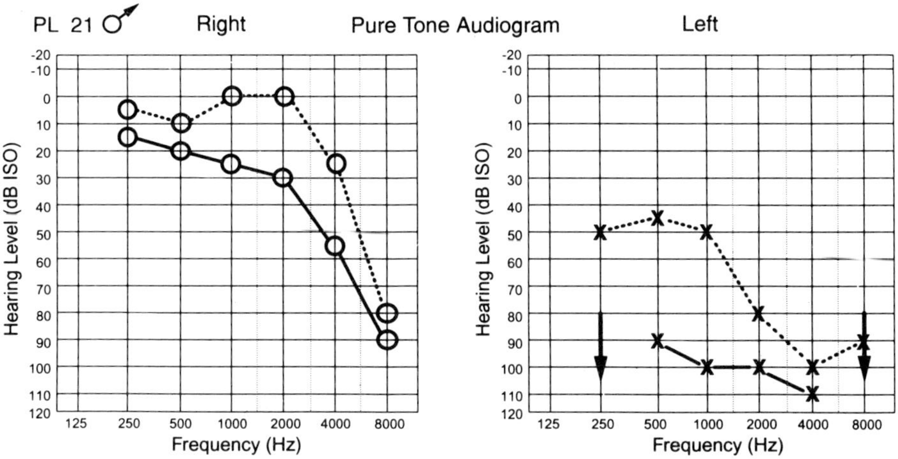

Figure 8 Audiometry of a 21-year-old man with bilateral autoimmune inner ear disease. He presented with sudden left hearing loss, distortion and vertigo 6 weeks previously, and a 10-day history of right hearing impairment and distortion. Solid line: pre-treatment May 1989; broken line: post-treatment October 1989. His improved hearing level has been maintained for more than 3 years on azathioprine and alternate-day low-dose steroids

Treatment

Many, but not all, patients respond to systemic steroids. Recommended regimens suggest enteric-coated prednisolone, 20 mg, four times daily for 2 weeks before reducing to a maintenance dose of 5–10 mg on alternate days for 3–6 months in the face of continuing clinical improvement and lack of toxicity. In the author's experience, much lower dosages can sometimes lead to improvement and reduce unwanted side-effects, such as weight gain and dyspepsia. Hughes et al.[39] found that 40% of their 47 patients who attended for long-term follow-up improved with steroids, whilst stabilization was achieved in 40%. Twenty per cent continued to deteriorate. Failure to respond to steroids may be an indication for immunosuppressive treatment with azathioprine or cyclophosphamide, but each case must be considered on its merits. Ethically, it may be difficult to justify potentially hazardous immunosuppressive therapy in the absence of precise diagnostic criteria unless warranted by the severity of the clinical symptoms, usually marked bilateral hearing loss or rapid loss in an only hearing ear. Hughes et al.[39] only treated less than 10% of their cases with cytotoxic therapy. The author has, however, preferred to use the well-established cytotoxic drug, azathioprine (2 mg/kg body weight daily) at an early stage of active disease and when the diagnosis has been established. This has enabled steroid maintenance to be continued at a low alternate-day dosage, thereby avoiding long-term side-effects. Figure 8 shows the efficacy of this combined regimen in a young man who presented with a short history of severe bilateral sensorineural hearing loss and positive inner ear autoantibodies. Certain patients may show improvement with plasma exchange. This is an expensive therapeutic modality which is not widely available and whose beneficial effects are of a relatively temporary nature, lasting at the most 3 months. It may, however, 'buy time' in the management of problem cases[44,45].

MENIERE'S DISEASE

Meniere's disease is an inner ear disorder which typically presents as a symptom complex of episodic vertigo, fluctuating hear loss, tinnitus and aural pressure. The natural history is unpredictable and characterized by symptomatic relapses and remissions, whilst the precise aetiology is still unknown. In 1938, the classic descriptions of Hallpike and Cairns[46] established that the underlying histopathological feature is distension of the endolymphatic system associated with an excess of endolymph – termed endolymphatic hydrops. This feature may occur in other disorders involving the inner ear, such as late syphilis, otosclerosis and Paget's disease. The term 'Meniere's disease' is, however, reserved for idiopathic hydrops when investigations have excluded other possible primary conditions.

Soon after McCabe's work on autoimmune sensorineural hearing loss, evidence began to accumulate implicating immune mechanisms in the aetiology or pathogenesis of classical Meniere's disease. Involvement of both cellular[36] and humoral[47] mechanisms was reported. Recognition of the prime importance of the endolymphatic sac as the major site of endolymph absorption had already focused attention on this structure. Kimura and Schuknecht[48] demonstrated the consistent development of endolymphatic hydrops histopathologically after obstruction of the endolymphatic duct and sac in guinea-pigs. Many other groups subsequently confirmed disturbance of the smoothly regulated normal inner ear fluid balance by sac ablation, and used this animal model extensively in various experimental situations, even though none of the animals appeared to experience vestibular symptoms. The increasing evidence of the special role of the endolymphatic sac in inner ear immunity alluded to previously[3,9,17,18] served to reinforce earlier hypotheses.

In an attempt to evaluate both humoral and cellular immune responses, Hughes et al.[36] ran a battery of tests on 11 patients with Meniere's disease. Cell-mediated lymphocyte responses to inner ear tissue were assessed by migration inhibition and transformation tests. Positive results were obtained in a small fraction (10–20%) of cases. Circulating immune complexes, assayed by a cryoprecipitation technique, were elevated in one patient. These same authors in a later study reported that 52% of 52 patients with autoimmune inner ear disease, as diagnosed by positive lymphocyte transformation studies, showed endolymphatic hydrops which was usually bilateral. Although cochleovestibular involvement was present, the vast majority of cases did not display typical Meniere's features. However, in one third, the progressive hearing loss was halted by a medical regimen of systemic steroids, diuretics, low salt diet and vestibular suppressants. Harris and Ryan[49] conducted a similar preliminary study in 14 Meniere's patients, but did not find any instances of positive lymphocyte transformation.

Evidence of humoral responses in the inner ear in Meniere's disease includes the finding by Arnold et al.[6,40] of IgG and IgA in the epithelial cells and lumen of the endolymphatic sac. Elies and Plester[50] reported similar findings in Meniere's patients. The author has studied general humoral immune factors in a large series of 66 patients with Meniere's disease and 36 normal controls[51]. Circulating immune complexes (CICs), serum immunoglobulin assays, an autoantibody screen to a battery of 10 general tissue antigens, excluding the inner ear, and acetate electrophoresis measurements were made. Using the more sensitive polyethylene glycol (PEG) assay, significantly increased CICs were found in 55% of the Meniere's group compared with 3% of the controls, using laboratory reference data. It was of interest that the mean levels of CICs in the control subjects were significantly lower than the reference values of the laboratory which provided the reactants. The proportion of elevated complex-specific immunoglobulins identified were: IgM in 86%, IgG in 44%, and IgA in 3%. There was also a statistically significant increased incidence of general autoantibodies in Meniere's patients, the commoner ones being antinuclear factor (ANF), thyroid thyroglobulin and smooth-muscle antibody. There was a distinct trend for raised levels of complexes to be associated with increased disease activity.

Subsequently, two other groups have conducted a similar study of immune complexes in Meniere's disease. Perez-Garrigues et al.[52] found a 21% incidence of raised CICs in a series of 40 cases. A few patients were studied serially, and it was found that elevated levels of complexes were more likely to be obtained during or near the time of a vertigo attack. Perhaps part of the difference in the incidence of raised CICs between these two series can be attributed to differences in the type of patient population. In the author's earlier series, the cases were almost exclusively problem patients who had been referred by other otolaryngologists for surgical management. Nearly one third had bilateral involvement, a reflection of disease severity.

Derebery et al.[53] found that 96% of 30 Meniere's patients attending the House Ear Clinic had significantly raised CICs compared with controls. The population was rather heterogeneous in that half had known inhalational or food allergies, whilst 47% had undergone previous surgery. Interestingly, the mean levels of CICs were lower in the surgical group than in the unoperated cases. These studies strongly suggest that humoral immune factors are important in a proportion of patients with Meniere's disease. Deposition of complexes in either the stria vascularis or endolymphatic sac capillaries may be responsible for the end-organ damage which is known to occur in this disorder (Figure 7). Direct confirmatory evidence for the role of CICs would be the finding of tissue-bound complexes, but definitive proof is still lacking. The inner ear cannot be biopsied without causing hearing and vestibular impairment, and postmorten studies are only likely to be examining tissues in the final stages of disease, when any active inflammatory stage has long since resolved.

Some indirect evidence has been reported by Futaki and associates[54] who removed endolymph from the endolymphatic sac during surgery. Specific concentrations of IgG were higher in Meniere's patients than in normal patients who were undergoing surgery for temporal bone fractures. It is known that high levels of IgG are present at the site of lesions in other autoimmune disorders.

Harada and colleagues[55] have studied the Type III reaction and its relationship to endolymphatic hydrops in research animals. An antigen–antibody reaction at the level of the stria leads to an increased permeability of Reissner's membrane and alters the physiological function of the stria in guinea-pigs. Since other animal studies do show the presence of IgG and complement within endolymph, these authors suggest that invasion of antigens into the endolymphatic fluid may lead to a Type III reaction after the formation of immune complexes. As mentioned before, Yoo et al.[56,57], on the other hand, investigated Type II collagen reactions. They found that the antibodies to Type II collagen are significantly higher in Meniere's disease, and especially when otosclerosis coexists. The clinical significance of their findings is not understood but serum transfer has produced hearing loss in animals, suggesting a Type II or Type III injury.

DELAYED ENDOLYMPHATIC HYDROPS

Delayed endolymphatic hydrops (EH) is an uncommon, though now well-recognized, subgroup of the spectrum of Meniere's disorders. The clinical manifestations consist of an early phase characterized by profound hearing loss in one ear and a late phase in which active symptoms of endolymphatic hydrops develop, either in the same ear or in the opposite ear. Meniere's disease, on the other hand, differs in that hydrops occurs in one or both ears that previously had normal auditory and vestibular function. The ipsilateral form of delayed EH in which episodic vertigo results from hydrops in the deaf ear is distinct from the contralateral type. In contralateral EH, the fluctuating hearing loss, sometimes with episodic vertigo, results from hydrops in the opposite ear that previously had normal hearing.

The primary profound or total hearing loss may be due to specific infections, such as mumps or measles in early childhood, non-specific viruses causing upper respiratory tract infections, or temporal bone trauma. In the majority of cases, however, the onset is congenital or neonatal and of unknown cause. Whilst one can readily understand how infection or trauma resulting in severe cochlear damage may also subsequently interfere with delicate inner ear fluid balance mechanisms in the same ear, it is somewhat more difficult to explain the mechanism of contralateral otological symptoms. The distinction between the two forms is therefore fully justified.

Schuknecht drew the attention of otologists to contralateral delayed EH in 1978[58], when he reported 6 cases, and has recently expanded his experience to 31 cases[59]. The mean age of onset of hearing loss was 8.5 years, with a mean time delay to the occurrence of contralateral symptoms of 20 years. The hearing loss was frequently fluctuant initially, like classical Meniere's disease, and involved the low and high frequencies. Aural pressure and tinnitus were usually present, and half developed vestibular symptoms. Histopathological features have been described in two cases[59]. Both deaf ears showed atrophy of cochlear and vestibular sensory neuroepithelium with retrograde neuronal degeneration, changes which are consistent with viral labyrinthitis, such as mumps and measles. The contralateral ears, however, showed the classical features of EH, with little or no atrophy of the sense organs or neurones. It was suggested that subclinical viral disease may be the underlying mechanism. Williams and his associates[60] have indeed reported evidence of persistent viral infection in Meniere's disorder. They found significant elevations in both humoral and cellular immune responses to viral antigens of herpes simplex I, varicella–zoster, rubella and cytomegalovirus. Serum immunoglobulins were quantitatively abnormal in 24 out of 25 patients. Both increased and decreased amounts of the three major Ig types were found in Meniere's serum, with no consistent pattern, which the authors suggested could be related to infection. They were, unfortunately, not able to determine whether the altered Ig content preceded or followed the onset of inner ear disease.

The association of sensorineural hearing loss with active chronic suppurative otitis media (CSOM) has been recognized for many years, and, in general, the frequency and severity correlates with the duration of active disease and presence of cholesteatoma[61]. Paparella suggested that enhancement of the semipermeable nature of the round window membrane by active inflammation enables the passage of toxic materials that cause biochemical changes in the inner ear fluids, resulting in destruction of the organ of Corti. In a later animal experiment from the same department, Goycoolea et al.[62] were able to demonstrate the movement of large molecules through the round window membrane of cats with otitis media, and localized inflammatory changes of serous labyrinthitis in the adjacent basal turn. Related histopathological features have been described in human studies[63,64]. These included serofibrinous precipitation within the perilymph, inflammatory cells on the inner aspect of the round window membrane, and cochlear EH. Paparella and his colleagues[65] subsequently reported 37 patients with Meniere's syndrome in whom they believed the pathogenesis was related to chronic otitis media. Antigen in the middle ear can induce an inner ear immune response, though to a lesser degree than when it is introduced directly into the perilymph[15]. Enhanced permeability of the round window membrane, due to infection, may well result in a much greater antigenic stimulus to the inner ear and a greater immune response. In addition, chronic or recurrent infection could provide the necessary trigger for the generation of an amplified secondary response, resulting in large numbers of plasma cells and lymphocytes throughout the cochlea and in the endolymphatic sac wall and lumen, and causing significant structural and functional impairment at both these main sites.

Contralateral otological features are notable by their absence in these clinical studies. However, contralateral features were reported in one experimental animal study[65]. Chinchillas with acute purulent otitis media exhibited the major pathological finding of serous labyrinthitis without evidence of suppuration. In certain animals, however, similar serous labyrinthine changes were seen in the opposite non-inoculated control ear. The author has described a small series of 5 cases with active CSOM and mastoiditis who subsequently developed contralateral Meniere's disease[66], and three further cases have since been managed. Primary treatment was eradication of the chronic infection. This resulted in significant improvement of the otovestibular symptoms arising from the contralateral ear in all patients, though half eventually relapsed. Since that report, specific inner ear immune studies have been carried out in 3 patients and autoantibodies to various cochleovestibular tissues identified in every case. Cell-mediated studies still need to be completed but these patients, who probably represent a subgroup of delayed EH, may well be an example of 'sympathetic cochleolabyrinthitis'[34]. It is of interest that the author has also found inner ear autoantibodies in one case of delayed EH with contralateral hydrops, and two patients with similar contralateral pathology who had previously undergone acoustic tumour surgery.

CONNECTIVE TISSUE DISEASES

Certain systemic connective tissue diseases may affect the inner ear. There is now considerable evidence that many are immunologically mediated disorders, based largely on the presence of demonstrable autoantibodies. The conditions are characterized by inflammation and necrosis of blood vessels, which is believed to be due to local tissue reaction to the deposition of immune complexes. The varied features depend on the particular organs and blood vessel sites involved. There are several distinct types, though, as this is a disease spectrum, some overlap may occur. Table 3 summarizes the main features.

Systemic lupus erythematosus

Systemic lupus erythematosus is a multisystem connective tissue disorder in which an autoimmune aetiology is most certain. Widespread immune complex deposition is present in many organs. Although more than half the patients have central nervous system (CNS) involvement resulting in cranial neuropathies, otological features are uncommon. Sudden sensorineural hearing loss, which is usually bilateral, is a common feature in reported cases.

Hamblin et al.[44] described a 42-year-old female who developed sudden severe cochlear hearing loss 6 weeks after the onset of systemic symptoms. Prednisolone, 40 mg daily, resulted in general improvement but no hearing gain. Plasma exchange, however, effected immediate and complete restoration of hearing. A single plasma exchange was repeated at 6-monthly intervals to reverse the recurrent hearing loss which ensued. The dramatic response to plasma exchange implies a vascular mechanism, and it was suggested that CICs could cause sludging in the stria vascularis.

Caldarelli et al.[67] reported the onset of bilateral profound sensorineural hearing loss associated with mild unsteadiness over a period of 3 weeks. SLE was diagnosed, but, despite aggressive treatment with steroids and cyclophosphamide, the profound deafness remained. The authors postulated

Table 3 Features of main connective tissue diseases

Laboratory test	*Normal population*	*Systemic lupus erythematosus*	*Polyarteritis nodosa*	*Wegener's granulomatosis*	*Cogan's syndrome*
Full blood count (FBC)					
Haemoglobin	—	↓ Normochromic, normocytic	↓ Normochromic, normocytic	↓ Normochromic, normocytic	↓ In acute disease
White cell count	—	↓ Lymphocytes	↑ Neutrophils ± eosinophilia	↑ Neutrophils	↑ Lymphocytes ± eosinophils, neutrophils, monocytes (acute only)
Platelets	—	↓	Normal	↑	
Erythrocyte sedimentation rate	—	↑	↑	↑	↑
Lupus erythematosus cells	Negative	Positive	May be positive	Negative	Negative
Coomb's test	Negative	May be positive	Negative	Negative	Negative
Antinuclear factor (ANF)	Low titres with increasing age	Positive, often high titre	May be positive in low titre	Negative	Negative
DNA-binding	Negative	Raised	Usually negative	Negative	Negative
Complement levels	C3 0.69–1.30 g/L C4 0.12–0.27 g/L	Low levels, C3 may be high	Normal or raised	Normal or raised	Normal C3 and C4 may be raised acutely
Extractable nuclear antigen (ENA) (type RNP S_m, R_o, La)	Negative	May be positive (S_m is most specific type)	Negative	Negative	Negative
C-reactive protein (CRP)	<0.8 mg/dl	Only slightly raised unless infection present	Raised	Raised	Raised
Syphilis serology (RPR, TPHA)	Negative	RPR positive, low titre TPHA negative	Negative	Negative	Negative

After Brookes and Booth, 1987[81]

that the pathogenesis was microinfarction of inner ear capillaries or arterioles, a mechanism responsible for CNS features. A little later, Bowman and Nelson[68] reported their experience of 9 patients with SLE and associated hearing loss. It is of interest that the diagnosis was made prior to the onset of otological symptoms in four patients. The same authors carried out a prospective study of 30 further SLE patients and found an 8% incidence of substantial previously unrecognized hearing loss without any other attributable cause, and strongly suspected a causal correlation.

Polyarteritis nodosa

Polyarteritis nodosa is a systemic necrotizing vasculitis of small and medium-sized arteries which demonstrates a 3:1 male to female predominance. Frequently, there is involvement of the renal, coronary, hepatic and visceral circulations. Deafness is unusual but invariably involves the inner ear. Occasionally, middle ear granulation tissue may be present, causing a conductive component. The onset is often sudden and typically bilateral and symmetrical. Significant hearing improvement following treatment with systemic steroids and in conjunction with the immunosuppressive drug, chlorambucil, has been reported[69,70].

Wegener's granulomatosis

Wegener's granulomatosis is a discrete syndrome of necrotizing granulomatosis, vasculitis of the small arteries and veins of the upper and lower respiratory tract and kidney with less frequent involvement of other organs. There may be difficulties in differentiating this disorder from PAN before the full complex develops. Patients will usually present with persistent epistaxis, and associated systemic features include weight loss, pyrexia, anaemia, leukocytosis and an elevated ESR. The average duration of untreated disease is about 8 months and death is usually due to renal failure.

Ear involvement occurs in 15–35% of cases and may be the presenting feature[71,72]. Seromucinous otitis media is an early feature, and, on occasions, the middle ear cleft becomes filled with granulomatous tissue. This may spread to involve the inner ear. Feghali and Linthicum[73] described the temporal bone features in a patient who died of Wegener's granulomatosis. They found preferential involvement of the capillaries of the endolymphatic sac, but not those of the cochlea, and suggested that a similar pathophysiology may well occur in other types of immune-complex-mediated autoimmune disease, resulting in Meniere-like symptoms. Although Wegener's granulomatosis has a sinister reputation, there is growing optimism for survival using combination regimens of steroids and cytotoxic immunosuppressant drugs.

Temporal arteritis

Pyrexia, bitemporal headaches, and tender palpable thickening of the temporal arteries are the main features of this condition which occurs in older age groups. The underlying vasculitis is primarily confined to the extracranial arteries. Blindness occurs in about 30% of untreated cases. Rapidly progressive hearing loss with vertigo which responds to steroids has been described, presumably due to involvement of the internal auditory artery.

Cogan's syndrome

Cogan's syndrome is a rare condition in which a non-syphilitic interstitial keratitis is associated with fluctuant but aggressive cochleovestibular damage. It usually affects young adults, and the ocular and otological symptoms commence suddenly and often simultaneously. The hearing loss is sensory in type and invariably bilateral. It progresses rapidly, though fluctuations may occur, and is associated with episodic vertigo, tinnitus and aural pressure, constituting a Meniere's syndrome. Ultimately, the deafness becomes profound and may be total. Vestibular assessment reveals significantly reduced or absent caloric responses. In contrast, the ophthalmic features, consisting of irritation, lacrimation, photophobia and blurred vision, typically progress more slowly.

There is now considerable evidence to support an autoimmune aetiology[2,25,31,37]. Hughes et al.[37] studied two cases and found evidence of cell-mediated autoimmunity. The author studied two cases who were found to have very high levels of CICs, which fluctuated with disease activity[31]. Arnold and Gebbers[25], using indirect immunofluorescent techniques, demonstrated IgG and IgA antibodies against human cornea and IgG antibodies against human inner ear tissue in the serum of a patient with Cogan's syndrome. These reactions were observed in the stria vascularis, Reissner's membrane, spiral ligament and dark cell areas. The main histopathological temporal bone features include endolymphatic hydrops, degeneration of the organ of Corti and severe neuronal loss with infiltration of lymphocytes and plasmacytes in the region of the spiral ligament. Systemic steroids alone do not usually prevent the relentless progression towards severe cochleovestibular dysfunction, and, in the author's experience, immunosuppressive drugs are indicated at an early stage.

Behçet's disease

Behçet's disease is a very uncommon chronic relapsing inflammatory disorder. The original classic symptom triad of uveitis and orogenital ulceration is now recognized as part of a multisystem vasculitic disorder which is very probably immunologically mediated. Little attention has been given to otological aspects. Brama and Fainaru[74] investigated 16 consecutive patients and found that 62% had features of inner ear involvement which typically commenced about a decade after the initial manifestations of the disease. Hearing loss is almost always bilateral and sensory in type, though only slowly progressive. It is frequently associated with vestibular symptoms.

Relapsing polychondritis

This disease is characterized by an inflammatory reaction occurring in the cartilage of several different organs. Early features include tender swelling of the nasal septum and costal cartilages, perhaps associated with an underlying cough and dyspnoea from involvement of the larynx and trachea. The auricles are affected first in about 90% of cases, resulting in pain, swelling and erythema. Chondritis of the cartilage of the Eustachian tube may lead to serous otitis media. Sensorineural hearing impairment can occur independently or in conjunction with a conductive loss. Cody and Sones[75] found that 80% of patients had a sensory hearing loss which was usually bilateral and either of sudden onset or progressed over a period of a few weeks. Many had vestibular symptoms with abnormalities on electronystagmography and caloric testing.

The condition has been considered an autoimmune disorder for some years, mainly because of the efficacy of corticosteroids. Cody and Sones[75] reported some recovery of hearing in patients with early sensorineural involvement, although relapses tended to occur when drug therapy was discontinued. Direct immunofluorescent examination of auricular cartilage, obtained from patients with the disease, has demonstrated deposits of immunoglobulins and the C3 component of complement at the chondrofibrous junction[76].

GENETIC ASPECTS OF AUTOIMMUNE INNER EAR DISEASE

The discovery of associations between certain diseases and the major histocompatibility complex or human leukocyte antigen (HLA) locus represents one of the most important advances in clinical medicine in the last two decades. A number of striking associations of particular HLA haplotypes and diseases with a suspected or presumed autoimmune aetiology have been found. Certain haplotypes are known to be associated with susceptibility to disease, whilst others are associated with resistance. Haplotype correlations are invariably incomplete, however, probably largely reflecting a multifactorial pathogenesis. Other recognized factors in these disorders include the influence of other genes or environmental factors, such as trauma, bacterial or viral damage, drugs or toxins. Stress can also inhibit immune defences and lead to exacerbation of symptoms in autoimmune disease. It has usually been possible, however, to define the risk of developing a disease when an antigen is present, relative to the risk when it is lacking.

All chronic autoimmune diseases studied have shown a correlation with one or several of the HLA antigens compared with an appropriate control population. Indeed, failure to identify an association is very significant evidence against an autoimmune pathogenesis. An increased tendency for other autoimmune diseases should also be established in the same patient population, and in close family members. Immune disorders characteristically also display an hereditary predisposition, yet the familial distribution of cases is such that they do not follow classical Mendelian laws.

Morrison and Xenellis[77] studied the detailed medical history of 671 patients with Meniere's disease and 689 controls. In the Meniere's group, 10.3% had another autoimmune disorder compared with 4.0% of controls. The increased incidence of general autoantibodies in Meniere's cases mentioned earlier[51] is entirely compatible with this population statistic. In the Meniere's group, 5.4% had a first-degree relative with Meniere's disease, and a recognized autoimmune disorder was present in 9.7% of relatives. In the control group, only 0.6% had a first-degree relative with Meniere's disease, and a recognized autoimmune disorder was present in 3.9% of relatives. These differences were all highly significant.

Bowman and Nelson[68] studied 39 patients with a clinical diagnosis of autoimmune inner ear disease, 28% of whom had other non-otological systemic autoimmune disease. They reported an increased frequency of the CW7 haplotype, which occurred in 51% of patients compared with 21% of 627 matched controls. A possible reduced frequency of DR4 was reported as well. Xenellis et al.[78] reported the results of an investigation of 41 patients with Meniere's disease. Cases were selected with the intention of maximizing any possible association. There was, therefore, a very high incidence of bilateral involvement constituting nearly two thirds of the cases. These patients were exclusively a tertiary referral population who were refractory to medical treatment and were severely disabled. The Class I HLA allele, CW7, was found in 75% of Meniere's patients, a highly significant association ($p < 0.01$) when compared with controls. The frequencies of the HLA alleles A1 and B8 were also increased but this was not significant after corrections were made for the number of antigens tested. No association was found with Class II DR3. In addition, no differences were found between males and females, or unilateral and bilateral cases.

The author has recently reported the results of a further collaborative HLA study in a more balanced and representative population of 60 Caucasian patients with Meniere's disease, conforming to AAOO criteria[79]. The first 50 cases were seen consecutively, and included early, established and late stages of the disease activity spectrum. In the light of our findings, a further 10 patients with bilateral disease were added. There was an equal sex incidence, whilst the disorder was bilateral in 20 cases. Distinct differences were found between Meniere's subjects with bilateral disease and unilateral cases. A highly significant ($p < 0.01$) positive correlation with the CW7 antigen was found in the bilateral group, and a highly significant ($p < 0.01$) negative association with B12. In fact, B12 was never observed in the bilateral disease patients though the incidence in controls was 28%. In contrast, in the unilateral disease group, there was only an association trend with CW7 ($p < 0.1$), but a statistically highly significant ($p < 0.01$) positive correlation with B12. The B12 antigen was identified in 43% of unilateral cases. The allele CW5 was also never found in the bilateral group though the numbers are insufficient to reach significance.

These three studies strongly support the contention that the Class I allele CW7 is a genetic marker for susceptibility to the development of autoimmune inner ear disease. The last study suggests that the B12 antigen may well exert a protective influence, or alternatively its absence increases susceptibility to the development of Meniere's disease. Autoimmune mechanisms may well be important in the pathogenesis of Meniere's disease or other inner ear disorders in some patients. Early genetic screening may predict this at-risk population and could therefore have significant management implications.

REFERENCES

1. Lehnhardt E. Plotzliche Horstorungen auf beiden Sieten gleichseitig oder nacheinander aufgetrete. Zeitschrift Laryngologie Rhinologie. 1958;37:1–16.
2. McCabe BF. Autoimmune sensorineural hearing loss. Ann Otol Rhinol Laryngol. 1979;88:585–9.
3. Rask-Anderson H, Stahle J. Immunodefence of the inner ear. Acta Otolaryngol. 1980;89: 283–94.
4. Morganstein C, Amano H, Orsulakova A. Ion transport in the endolymphatic space. Am J Otolaryngol. 1982;3:323–7.
5. Lim D, Silver P. The endolymphatic duct system. A light and electron microscopic investigation. In: Pulec J, ed. Proceedings of Barany Society Meeting, Anaheim, California. 1974:390.
6. Arnold W, Altermatt HJ, Gebbers JO. Demonstration of immunoglobulins (IgA and IgG) in the human endolymphatic sac. Laryngol Rhinol Otol. 1984;63:464–7.
7. Palva T, Raunio V. Disc electrophoretic studies of human perilymph and endolymph. Acta Otolaryngol. 1967;63:128–37.
8. Mogi G, Lim DJ, Watanabe N. Immunologic study of the inner ear: Immunoglobulins in perilymph. Arch Otolaryngol. 1982;108:270–5.
9. Harris JP. Immunology of the inner ear: response of the inner ear to antigen challenge. Otolaryngol Head Neck Surg. 1983;91:18–23.
10. Arnold WJ, Altermatt HJ. Presence of immunoglobulins (IgA, IgG) and secretory component in the human endolymphatic sac. In Myers EN, ed. New dimensions in otolaryngology – head and neck surgery, Vol. 2. Amsterdam: Elsevier Biomedical; 1985:128–9.
11. Beickert P. Zur Frage der Empfindungs-schwerhorigkeit und Autoallergie. Zeitschrift Laryngol Rhinol Grenzgebiete. 1961;40:837–42.
12. Terrayama Y, Sasaki Y. Studies on experimental allergic (isoimmune) labyrinthitis in guinea pigs. Acta Otolaryngol. 1968;58:49–56.
13. Yoo TJ, Stuart JM, Cremar MA, Ownes AS, Kawk AH. Type II collagen-induced autoimmune sensorineural hearing loss and vestibular dysfunction in rats. Ann Otol Rhinol Laryngol. 1983;92:267–71.
14. Yoo TJ, Yazawa Y, Tomada K, Floyd R. Type II collagen-induced autoimmune endolymphatic hydrops in the guinea pig. Science. 1983;222:65–7.
15. Harris JP, Tomiyama S. Experimental immune system of the inner ear. In: Immunobiology, histophysiology and tumour immunology in otolaryngology. Proceedings of the 2nd International Conference, Utrecht. Amsterdam/Berkeley: Kugler Publications; 1987: 113–21.
16. McCabe BF. Treatment of autoimmune inner ear disease. In: Proceedings of the Sixth Shambaugh International Workshop on Otomicrosurgery and Third Shea Fluctuant Hearing Loss Symposium. Huntsville: Strode; 1981:289–90.
17. Harris JP. Immunology of the inner ear: evidence of local antibody production. Ann Otol Rhinol Laryngol. 1984;93:157–62.
18. Tomiyama S, Harris JP. The endolymphatic sac: its importance in inner ear immune response. Laryngoscope. 1986;96:685–91.
19. Woolf NK. Harris JP. Cochlear pathophysiology associated with inner ear immune responses. Acta Otolaryngol (Stockh). 1986;102:353–64.
20. Harris JP, Woolf HK, Ryan AF, Butler DM, Richman DD. Immunologic and electrophysiologic response to cytomegalovirus inner ear infection in the guinea pig. J Infect Dis. 1984;150:523–30.
21. Gell PGH, Coombs RRA. Clinical aspects of immunology. 2nd edn. Oxford: 1984.
22. Boyles JH. Allergy testing in otology. Am J Otol. 1980;5:450–5.

23. Clemis JD. Cochleovestibular disorders and allergy. Otolaryngol Clin N Am. 1974;7: 757–80.
24. Shambaugh GE Jr. Allergic causes for fluctuant hearing loss. In: Proceedings of the Sixth Shambaugh and Third Shea International Workshop in Otology. Huntsville: Strode; 1981.
25. Arnold, W, Gebbers JO. Serum antibodies which bind to human cornea and inner ear tissues in a patient with Cogan's syndrome. Laryngol Rhinol Otol. 1984;63:428–32.
26. Juhn SK, Rybar L. Nature of the blood–labyrinth barrier. In: Vosteen KH, Schuknecht HF, Pfaltz ER, et al. eds. Meniere's disease: pathogenesis, diagnosis and treatment. New York: Thieme Verlag; 1981:59–67.
27. Lundquist PC. Aspects of endolymphatic sac morphology and function. Arch Otolaryngol. 1976;212:231–40.
28. Solling J, Solling K, Jacobsen KU, Olsen S, From L. Circulating immune complexes in syphilis. Acta Dermato-Venereol. 1978;58:263–7.
29. Engel S, Diezel W. Persistent serum immune complexes in syphilis. Br J Vener Dis. 1980;56:221–2.
30. Baughn RE, Tung KSK, Musker DM. Detection of circulating immune complexes in the sera of rabbits with experimental syphilis: possible role in immune regulation. Infect Immun. 1980;29:575–82.
31. Brookes GB. Immune complex associated deafness: preliminary communication. J R Soc Med. 1985;78:47–55.
32. Kanzaki J, Ouchi T. Steroid-responsive bilateral sensorineural hearing loss and immune complexes. Arch Otolaryngol. 1981;230:5–9.
33. Stephens SDG, Luxon LM, Hinchcliffe R. Immunological disorders and auditory lesions. Audiology. 1982;21:128–48.
34. Harris JP, Low NC, House WF. Contralateral hearing loss following inner ear injury: sympathetic cochleolabyrinthitis? Am J Otol. 1985;6:371–7.
35. Glynn LE, Holborrow EJ. The eye. In: Autoimmunity and disease. Oxford: Blackwell Scientific Publications; 1965:320–40.
36. Hughes GB, Kinney SE, Barna BP, Calabrese LH. Autoimmune reactivity in Meniere's disease – a preliminary report. Laryngoscope. 1983;93:1153–4.
37. Hughes GB, Kinney SE, Barna BP, Tomsak RL, Calabrese LH. Autoimmune reactivity in Cogan's syndrome: a preliminary report. Otolaryngol Head Neck Surg. 1983;91:24–8.
38. Hughes GB, Kinney SE, Barna BP, Calabrese LH. Autoimmune inner ear disease: Five year review. In: Immunobiology, histopathology and tumour immunology in otolaryngology. Proceedings of the 2nd International Conference, Utrecht. Amsterdam/Berkeley: Kugler Publications; 1987:23–32.
39. Hughes GB. Is surgery ever needed for immune inner ear disease? Paper presented to Politzer Society International Conference on Reality in Ear Surgery and Otoneurosurgery. Maastricht, 1991.
40. Arnold W, Pfaltz R, Altermatt HJ. Evidence of serum autoantibodies against inner ear tissues in the blood of patients with certain sensorineural hearing disorders. Acta Otolaryngol (Stockh). 1985;99:437–44.
41. Harris JP, Sharp PA. Inner ear autoantibodies in patients with rapidly progressive sensorineural hearing loss. Laryngoscope. 1990;100:516–24.
42. Harris JP. Experimental autoimmune sensorineural hearing loss. Laryngoscope. 1987;97:63–76.
43. Orozco CR, Niparko JR, Richardson BC, Dolan DF, Ptok MU, Altschuler RA. Experimental model of immune-mediated hearing loss using cross-species immunisation. Laryngoscope. 1990;100:941–7.
44. Hamblin TJ, Mufti GJ, Bracewell A. Severe deafness in SLE: its immediate relief by plasma exchange. Br Med J. 1982;284:1374–5.
45. Brookes GB, Newland AC. Plasma exchange in the treatment of immune complex associated sensorineural deafness. J Laryngol Otol. 1986;100:25–33.
46. Hallpike CS, Cairns H. Pathology of Meniere's syndrome. J Laryngol Otol. 1938;53:625–55.
47. Yoo TJ, Stuart JM, Kang AH, Townes AS, Tomada K, Dixit S. Type II collagen autoimmunity in otosclerosis and Meniere's disease. Science. 1982;217:1153–5.
48. Kimura RS, Schuknecht HF. Membranous hydrops in the inner ear of the guinea pig by

obliteration of the endolymphatic sac. Pract Otorhinolaryngol. 1965;27:343–54.
49. Harris JP, Ryan AF. Autoimmunity in the pathogenesis of Meniere's disease. 1987.
50. Elies W, Plester D. Sensorineural hearing loss and immunity. In: Veldman JE, McCabe BF, Huizing EH, Mygind N, eds. Immunobiology, autoimmunity, transplantation in otorhinolaryngology. Amsterdam/Berkeley: Kugler Publications; 1985:111–7.
51. Brookes GB. Circulating immune complexes in Meniere's disease. Arch Otolaryngol. 1986;112:536–40.
52. Perez-Garrigues H, Enguidanos MJ, Morera C. Immunological disturbance in Meniere's disease. In: Sacristan T, Alvarez-Vicent JJ, Bartual J, Antoli-Candela F, et al. eds. Proceedings of the XIV World Congress of Otorhinolaryngology, Head and Neck Surgery. Amsterdam, Berkeley: Kugler & Ghedini Publications; 1990:769–71.
53. Derebery MJ, Rao VS, Siglock TJ, Linthicum FH, Nelson RA. Meniere's disease: an immune complex-mediated illness? Laryngoscope. 1991;101:225–9.
54. Futaki T, Yamane M, Shirahata et al. Immunological analysis of IgG and other protein fractions in endolymph obtained from endolymphatic sac of Meniere's patients and a control. Acta Otolaryngol (Suppl) (Stockh). 1984;419:71–8.
55. Harada T, Matsunaga T, Hong K, Indue K. Endolymphatic hydrops and type III allergic reaction. Acta Otolaryngol (Stockh). 1984;97:450–9.
56. Yoo TJ. Etiopathogenesis of Meniere's disease: a hypothesis. Ann Otol Rhinol Laryngol (Suppl.) 1984;113:6–12.
57. Yoo TJ, Floyd R, Ishibe T et al. Immunologic testing of certain ear diseases. Am J Otol. 1985;6:96–101.
58. Schuknecht HF. Delayed endolymphatic hydrops. Ann Otol Rhinol Laryngol. 1978;87:743–8.
59. Schuknecht HF, Suzuka Y, Zimmermann CF. Delayed endolymphatic hydrops and its relationship to Meniere's disease. Ann Otol Rhinol Laryngol. 1990;99:843–53.
60. Williams L, Lowery M, Shannon B. Evidence of persistent viral infection in Meniere's disease. Arch Otolaryngol. 1987;113:397–400.
61. Paparella MM, Brady DR, Hoel R. Sensorineural hearing loss in chronic otitis media and mastoiditis. Trans Am Acad Ophthalmol Otolaryngol. 1970;74:108–15.
62. Goycoolea MV, Paparella MM, Goldberg B, Carpenter AM. Permeability of the round window membrane in otitis media. Arch Otolaryngol. 1980;106:430–3.
63. Paparella MM, Goycoolea MV, Meyerhoff WL, Shea D. Endolymphatic hydrops with otitis media. Laryngoscope. 1979;89:43–54.
64. Stewart TJ, Belal A. Surgical anatomy and pathology of the round window. Clin Otolaryngol. 1981;6:45–62.
65. Paparella MM, Morizono T, Le CT, Mancini F, Sipila P, Choo YB, Liden G, Kim CS. Sensorineural hearing loss in otitis media. Ann Otol Rhinol Laryngol. 1984;93:623–9.
66. Brookes GB. Meniere's disease and contralateral chronic suppurative otitis media – an aetiological link? In: Saccristan T, Alvarez-Vincent JJ, Bartual J, Antoli-Candela F, Rubio L, eds. Proceedings of the XIV World Congress of Otorhinolaryngology. Amsterdam: Kugler & Ghedini Publications; 1990:725–30.
67. Caldarelli DD, Rejowski JE, Corey JP. Sensorineural hearing loss in lupus erythematosus. Am J Otol. 1986;7:210–3.
68. Bowman CA, Nelson RA. HLA antigens in autoimmune sensorineural hearing loss. Laryngoscope. 1987;97:7–9.
69. Peitersen E, Carlsen BJ. Hearing impairment as the initial sign of polyarteritis nodosa. Acta Otolaryngol. 1966;61:189–93.
70. Wing L, Bulteau V. Deafness in Wegener's granulomatosis. J Otolaryngol Aust. 1967;2: 91–2.
71. Blatt I, Seltzer H, Rubin P, Furstenberg A, Maxwell J, Schull W. Fatal granulomatosis of the respiratory tract – Wegener's granulomatosis. Arch Otolaryngol. 1959;70:707–11.
72. Kornblut AD, Wolff SM, Fauci AS. Ear disease in patients with Wegener's granulomatosis. Laryngoscope. 1982;92:713–7.
73. Feghali and Linthicum (1984).
74. Brama I, Fainaru M. Inner ear involvement in Behçet's disease. Arch Otolaryngol. 1980;106:215–7.
75. Cody DT, Sones DA. Relapsing polychrondritis: audiological manifestations. Laryngoscope. 1971;81:1208–22.

76. Valenzuela R. Relapsing polychondritis: immunomicroscopic findings in cartilage ear biopsy specimens. Hum Pathol. 1980;11:19–26.
77. Morrison AW, Xenellis J. Immunological aspects of Meniere's disease. In: Immunobiology, histophysiology and tumour immunology in otolaryngology. Proceedings of the 2nd International Acad Conference, Utrecht. Amsterdam: Kugler Publications. 1987:9–14.
78. Xenellis J, Morrison AW, McClowsky D, Festenstein H. HLA antigens in the pathogenesis of Meniere's disease. J Laryngol Otol. 1986;100:21–4.
79. Brookes GB, Davey N, Batchelor JR. Is Meniere's disease an autoimmune disorder? Otology in the 90s: trends and perspectives. In: Proceedings of the Politzer Society International Conference. 1992:76.
80. Hughes GB, Barna BP, Calabrese LH. Immune mechanisms in auditory and vestibular disease. In: Cummings CW, et al., eds. Otolaryngology – head and neck surgery. Vol. 4. Ear and skull base. St. Louis: C V Mosby.
81. Brookes GB, Booth JB. Diseases of the temporal bone. In Kerr AG, ed. Scott-Brown's Otolaryngology, 5th Edn. London: Butterworth; 1987.
82. Lim DJ. Scanning electron microscopic morphology of the ear. In: Paparella MM, Shumrick CA, eds. Textbook of Otolaryngology. Vol. 1. Basic Sciences and Related Disciplines. Philadelphia: W B Saunders; 1980:439–69.

12
Middle Ear Disorders

G. B. BROOKES

INTRODUCTION

Immunological responses fulfil a vital protective role in the middle ear cavity. This is most evident with the onset of bacterial or viral infections from the upper respiratory tract. On occasions, however, incomplete resolution of these infections occurs, and immune mechanisms may inadvertently cause or contribute to the development of secondary disorders. Commonest, and hence most important, of these conditions is otitis media with effusion. There is accumulating evidence to suggest that protective immune mechanisms may contribute to enhanced local bone resorption in acquired cholesteatoma, and the pathogenesis of otosclerosis in genetically susceptible individuals. In addition, 'immune protection' is an unwanted phenomenon when allograft tissues or synthetic materials are implanted during tympanomastoid reconstructive surgery, and may compromise functional results. This chapter presents an overview of the role of immune processes in these various middle ear disorders.

APPLIED ANATOMY AND PHYSIOLOGY

The middle ear and Eustachian tube, or tubotympanum, can be considered as a single functioning unit of the upper respiratory tract. They are lined by pseudostratified ciliated columnar epithelium and, in addition, both non-secretory and secretory cells are present. The latter produce mucus or protein-rich serous fluid. The subepithelial connective tissue contains a rich supply of blood vessels and lymph capillaries, as well as occasional mast cells, macrophages and plasma cells. The density of the mucus-producing ciliated cells is very much greater in the Eustachian tube, where they comprise more than 80% of the constituent cells, compared with the hypotympanum or inferior part of the middle ear cavity, where their concentration varies

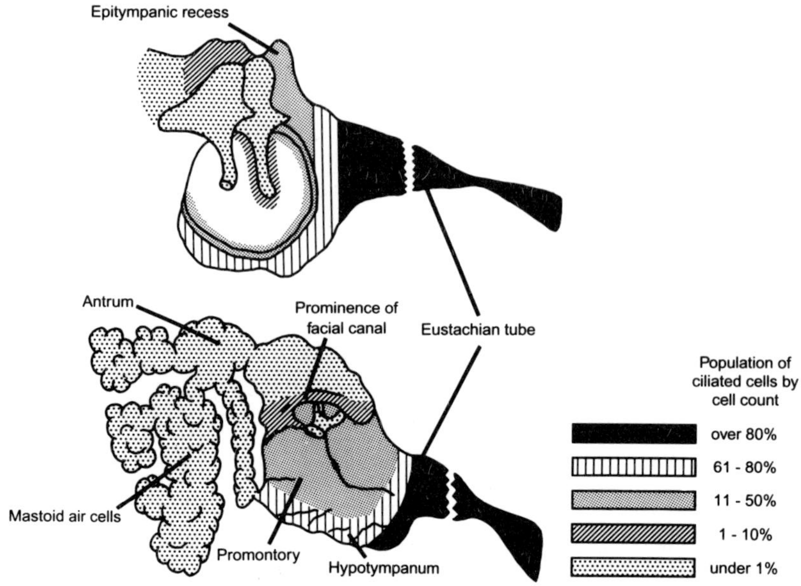

Figure 1 Distribution of ciliated mucus-secreting cells in the middle ear and mastoid. (From Reference 68)

between 50 and 80%. The proportion of these cells is even less on the promontory region or medial wall of the middle ear space and in the mastoid itself (Figure 1).

Mucus and serous secretions form a 'mucus blanket' which is cleared by the ciliated cells down the Eustachian tube. This mucus ciliary transport system is a major biological defence mechanism in protecting the tympanic cavity from infection. Cilial dysfunction in the tubotympanum is an invariable precursor of otitis media. Certain viruses appear to have a specific propensity for damaging cilia and enable secondary bacterial invasion to occur. The normal tympanic cavity is, however, sterile, and has a very limited opportunity to receive antigenic stimulation from the nasopharynx via the Eustachian tube. Apart from the paucity of lymphocytes, morphological studies show that the middle ear mucosa does not contain well-defined associated aggregates of lymphoid tissue which are typical of other mucosal sites such as the pharynx and lower respiratory tract that are readily capable of producing a local immune response[1]. It has been known for many years that systemic immune systems afford significant protection mediated by regional drainage lymph nodes which rapidly produce antibodies following antigenic stimulation of the ear. The middle ear can, however, be regarded as a 'potential site' of immune reactivity, as there is now good clinical and experimental evidence suggesting that it is also protected by both local humoral and cellular immune mechanisms.

OTITIS MEDIA WITH EFFUSION

Otitis media, a very common disease in infancy and early childhood, is acquired from the nasopharynx via the Eustachian tube. A recent review of several worldwide studies concludes that up to 65% of infants will develop otitis media by two years of age[2]. Perhaps more importantly, 25% of infants have already had at least one episode of otitis media before they are six months old, sometimes within a day or so of birth. Such children frequently progress to chronic or recurrent suppurative middle ear disease and persistent effusions. The possible association of allergy and otitis media has been appreciated for many years. Estimates of the frequency of an allergic predisposition as a primary causative factor in otitis media with effusion (OME) range from 25–80%[3–5]. In the mid 1970s, immune responses associated with middle ear disease were documented by several groups, and, since then, evidence has increased to confirm their important role in the pathogenesis of OME[6–8].

Study of the protein content of middle ear effusions (MEE) have been carried out to establish their origin. As there is little qualitative or quantitative difference between the major proteins in middle ear fluid and serum, apart from immunoglobulins and their secretory component, it is known that the effusion is a serum transudate[6]. The increased concentration of immunoglobulins, however, results from local synthesis by plasma cells in the middle ear mucosa[6,7]. These cellular features are typical of the common immune mucosal systems at other anatomical sites, when a transformation of lining mucosa also takes place. *Streptococcus pneumoniae* and *Haemophilus influenzae* are the primary pathogens in acute suppurative otitis media, though approximately 25% of effusions are sterile. Specific secretory IgA antibodies to these and other upper respiratory tract bacteria and viruses have been demonstrated in the effusion of patients with OME, and reflect the protective role of the local immune system[6,8,9]. The secretory component protein is only present in very small amounts in normal serum; Mogi et al.[7] found that it was present in more than 80% of middle ear effusions, particularly the thicker mucoid variety. The mode of action of secretory IgA remains uncertain. It may prevent bacteria adhering to mucosal surfaces, a mechanism termed immune adherence[10]. Alternatively, it has been proposed that it may act as a blocking antibody, and actually prevent bacterial opsonization by IgG antibodies and subsequent phagocytosis. The immune system may be relatively immature in younger children, and it has been suggested that this may explain the clinical finding of an increased frequency of recurrent disease with early primary infection.

There is some evidence for minor immune deficiency amongst the otitis-prone population, i.e. those children with 8 or more episodes of otitis media. Rynnel et al.[11] showed, in a population study, that such children were more likely than healthy ones to be IgG_2 deficient. IgG_2 is the subclass of IgG which is mainly directed against bacteria with external carbohydrate antigens, such as *S. pneumoniae* and *H. influenzae*. Antibodies against pneumococcal capsular antigens were decreased in an otitis-prone group[12,13]. Furthermore, immunization against *Pneumococcus* antigen produced antibody levels which correlated with prevaccination serum IgG_2 levels[14]. An inverse correlation has also been demonstrated between IgG_2 subclass levels for *Staphylococcus epidermidis* and the number of episodes of acute otitis media[15]. A lower postvaccination response to one protein antigen (rubella) has also been noted in a small group of children with recurrent otitis media when compared with age-matched controls without ear infections[16]. Unfortunately, a more recent study failed to confirm IgG_2 deficiency in a further group of children with repeated ear infections and did not show any reduction in otitis frequency in those treated with γ-globulin replacement therapy[17].

It has been proposed that the proportion of otitis-prone children with mannan-binding protein deficiency is greater than the normal 5% occurrence[18]. Mannan-binding protein has opsonizing properties; that is, it aids the adherence of neutrophils to bacteria[19], thus facilitating their subsequent phagocytosis. It is probably most important under 2 years of age when antibodies such as those of the IgG_2 subclass, which are also opsonins, have not fully developed.

Deficiency of C1q, an early complement component, is found in the serum of practically all children with recurrent purulent, but not chronic secretory, otitis media. This is not due to classical pathway activation because C1r and C1s levels are normal[20]. It may reflect a genetic abnormality. Middle ear mucous-type effusions can also decrease ciliary beat frequency in vitro[21], suggesting a disturbance of the intrinsic defence mechanisms.

Middle ear effusions cannot, however, be regarded as a specific diagnostic entity. Clinically, it has been recognized for many years that the condition is likely to be multifactorial, and variables such as adenoidal hypertrophy, an allergic predisposition or general impaired immunity, may all compromise Eustachian tube function or enhance the likelihood of tubal transmission of infective agents. In addition, many immune studies have been conducted in rather heterogeneous patient populations at different stages of the disease and following various previous treatment modalities. Such variable factors will undoubtedly have a significant impact on immunological results[22,23]. Thus, effusion samples collected for analysis may have been obtained from children who have suffered from recurrent suppurative otitis media, chronic OME and those who have received multiple courses of antibiotics. Because OME may often be asymptomatic, it cannot even be assumed that the first clinically apparent episode is the actual commencement of the disorder, which may, in fact, have passed unnoticed in early infancy. These variations have inevitably resulted in difficulties in the interpretation of results and their synthesis into consistent theories.

These problems in study design have been largely overcome by Ogra, Bernstein and colleagues[24]. They have conducted long-term investigations on groups of healthy neonates recruited at birth in order to define the developmental characteristics of immune competence in the middle ear. The subjects were closely monitored until two years of age and the occurrence of the first episode of OME. Some were asymptomatic, but all cases were followed up subsequently for a further two-year period. They found that approximately one third of a population of 150 children developed OME. Sixty per cent of cases were asymptomatic and tended to be eight months

Table 1 Relationship of immune status to bacteriological status of middle ear effusions

	Present in MEE in % subjects during 1st episode of OME				
Clinical and bacteriological status	*SIgA*	*IgM*	*IgE*	*IgG*	*CIC C1q or PEG*
Symptomatic					
Culture positive	100	100	14.2	100	100
Culture negative	0	Few	100	100	100
Asymptomatic					
Culture positive	83.3	0	16.6	100	100
Culture negative	0	0	100	100	100

CIC – circulating immune complexes; SIgA – secretory IgA; C1q or PEG – polyethylene glycol precipitate as the assays employed. From Reference 24

old or less. Those with symptoms, consisting of otalgia, fever, irritability or other features of systemic illness, were usually more than nine months old. Fluid was obtained as soon as the diagnosis of an effusion had been made and invariably prior to commencement of antibiotic treatment. Tests were carried out for bacterial and viral cultures. In two thirds of cases, pathogenic bacteria were cultured, whilst one third was sterile.

The immune results are shown in Table 1. Important findings were that secretory IgA antibodies were generally only found in ears where active bacterial infection could be demonstrated, whereas IgG and circulating immune complexes were always found regardless of bacteriological status. Low levels of IgE were detected in a few culture-positive fluids, but were always present in culture-negative cases. Further follow up showed that approximately 20% of culture-positive cases developed a recurrence, whereas 80% of culture-negative episodes were associated with either a persistent effusion or a recurrence.

This study gives further confirmatory data to support the hypothesis that the development of secretory IgA is indeed a local protective phenomenon. Evidence of a recent viral infection based on nasopharyngeal secretion analysis has been documented by other workers in about 25% of cases[25,26], and may be an important additional factor accounting for other immunomodulatory disturbances which may predispose to bacterial and recurrent otitis media. A plausible 'allergic' theory proposes the middle ear as a target organ for an IgE-mediated response following access of an allergen to the middle ear cleft. Ogra et al.[24] also speculate that an individual's constitutional predisposition to IgE hypersensitivity reactions could determine the development of subsequent recurrences. Another possibility is that the intranasal swelling of perennial allergic rhinitis compromises Eustachian tube function and hence middle ear ventilation.

The role of IgG, which is uniformly found in MEE, has been clarified by a number of experimental animal studies. Catanzaro and colleagues[27] studied the middle ear and serum response to the introduction of antigens in guinea-pigs. The initial response consists of a mild degree of mucosal hyperplasia and leukocytic infiltration of both the middle ear cavity and the mucosa. There are very few plasma cells and almost no specific immunoglobulin in

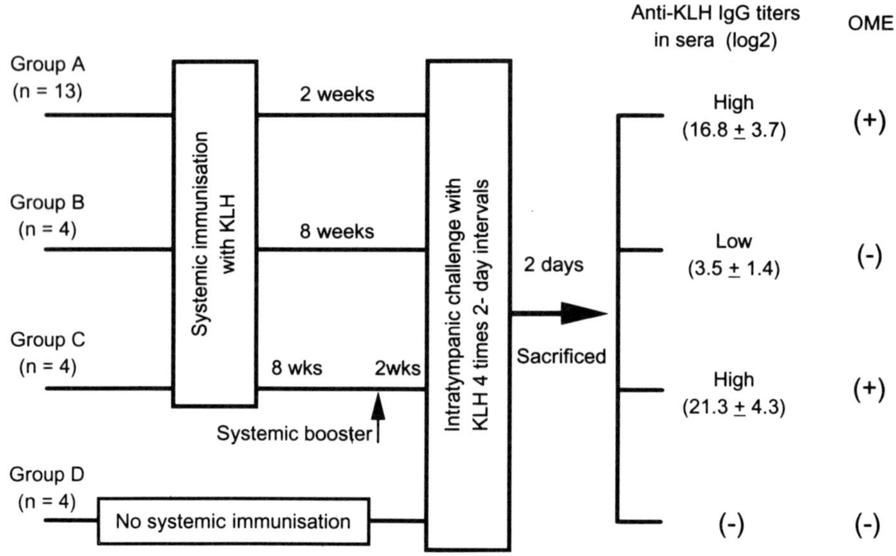

Figure 2 Effect of serum IgG antibody on the induction of otitis media with effusion in chinchilla. W = week; Ag = antigen; KLH = keyhole limpet haemocyanin. (From Reference 30)

the middle ear. There is also a very limited serum antibody response and the antigen does not sensitize circulating T cells[28]. In contrast, where an animal has been sensitized systemically by previous antigen exposure, middle ear challenge produces rapid mucosal hyperplasia and extensive MEE. Within two weeks, many plasma cells are found in the mucosa and high levels of specific immunoglobulin can be detected in the middle ear cavity[29]. Suzuki et al.[30] have conducted similar experiments in chinchilla, and their findings corroborate the thesis that a secondary immune response in the middle ear causes OME. Figure 2 summarizes these experimental findings. Consideration of aspects of local complement activation and immune complexes is necessary, however, to elucidate the mechanisms for the *maintenance* of chronic OME.

Veltry and Sprinkle[31] identified soluble immune complexes in middle ear fluids and first suggested that OME may represent an immune complex-mediated disorder. Their theory was initially supported by other groups[32,33]. However, soluble immune complexes are an inevitable component of inflammatory disease and represent an important mechanism of clearing bacteria or foreign antigens. It has not been demonstrated that immune complexes are bound in the basement membrane of middle ear epithelium or in local blood vessels, and the consensus is that they do not, in themselves, reflect direct immunopathological tissue damage.

Serum proteins of the complement system actively participate in the induction of acute inflammatory responses, both to limit spread of noxious agents and to facilitate their destruction by phagocytosis and/or lysis. Sequential activation generates complement component complexes and the

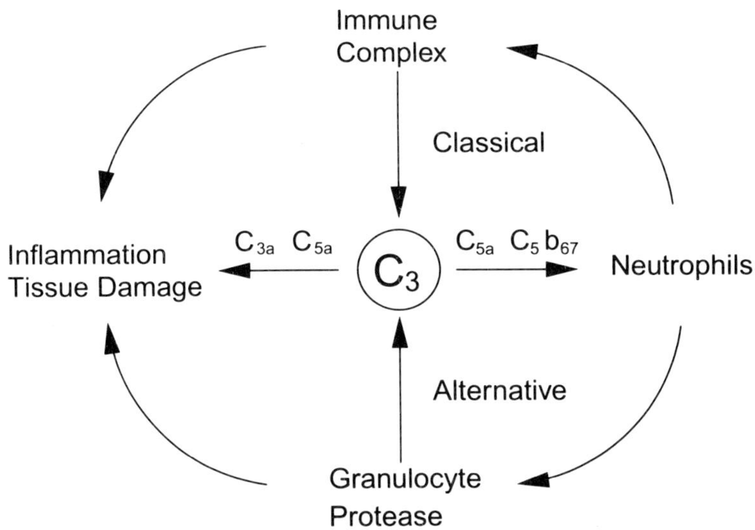

Figure 3 Immune cycle that maintains inflammatory change in the middle ear affected by OME. (From Reference 69)

release of biologically active peptides. It thus has an essential protective role in the humoral immune response. There are two main types of complement activation and evidence for both mechanisms exists in experimental studies of OME[34,35]. Immune complexes are well-documented activators of the classical pathway as are individual unbound immunoglobulins and viruses. The alternative complement activation system does not require antibody but may be achieved by various substances, particularly bacterial capsular antigens or endotoxins in the present context. Breakdown complement components, C2, C4 and particularly C3a and C5a, have all been found in the middle ear and are at mean concentrations which are significantly greater than those found in corresponding sera. Mean histamine levels are also significantly raised in OME. It is believed that complement breakdown products result in the activation of mast cells, releasing histamine and other inflammatory mediators which produce vasodilatation, occasional oedema and neutrophil chemotaxis. Furthermore, the ingestion of immune complexes by these neutrophils causes the release of lysozyme enzymes, granulocytic proteases which produce tissue injury. It therefore appears that chronic OME is maintained by a vicious cycle of inflammatory mediators (Figure 3).

Watanabi et al.[36] have recently applied the results of these immune studies to the feasibility of enhancing mucosal immunity to protect the middle ear from bacterial invasion and suppress the occurrence of OME. Animals were systemically primed and the derived specific antigen was then inoculated into the duodenal or tracheal lumen. Many antigen-specific IgA-forming cells were induced in various secretory sites, including the middle ear mucosa, Eustachian tube and nasopharynx. With antigenic challenge into the tympanic cavity, they found that only 20% of these animals developed OME, which was, however, universally present in animals without mucosal immunization. They have postulated that this type of mucosal immunization may be particularly effective because of the induction of regulatory T cells. Thus, T helper cells may stimulate a local IgA response, whilst T suppressor cells may, at the same time, suppress IgG-mediated inflammatory reactions in the middle ear. This study raises the possibility that an oral vaccine may one day be produced which would prevent OME.

As yet, however, the prospect of primary management of OME by neonatal vaccination is purely speculative. Contemporary clinical management of OME will continue to consist of antibiotics in conjunction with systemic and possibly nasal decongestants. Persistence of OME with hearing loss has conventionally been managed by incising the tympanic membrane (myringotomy) to drain the fluid and inserting a grommet to allow ventilation of the middle ear cleft. It may well be that middle ear ventilation, whether by temperature change, exposure to a sudden increase in oxygen tension or the physical effects of acute dehydration, has a strong inhibitory influence on immune responses which may be very sensitive to these rapid and dramatic in vivo changes.

OTOSCLEROSIS

Otosclerosis is a localized disease of the bony labyrinth which most frequently causes ankylosis of the stapes footplate and a conductive hearing loss. Less commonly, the bone surrounding the cochlea is affected, causing sensorineural hearing impairment. The mature hard lamellar bone of the otic capsule becomes replaced by immature woven bone of increased thickness, vascularity and cellularity, similar to that seen elsewhere in healing fractures. The new bone is initially spongy, hence the descriptive term otospongiosis, but these foci subsequently become denser and sclerotic.

The disease is unique to the human species. The incidence is probably slightly greater in females than males and may be accelerated by hormonal influences during pregnancy. A positive family history is obtained in 35–50% of cases. Genetic studies by Larsson[37] suggested an autosomal dominant inheritance with incomplete manifestation. Morrison[38] found a similar mode of inheritance and concluded that the condition was a hereditary disorder of collagen. Several studies have subsequently investigated a possible association with major histocompatibility (HLA) antigens, but the results have been inconsistent and do not support a genetic control of otosclerosis regulated by HLA antigens of the A and B loci[39–42].

Although the aetiology of otosclerosis is unknown, there is increasing evidence to suggest that immunological factors may well be important. Anson and Bast[43] first suggested that embryonic cartilage remnants in the endochondral layer of the otic capsule could play a significant role. A subsequent histopathological study by Nager[44] confirmed that bone resorption activity commenced at the interface between this incompletely differentiated endochondral layer and the completely differentiated periosteal layer of the labyrinthine capsule. Active vascular connective tissue, which is possibly derived from the submucosa overlying the stapes footplate, grows into bony lacunae and inflammatory changes of basement membrane thickening, endothelial oedema and vascular obliteration occur[45]. The mechanism which controls the osteolytic process of the transformed osteocytes is unclear. Local lymphocytes, granulocytes, macrophages and mast cells are present in these areas, and are believed to release mediators which stimulate osteoclastic activity[46].

The possibility that such inflammatory activity was immune mediated led some workers to search for comparable reactions in animal models. Cartilage contains mainly Type II collagen, and Yoo et al.[47] hyperimmunized rats with this antigen. They reported 'otoslerosis-like' lesions in the otic capsule and external ear canal within one month, though changes were not seen in association with the stapes footplate, the typical site of predeliction for otosclerosis in humans. An antibody-mediated pathogenesis was hypothesized. Huang et al.[48] also studied bovine collagen-induced resorption in rat temporal bones and found otic capsule lesions appearing six months after immunization. Similar studies by Bretlau et al.[49] found spongiotic areas exclusively in the endochondral layer of the otic capsule close to the middle ear after six weeks. The changes were only present in both temporal bones of one case. In these lytic areas, mononuclear cells were seen together with avascular fibrotic spaces. However, similar, though less pronounced, findings occurred in two control animals. In a parallel experiment using NZB mice, animals which spontaneously develop autoimmune diseases, no such lesions were found. However, Harris et al.[50] conducted similar experiments in rats inducing Type II collagen autoimmunity. Although severe arthritis was produced, they did not find any middle or inner ear abnormalities. Bretlau and colleagues[49] suggested that weakness of the antigenic immunizing preparation given over too short a period may explain some of the variations in these results, whilst strain differences in the rats used may also explain other apparent discrepancies in the data.

Other workers have conducted immunological and viral studies of stapes footplates removed at stapedectomy surgery to explore alternative aetiological factors. Thus, Schrader et al.[51] examined 122 surgical footplate specimens and applied the PAP–immunoperoxidase technique for IgG and IgM. The foci were differentiated histologically into active (33%) and inactive (67%) types. In 75% of the active foci, IgG deposits could be demonstrated, though IgM antibodies were not found. In specimens with inactive otosclerosis, neither IgG nor IgM were present. To prove the specificity of antibodies, sera of four patients with active otosclerosis were incubated on cryostat sections of fetal human cochleas. A positive immunofixation reaction at the junction of bone and cartilage was obtained. Arnold and Friedmann[52] also conducted immunofluorescent studies of stapes footplates for IgG, IgM, IgA and IgD antibodies, and, in addition, looked for viral antigens to measles, mumps and rubella viruses. In the active resorptive otospongiotic phase, a cell population reflecting chronic inflammation was found. Lymphocyte typing showed that 81% were T cells and 7% B-lymphocytes, indicating a cellular immune reaction. Deposition of IgG immunoglobulins was present on capillary walls, supporting cells and connective tissue fibres of the resorption lacunae and on osteoclasts, indicating a humoral response as well. IgA and IgM antibodies were only seen infrequently. They concluded that otosclerosis is unequivocably an immunological reaction characterized by the presence of immunocompetent cells and immunoglobulins. These features were never seen in healthy ears.

It is well established that certain viruses have an affinity for the inner ear. McKenna et al.[53] found ultrastructural evidence for a viral infection in otosclerosis. Arnold and Friedmann[52] used polyclonal and monoclonal antibodies against measles, mumps and rubella viruses, and showed that an expression of viral antigens takes place preferentially at the active otospongiotic stage. None of the patients tested showed serological evidence of a recent or acute infection with these viruses. Attempts to culture the viruses from otosclerotic tissue were unsuccessful. The immunohistochemical detection of viral antigens in these lesions suggests that they probably induce an immune reaction with a consequent inflammatory response. They also found a direct correlation between the activity of the otosclerotic focus, the signs of cellular reaction and the intensity of the immunohistochemical reactions. Thus, with increasing degrees of sclerosis, weaker reaction products were obtained. Arnold and Friedmann further suggest that genetic predisposition confers a particular susceptibility of the endochondral–periosteal layer to viral infection.

It is difficult to envisage the impact that these contemporary findings may exert on future clinical management of otosclerosis. Stapes footplate fixation represents the end-stage of an active process, and, once established, cannot, therefore, be modified by medical intervention. Systemic steroids may, however, need to be considered as adjunctive therapy with fluorides in the treatment of actively progressive hearing impairment due to cochlear involvement. One may also speculate about the future possibility of vaccination in genetically susceptible individuals with a strong family history of otosclerosis.

CHOLESTEATOMA

Acquired aural cholesteatoma is still an incompletely understood sequel to chronic otitis media. It is characterized by the invasion of keratinizing stratified squamous epithelium into the middle ear, attic or mastoid regions. These sites are aerated in the normal ear, but Eustachian tube obstruction and reduced oxygenation is invariably present in association with cholesteatoma formation. Localized bone absorption is a frequent finding and the disease requires surgical intervention to reduce the risk of progressive tissue destruction, increased functional disability and possible life-threatening intracranial complications.

Acquired aural cholesteatomas arise as sac-like structures in the superior pars flaccida region or the posterosuperior quadrant of the tympanic membrane. The accumulation of debris within the cholesteatoma sac often leads to secondary infection with both aerobic and anaerobic organisms, causing offensive purulent discharge. Histologically, the cholesteatoma wall or matrix consists of a layer of keratinizing stratified squamous epithelium overlying subepithelial connective tissue, which separates the matrix from bone.

The subepithelial region is very vascular and contains an extensive mononuclear chronic inflammatory cell infiltrate, consisting of macrophages, lymphocytes and plasma cells. These mononuclear cells are prevalent at areas of bone resorption. Although multinucleated osteoclasts are primarily responsible for bone resorption in other sites, they can only be identified infrequently in human cholesteatoma[54,55]. However, in cholesteatoma there is a markedly increased number of epidermal Langerhans cells compared with tympanic membrane and ear canal epithelium[55]. Gantz[56] and Veldman[57] have both confirmed this by applying monoclonal antibody staining techniques. These Langerhans cells have relatively prominent endoplasmic reticulum, and increased Golgi apparatus and lysozymes, features reflecting increased secretory activity.

The mesenchymal Langerhans cells are derived from precursor cells which originate in the bone marrow and are known to play an important role in the cutaneous immune surveillance system. They possess similar receptors, Fc-IgG and C3b, as macrophages and are accordingly able to recognize antigen and present it to T lymphocytes as part of the afferent limb of the cutaneous immune response. They are believed to produce lymphokines, lysosomal enzymes and prostaglandins at sites of contact sensitivity, and also interleukin-1[58], and consequently participate in a non-specific effector response to antigen by inducing localized inflammation. The features of lymphocytes in the subepithelial granulation tissue has also been studied using monoclonal antibodies[57,59]. T lymphocytes have been demonstrated in large numbers, indicating that cell-mediated immune mechanisms are active in acquired cholesteatoma. In contrast, B lymphocytes were only rarely found.

The accumulation of keratin debris in the cholesteatoma sac frequently leads to secondary bacterial infection because of stasis. Gantz and Hart[60] have suggested that the immune response is generated against these secondary infective agents and the retained debris in an attempt to eliminate them. This is unfortunately impossible due to the anatomical constraints of the sac matrix, and he further postulates that the continued presence of antigen activates a contact hypersensitivity state (Figure 4). Lymphokine production in the effector limb of the immune response (Figure 5) attracts macrophages, thereby enhancing the local inflammatory response. Further tissue destruction by hydrolytic enzymes potentiates these processes, which readily explain the aggressive local nature of CSOM and cholesteatoma.

ALLOGRAFTS

Tympanic membrane perforation and erosion of middle ear ossicles is a frequent sequel to CSOM with or without cholesteatoma. Ear drum repair and ossicular chain reconstruction is the second priority of contemporary

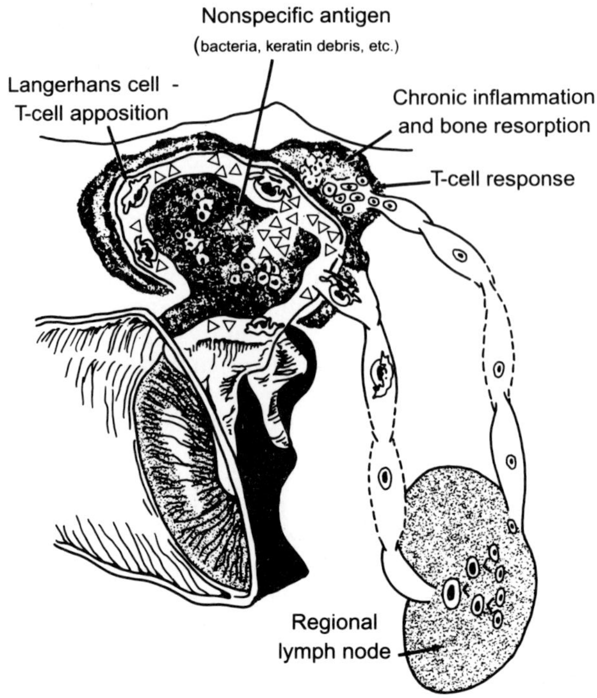

Figure 4 Theoretical immunological mechanisms in acquired cholesteatoma. (From Reference 60)

Inflammatory Reaction

EFFECTOR SYSTEM

T-Lymphocyte —Lymphokine Production→ Macrophage, Osteocyte, Osteoclast —Enzyme Release→ Antigen Elimination

Lysozyme
Neutral Proteases
- Collagenase
- Elastase

Acid Hydrolases
- Acid Phosphatase
- Cathepsins

Arachidonic Acid
- Prostaglandin

↓

Connective Tissue Breakdown
(Bone Resorption)

Figure 5 Effector phase of the cell-mediated immune response in acquired cholesteatoma. (From Reference 61)

Table 2 Effect of current preservation techniques on transplantation antigens in human tympanomeatal and dura mater allografts

	Transplantation antigens	
	Class I	*Class II*
Unpreserved grafts		
Controls	+	+
Preserved grafts		
Freeze-dried	+	+
Cialit	+	+
Alcohol	−	−
Formaldehyde	−	−
Formaldehyde/Cialit	−	−
Glutaraldehyde/Cialit	−	−

From Reference 66

otological surgery after eradication of disease. Numerous materials and reconstructive techniques have been described and, on occasions, lack of suitable host tissues have resulted in the use of allografts.

House et al.[61] introduced the incus allograft, formerly termed 'incus homograft'. These were acquired from the healthy middle ears of patients undergoing translabyrinthine surgery for acoustic neuroma removal. They were preserved in 70% alcohol prior to use, and histological studies on transplanted ossicles removes 9–21 months postoperatively showed no evidence of an associated inflammatory response[62]. Kerr and Smyth[63] examined and compared 19 autografts and alcohol-preserved allografts removed at revision surgery after periods of 3–39 months. Histologically, both allografts and autografts were similar with vascularization and plasma cell infiltration of marrow spaces, together with small areas of new bone formation. They also concluded that there was no evidence of allograft ossicular bone rejection in the middle ear. This apparent absence of overt immune rejection responses to preserved allogenic tissues initially led otologists to believe that the middle ear was a privileged site, where rejection responses did not occur, and/or that tissue allografts were not immunogenic.

Although autologous temporalis fascia is probably the commonest tissue used for tympanic membrane repair, acceptance of these previous conclusions supported the feasibility of using preserved cadaveric dura for ear drum reconstruction, or even autologous composite tympano-ossicular grafts, also obtained from cadavers. Kuijpers and Van Den Broek[64], however, established the antigenicity of allograft tissues, so that scientific attention moved to investigate other factors. Two of the most important features in graft immunogenicity concern the effect of preservation techniques on donor tissue antigens, and the degree of incompatibility of antigens of the HLA major histocompatibility complex (MHC). Veldman and Kuijpers[65] and Frootko[66] have conducted important experimental investigations in these spheres.

Various methods of preservation of grafts have been described (Table 2). Frootko[66] studied the effects of preservation of both human tympanomeatal and dural allografts on HLA or transplantation antigens. The HLA antigens are divided into Class I (HLA-A,B,C) and Class II (HLA–DR), and donor–

recipient incompatibility of these is thought to be responsible for early foreign tissue rejection. Unpreserved and freeze-dried grafts were found to express both Class I and Class II antigens. In both types of graft, transplantation antigens were partially destroyed by Cialit, and appeared to be totally destroyed or altered by alcohol, formaldehyde, formaldehyde–Cialit, and glutaraldehyde–Cialit preservation techniques.

Veldman and Kuijpers[65] studied the immune responses to viable and preserved tympano-ossicular allografts in animal models. Tympanic membrane and ossicular complexes were transplanted into non-sensitized animals and those who had been previously sensitized by donor skin grafting. A plasma cell reaction was seen in the outer cortical region of the draining lymph nodes following implantation of allografts. This immunoblast reaction was more pronounced on viable and formaldehyde-treated specimens. The ossicular transplants showed no signs of graft rejection during the primary response, but transplanted tympanomeatal flaps showed a mononuclear cell infiltration and tissue resorption within 6 weeks, with clear signs of rejection. When animals had been sensitized, a vigorous cell-mediated reaction was observed in the draining lymph nodes.

Frootko[66] explored the possibility that postgrafting myringitis may be an immune-mediated disorder. Myringitis is an inflammatory reaction involving the tympanic membrane which becomes vascular, and may be associated with impaired epithelialization. The thickened tissue is likely to secrete excessive mucus, resulting in persistent otorrhoea and impaired hearing improvement. Myringitis and perforation without apparent cause were observed by Frootko[66] in a small number of patients in whom primary Cialit-preserved dural allografts were used to repair the tympanic membrane, and also in revision cases and when surgery was undertaken to the contralateral ear with the same donor graft tissue. He therefore investigated the donor specific lymphocytotoxic antibody (DSLA) response and the clinical behaviour of primary dural allografts in 40 patients undergoing myringoplasty. All ears were free of infection preoperatively and were subsequently followed up for 6 months. The recipients and single dural donor were tissue typed prior to surgery. A preoperative and 4 month postoperative blood sample was obtained for antibody assays, whilst no attempt was made to select recipients on the basis of tissue compatibility with the donor. Donor splenic lymphocytes were separated into T and B cell types, and subsequently incubated with the recipient sera in turn. DSLAs were demonstrated by a dye exclusion technique.

Myringitis developed in 5 grafts between 3 and 5 weeks postoperatively. Although there was no apparent correlation between DSLA response and graft perforation, there was a statistically significant correlation with the occurrence of myringitis (Table 3). This strongly suggested that myringitis is an immunological rejection phenomenon. These results were independent of the graft preservation technique used, and 85% of these large perforations were successfully repaired despite clear mismatch for both Class I and Class II antigens. The author has never utilized autologous tissues for tympanic membrane grafting, but, nevertheless, myringitis still occurs on occasions. If this just represented a local tissue response to chronic inflammation, one

Table 3 Correlation of graft perforation and myringitis and the production of DSLAs

Donor-specific B-lymphocyte antibodies		*No. cases*	*Perforation*		*Myringitis*	
Preop	*Postop*		*Yes*	*No*	*Yes*	*No*
+	+	3	0	3	0	3
–	+	5	1	4	1	4
–	–	32	5	27	5	1
			$\chi^2 = 0.16$		$\chi^2 = 15.78$	
			$p = \text{NS}$		$p < 0.001$	

From Reference 66

would expect rapid resolution when the local infection had been eradicated. In fact, myringitis frequently becomes chronic, and management often necessitates intensive local toilet and treatment with topical steroids. Occasionally, revision surgery must be undertaken to remove the inflamed tissue before proper healing can take place. Perhaps then, the chronic inflammation sensitizes the individual to develop a secondary 'autoimmune' phenomenon.

Despite these experimental finding, otological grafting of allografts is generally very successful[67]. Veldman and Kuijpers[65] have suggested that a degree of immunotolerance to the remnants of the donor antigens occurs. Nonetheless, it must be appreciated that if a host–graft tissue reaction does occur, and the grafted tympanic membrane becomes a connective tissue scar, it can still fulfil its function as a flexible sound transmitting barrier. Perhaps the fact that the transplanted tissues are surrounded by air also has an inhibitory effect on the in vivo immune mechanisms.

REFERENCES

1. Lim DJ. Functional morphology of the lining membrane of the middle ear and Eustachian tube. Ann Otol Rhinol Laryngol. 1974;80 Suppl 11:1–22.
2. Lim DJ, Bluestone CD, Klein JO, Nelson JD, eds. Recent advances in otitis media with effusion. Philadelphia: BC Becker Inc.; 1985.
3. McGovern JP, Haywood TJ, Fernandes A. Allergy and secretory otitis media. J Am Med Assoc. 1967;200:124–8.
4. Viscomi GJ. Allergic secretory otitis media: an approach to management. Laryngoscope. 1974;85:751–8.
5. Phillips MJ, Knight NJ, Manning H, Abbott AL, Tripp WG. IgE and secretory otitis media. Lancet. 1974;2:1176–8.
6. Bernstein JM, Tomasi TB, Ogra P. The immunochemistry of middle ear effusions. Arch Otolaryngol. 1974;99:320–6.
7. Mogi G, Honjo S, Maeda S, Yoshida T, Watanabe N. Quantitative determination of secretory immunoglobulin A (SIgA) in middle ear effusions. Ann Otol Rhinol Laryngol. 1974;83:239–46.
8. Liu YS, Lim DJ, Lang RW, Birck HG. Chronic middle ear effusions: immunochemical and bacteriological investigation. Arch Otolaryngol. 1975:101:278–86.
9. Juhn SK, Giebink GS, Huff JS, Mills EL. Biochemical and immunochemical characteristics of middle ear effusions in relation to bacteriological findings. Ann Otol Rhinol Laryngol. 1989;89,Suppl 68:161–8.
10. Mogi G, Maeda S, Umehara T, Fujiyoshi T, Kurono Y. Secretory IgA, serum IgA and

secretory component in middle ear effusions. In: Lim DJ, Bluestone CD, Klein JO, Nelson JD, eds. Recent advances in otitis media with effusion. Philadelphia & Toronto: Decker BC; 1985:147–9.

11. Freijd A, Oxelius VA, Rynnel-Dagoo B. A prospective study demonstrating an association between plasma IgG concentrations and susceptibility to otitis media in children. Scand J Infect Dis. 1985;17:115–20.
12. Freijd A, Hammarstrom L, Persson MA, Smith CI. Plasma anti-pneumococcal antibody activity of the IgG class and subclasses in otitis-prone children. Clin Exp Immunol. 1984;56:233–8.
13. Prellner K, Kalm O, Pedersen FK. Pneumococcal antibodies and complement during and after periods of recurrent otitis. Int J Pediatr Otorhinolaryngol. 1984;7:39–49.
14. Siber GR, Schur PH, Aisenberg AC, Weitzman SA, Schiffman G. Correlation between serum IgG_2 concentrations and the antibody response to bacterial polysaccharide antigens. N Engl J Med. 1980;303:178–82.
15. Bernstein JM. Recent advances in immunologic reactivity in otitis media with effusion. J Allergy Clin Immunol., 1988;81:1004–9.
16. Prellner K, Harsen G, Lofgren B et al. Responses to rubella, tetanus and diphtheria vaccines in otitis-prone and non-otitis-prone children. Ann Otol Rhinol Laryngol. 1990;628–32.
17. Jorgensen F, Andersson B, Hanson LA et al. Gamma-globulin treatment of recurrent otitis media in children. Pediatr Infect Dis J. 1990;9:389–94.
18. Richardson VF, Larcher VF, Price JF. A common congenital immunodeficiency predisposing to infection and atopy in infancy. Arch Dis Child. 1983;58:799–802.
19. Super M, Thiel S, Lu J et al. Low levels of mannan binding protein underlay a common defect in opsonization. Lancet. 1989;1:1236.
20. Prellner K. Complement and other amplification mechanisms. In: Bernstein JM, Ogra PL, eds. Immunology of the ear, New York: Raven Press 345–61.
21. Takeuchi K, Saida S, Majima Y, Sakakura Y. The effect of middle ear effusions from children on in-vitro ciliary activity. Eur Arch Otorhinolaryngol. 1990;247:323–5.
22. Palva T, Taskinen E, Hayry P. T lymphocytes in secretory otitis media. In: Veldman JE, McCabe BF, Huizing EH, Mygind N, eds. Immunology, autoimmunity, transplantation in otorhinolaryngology. Amsterdam & Berkeley: Kugler Publications; 1985:45–50.
23. Cauwenberge PV, Plum J, De Smedt M. Analysis of T and B lymphocytes in middle ear effusions of children with OME. In: Immunobiology, histophysiology and tumour immunology in otolaryngology. Proceedings of the 2nd International Academic Conference, Utrecht. Amsterdam/Berkeley: Kugler Publications; 1987:247–52.
24. Ogra PL, Tsutsumi H, Bernstein JM, Okamoto Y, Brodsky L. Influence of immune mechanisms on the natural history of otitis media. In: Immunobiology, histopathology and tumour immunology in otolaryngology. Proceedings of the 2nd International Academic Conference, Utrecht. Amsterdam/Berkeley: Kugler Publications; 1987:235–40.
25. Sarkkinen HK, Halonen PE, Arstila PP et al. Detection of respiratory syncytial, parainfluenza type 2 and adenovirus antigens by radioimmunoassay and enzyme immunoassay on nasopharyngeal specimens from children with acute respiratory disease. J Clin Microbiol. 1981;13:256–65.
26. Chonmaitree T, Howie VM, Truant AL. Presence of respiratory viruses in middle ear fluids with nasal wash specimens from children with otitis media. Paediatrics. 1986;77:698.
27. Catanzaro A, Ryan AF, Robb J. Immune-mediated and non-specific inflammatory events in the middle ear. Clin Immunol Immunopathol. 1982;24:361–76.
28. Ryan AF, Cleveland PH, Hartman MT, Catanzaro A. Humoral and cell-mediated immunity in peripheral blood following introduction of antigen into the middle ear. Ann Otol Rhinol Laryngol. 1982;91:70–5.
29. Ryan AF, Catanzaro A, Wasserman SI, Harris JP. Secondary immune response in the middle ear: physiological, anatomical and immunological observations. Ann Otol Rhinol Laryngol. 1986;95:242–9.
30. Suzuki M, Kawauchi H, Mogi G. Immune-mediated otitis media with effusion. Am J Otolaryngol. 1988;9:199–209.
31. Veltri W, Sprinkle PM. Secretory otitis media: an immune complex disease. Ann Otol Rhinol Laryngol. 1976;85 Suppl 25:135–9.
32. Mravec J, Lewis DM, Lim DJ. Experimental otitis media with effusion: an immune-complex

mediated response. Trans Am Acad Ophthal Otolaryngol ORL. 1978;86:258–68.
33. Palva T, Lehtinen T, Rinne J. Immune complexes in middle ear fluid in chronic secretory otitis media. Ann Otol Rhinol Laryngol. 1983;92:42–4.
34. Bernstein JM, Shenkheim HA, Genco RJ, Bartholomew WR. Complement activity in middle ear effusions. Clin Exp Immunol. 1978;78:120–7.
35. Meri S, Lehtinen T, Palva T. Complement in chronic secretory otitis media. Arch Otolaryngol. 1984;110:774–8.
36. Watanabe N, Yoshimura H, Mogi G. Induction of antigen-specific-IgA forming cells in the middle ear mucosa. Arch Otolaryngol Head Neck Surg. 1988;114:758–62.
37. Larrson A. Otosclerosis. A genetic and clinical study. Acta Otolaryngol (Stockh). 1960;Suppl 154:1–86.
38. Morrison AW. Genetic factors in otosclerosis. Ann R Coll Surg. 1967;41:202–37.
39. Wayoff M, Chobaut JC, Raffoux C, Bertrand D. Systeme HLA et otospongiose. J Fr Otolaryngol. 1979;28:299–301.
40. Gregoriadis S, Zerras J, Varletzidis E, Toubis M, Pantazopoulos P, Fessas P. HLA antigens and otosclerosis. Arch Otolaryngol. 1982;108:769–71.
41. Majsky A, Novotny Z, Fajstarr Y. HLA antigens and otosclerosis. Tissue Antigens. 1982;20:306–7.
42. Dahlqvist A, Diamant H, Dahlqvist S, Cedergren B. HLA antigens in patients with otosclerosis. Acta Otolaryngol (Stockh). 1985;100:33–5.
43. Anson BJ, Bast TH. The temporal bone and the ear. Springfield, IL: Charles C. Thomas; 1949.
44. Nager GF. Histopathology of otosclerosis. Arch Otolaryngol. 1969;89:341–63.
45. Arnold W, Plester DW. Vascular degeneration in otosclerosis and its influence on the mesenchymal reaction of the mucoperiosteum. Arch Otol Rhinol Laryngol. 1975;209: 127–43.
46. Lim DJ, Robinson M, Saunders WH. Morphologic and immunohistochemical observation of otosclerotic stapes. Am J Otolaryngol. 1987;8:282–95.
47. Yoo TJ, Stuart JM, Kong AH, Townes AS, Tomada K, Dixit S. Type II collagen autoimmunity in otosclerosis and Meniere's disease. Science. 1982;217:1153–5.
48. Huang C-C, Saporta D, Abramson M. Type II collagen-induced bone resorption in the temporal bone of rats: histological and immunohistochemical studies. Arch Otorhinolaryngol. 1985;242:183–8.
49. Bretlau P, Balle V, Causse JB, Horsley-Petersen K, Sorensen CH, Solvsteen M. Is otosclerosis an autoimmune disease? In: Immunobiology, histophysiology and tumour immunology in otolaryngology. Proceedings of the 2nd International Academic Conference. Amsterdam: Kugler Publications; 1986:201–6.
50. Harris JP, Woolf NK, Ryan AF. A re-examination of experimental Type II collagen autoimmunity: middle and inner ear morphology and function. Ann Otol Rhinol Laryngol. 1986;95:176–80.
51. Schrader M, Poppendieck J, Plester D. Autoimmunologic aspects of otosclerosis. In: Immunobiology, histophysiology and tumour immunology in otolaryngology. Proceedings of the 2nd International Academic Conference, Utrecht. Amsterdam, Berkeley: Kugler Publications; 1987:433–4.
52. Arnold W, Friedmann I. Otosclerosis – an inflammatory disease of the otic capsule of viral aetiology? J Laryngol Otol. 1988;102:865–71.
53. McKenna MJ, Mills GB, Galey FR, Linthicum FH. Filamentous structures morphologically similar to viral nucleocapsids in otosclerotic lesions in two patients. Am J Otolaryngol. 1986;7:25–8.
54. Gantz BJ, Maynard J. Ultrastructural evaluation of the biochemical events of bone resorption in human chronic otitis media. Am J Otol. 1982;3:279–83.
55. Lim D, Saunders W. Acquired cholesteatomas. Ann Otol Rhinol Laryngol. 1972;81:1–12.
56. Gantz BJ. Epidermal Langerhans cells in cholesteatoma. Ann Otol Rhinol Laryngol. 1984;93:150–6.
57. Veldman JE. The Langerhans T-cell microenvironment in aural cholesteatoma. In: Veldman J, Huizing B, Mygind E, eds. Immunobiology, autoimmunity, transplantation in otorhinolaryngology. Amsterdam: Kugler Publications; 1985:69–79.
58. Sauder DN, Dinarello CA, Morhenn VB. Langerhans cell production of interleukin-1. J

Invest Dermatol. 1984;82:605–7.
59. Veldman JE, Van Dijk CM, Visser CE, Huizing EH. Aural cholesteatoma and immunity. In: Veldman JE, McCabe BF, eds. Otoimmunology. Amsterdam/Berkeley: Kugler Publications; 1987:69–79.
60. Gantz BJ, Hart MJ. Immunobiology of acquired aural cholesteatoma. In: Bernstein J, Ogra P, eds. Immunology of the ear. New York: Raven Press; 1987:391–402.
61. House WF, Patterson ME, Linthicum FH. Incus homografts in chronic ear surgery. Arch Otolaryngol. 1966;84:148–53.
62. Linthicum FH. Post-operative temporal bone histopathology. Laryngoscope. 1966;76: 1232–41.
63. Kerr AG, Smyth GDL. The fate of transplanted ossicles. J Laryngol Otol. 1971;85:337–47.
64. Kuijpers W, Van Den Broek P. Biological considerations for the use of homograft tympanic membranes and ossicles. Acta Otolaryngol. 1975;80:283–93.
65. Veldman JE, Kuijpers W. Antigenicity of tympano-ossicular homografts of the middle ear: analyses of immune response to viable and preserved grafts in animal models. Otolaryngol Head Neck Surg. 1981;89:142–52.
66. Frootko NJ. Immune responses in allograft tympanoplasty. In: Immunology, autoimmunity and transplantation in otorhinolaryngology. Proceedings of the 1st International Conference, Utrecht. Amsterdam: Kugler Publications; 1985:171–6.
67. Marquet J. Ten years experience in tympanoplasty using homologous implants. J Laryngol Otol. 1976;90:897–905.
68. Shimada T, Lim DJ. Distribution of ciliated cells in the human middle ear: electron and light microscopic observations. Ann Otol Rhinol Laryngol. 1972;81:203–11.
69. Mogi G. Experimental otitis media with effusion. Immunobiology, histophysiology and tumour immunology in otolaryngology. Proceedings of the 2nd International Academic Conference, Utrecht. Amsterdam/Berkeley: Kugler Publications; 1987:253–63.

13
Future Prospects for Immunological Involvement in ENT Disorders

G. K. SCADDING

INTRODUCTION

From the previous chapters, the contributions which immunological knowledge has made to the understanding, diagnosis and treatment of ENT disorders can be assessed. It is possible, even likely, that, over the next few decades, immunological methods will provide greater input into this sphere.

ALLERGIC RHINITIS

At present, the major focus of attention is upon the development of safer 'third-generation' corticosteroids with little or no gut absorption and extensive first-pass metabolism, for use in rhinitis and asthma[1]. There is a group of patients who do not show any response to corticosteroids, even when used orally. Recently, steroid-resistant genes have been identified in such patients, opening up possibilities for therapy.

In addition, the effects of antagonism or inhibitors of synthesis of various individual mediators, such as leukotrienes, platelet activating factor (PAF) and bradykinin[2], are currently being investigated. It is conceivable that a 'cocktail' of mediator inhibitors could prove therapeutically useful with minimal or no side-effects. Such a 'cocktail' could be tailored to individual needs by keeping each preparation separate.

Immunotherapy

Classical hyposensitization, although little practised in the UK at present, is still under investigation as a mode of treatment for those patients who fail to respond to conventional therapy. Other routes of allergen administration (oral, sublingual, nasal) have been tried but without great success. The use of very low doses, and even of homeopathic doses, will probably receive further attention in the United Kingdom. In the USA, limiting dilution desensitization, in which the dose of allergen which just fails to elicit a response when tested intradermally is chronically administered, is recognized as a treatment for allergic rhinitis. However its effectiveness has not been demonstrated sufficiently convincingly for generalized use here.

Liposomes for immunotherapy

The observation that specific IgE responses may be significantly lower with liposome adjuvants than with alum has been made independently in two different laboratries using different immunization schedules[3]. The mechanism underlying the adjuvant effect of liposomes is not clear. Allergen administered in liposomes is retained in the tissues for longer periods to be phagocytosed by the reticuloendothelial system. The route of entry seems to be important in determining antibody isotypes evolved: marked enhancement of IgA responses have been reported following ingestion of antigen in liposomes. Encapsulation of allergen by the liposomes seems likely to reduce activation of mast cells and basophils. Allergens are, by their very nature, soluble in aqueous solution and should be highly suitable for such encapsulation. Unfortunately, there is a tendency for the vesicles to aggregate and fuse on standing but recent technical advances are helping to overcome this problem. It seems that the use of liposomes should be considered in immunotherapy.

There is a possibility that immunization with a decapeptide sequence within the CH4 domain of human IgE may help to prevent mast cell degranulation in response to allergen exposure[4]. An antiserum obtained by immunizing rabbits with this decapeptide conjugated to keyhole limpet haemocyanin (KLH) was shown to inhibit histamine release from rat mast cells both in vitro and in vivo. Immunization of sensitized rats with the same peptide reduced IgE antibody formation and serum histamine concentration and abolished systemic anaphylactic reactions in response to allergen challenge. Further experiments are in progress with a view to eventual testing in man. If feasible, this approach would have the great advantage that a single type of injection would work in all allergic patients, regardless of their allergen sensitivity.

At present, the major focus of immunological attention is upon the T cell and upon cytokines which appear to exert control over IgE production. Various strategies have been proposed to prevent sensitization to allergens by immunological attack at the T cell–macrophage level of antigen presentation[5] (Figure 1). Immunogenic peptides from the major cat allergen, Ferl d1, which react with T cells, have been identified in vitro. Animal experiments are in progress and a trial in allergic subjects is planned. Recently, a trial of cyclosporin has been undertaken in patients with steroid-dependent asthma; this showed beneficial results. There are other T cell immunomodulators which are likely to be tested shortly.

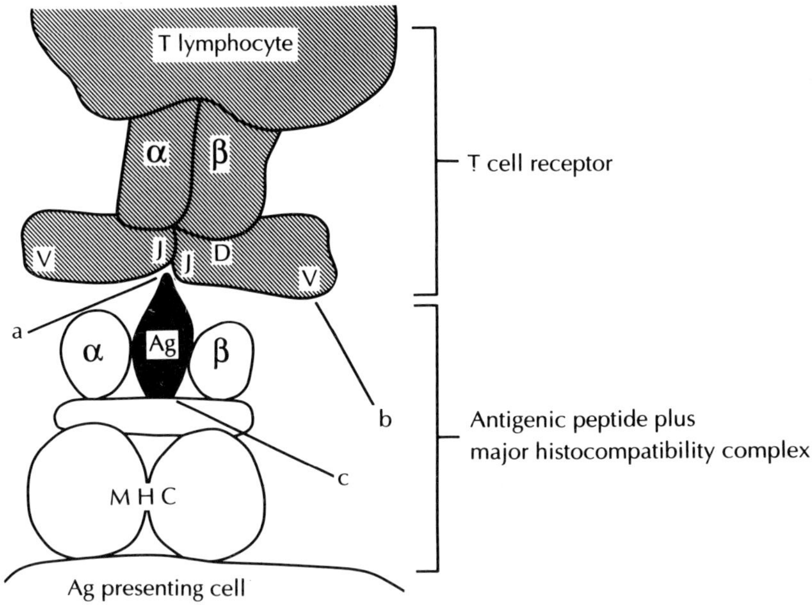

Figure 1 Diagrammatic representation of the ternary complex between the T cell receptor MHC Class II molecule and a peptide fragment of antigen. a, b and c are possible sites for inhibition of this reaction. Functional inactivation of individual clones of specific T cells (a), or subsets of T cells of different specificities, but expressing T cell receptors with shared characteristics (b) are possible. Alternatively (c), there could be displacement of 'disease-related' determinants from the antigen-combining site of MHC molecules by a non-stimulatory peptide. α and β in the shaded area are subunits of the T cell receptor. V = variable region, J = joining region, D = diversity region of the T cell receptor. Ag = antigen; MHC = major histocompatibility complex; α and β in the unshaded area are subunits of the MHC molecule. (After O'Hehir and Lamb, Clinical Experimental Allergy. 1992;22:7–11[5], with permission of Blackwell Scientific Publications.)

Cytokines are low-molecular-weight polypeptides produced by cells which act locally on the cells themselves or upon other nearby cells. They are short-lived and highly potent, being produced in response to induction signals and active via high-affinity cell-surface receptors, to effect cell growth and/or differentiation. Antibodies to relevant cytokines, such as IL-4, GM–CSF, and those to adhesion molecules, such as ICAM-1, are at present under trial in vitro and in animal systems. Future trials in asthma and rhinitis are awaited.

Genetic research into atopy could prove promising. A gene recently identified on chromosome 11 by Hopkin and colleagues[6] as being responsible for IgE responsiveness is under further investigation by other groups. As yet, there is no confirmation but, if this observation is confirmed and the relevant gene products identified, then a very basic attack on atopy at the genetic level could be mounted.

CHRONIC ENT INFECTIONS

Although anatomical factors undoubtedly underlie many cases of recurrent infection and are amenable to surgical intervention, there remains a group of patients who are not helped by operation. Some of these suffer from the defects outlined in Chapter 1: ciliary dyskinesia, mucus abnormalities, hypo-γ-globulinaemia or immunoglobulin subclass deficiencies. At present, of these, only the secondary ciliary dyskinesias and the immunoglobulin deficiencies are treatable, by removing the primary cause and by replacement therapy respectively. Although the latter undoubtedly improves the quality of life, it may not prove curative, especially if there have been several years of chronic infection prior to diagnosis. Unravelling of the cause of defective immunoglobulin production and treatment at this level would probably prove more satisfactory as well as obviating the need for transfer of blood products.

Even when patients with the above conditions are identified, there remains a group of sufferers from chronic infection, such as sinusitis, without any obvious underlying cause. It is likely that a proportion of these have a subtle immunological deficiency. Possibly this represents a defect in their antibody repertoire towards a specific micro-organism. With improved and simplified tests, it should be possible to detect defective specific immune responses to relevant pathogens and to organize either specific replacement (see designer antibodies) or vaccination in such a way that the immune system is enabled to respond protectively.

In some individuals, persistent infection of sinuses and/or bronchi is with organisms of low virulence which are not cleared because they exert adverse effects upon the mucociliary escalator[7]. The continued recruitment of inflammatory cells leads to local damage by neutrophil enzymes and potentiates the situation. Under these circumstances, immunosuppression may be helpful with or without continued low-dose antibiotics which can decrease the production of molecules harmful to cilia. Selective reduction of neutrophil influx by antiadhesion molecules may be a possible therapeutic option.

The formation of nasal polyps may occur under the influence of one or two major cytokines; if identified, then specific designer antibodies (vide infra) may prove helpful.

The minor immunological abnormalities found in children with recurrent otitis media may be amenable to treatment. If lack of mannan-binding protein is confirmed as a common deficiency, the effect of its replacement could be assessed. If significantly helpful, its eventual production on a large scale, e.g. in genetically altered sheep, would seem a possibility. It is of course much easier to replace a single protein than to replace antibodies of a particular class or subclass since these represent millions of different molecules.

Mucus

Abnormalities of mucus represent a largely unexplored area. There are several genes responsible for mucus production and it is hoped that the human genome project will lead to further information about these. The gene

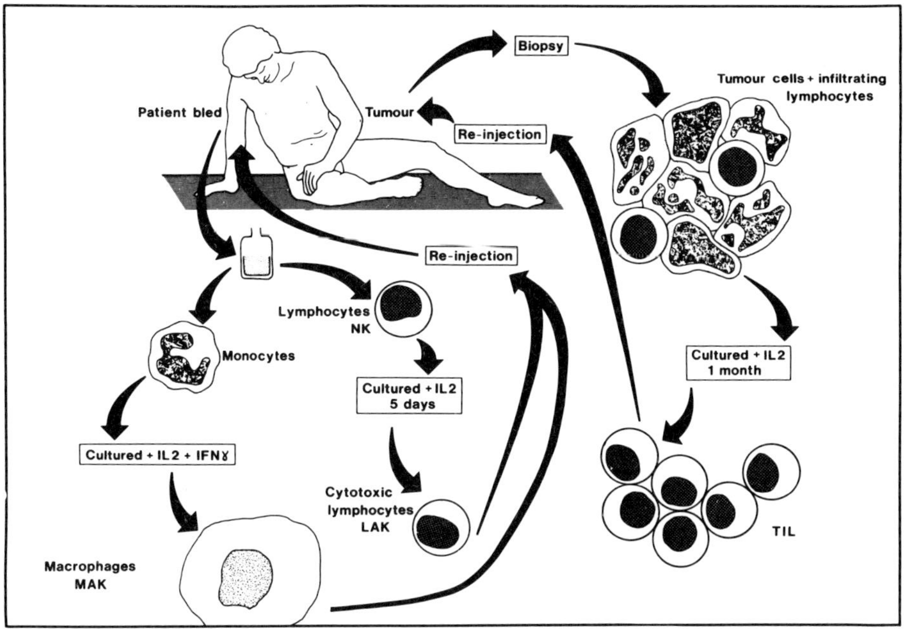

Figure 2 Enhancement of the immunological response to tumours is now being attempted by various means. Lymphocytes removed in biopsy samples are separated and cultured together with IL-2 in vitro for a month to increase their numbers and cause activation prior to re-injection at the tumour site. Alternatively, mononuclear cells can be separated from blood and then activated during 5-day in-vitro culture by addition of IL-2 (lymphocytes) or IL-2 plus interferon (monocytes). This results in the generation of killer cells which can then be reinjected

responsible for cystic fibrosis (cystic fibrosis transmembrane conductance regulator) was cloned in 1988 and the major mutation in white people, ΔF508, was characterized[8]. Attempts to insert a normal gene into the airways via a microbiological carrier will begin shortly.

MALIGNANCIES OF EAR, NOSE AND THROAT

Sadly, the prognoses of many malignant conditions of the upper respiratory tract remain poor despite advances in surgery and radiotherapy. Until recently, tumour-specific antigens and tumour immunotherapy have proved rather disappointing fields, but newer methods of treatment are beginning to show promise[9–11]. Figure 2 shows the basis for some of these.

Cytokine therapy is also proving useful in some cancer fields[12], e.g. interferon induces long-term remission in hairy cell leukaemia.

DESIGNER ANTIBODIES

Kohler and Milstein[13] showed eighteen years ago that individual murine B cells could be immortalized by fusing them with a myeloma cell line. The millions of identical monoclonal antibodies generated by this hybridoma technology have proved to be highly specific reagents for detecting many molecules of biological interest and have greatly enhanced the power and scope of laboratory diagnosis. Their therapeutic promise for the treatment of cancer, infection and autoimmunity has never been realized. One major reason is that murine antibodies have a short half-life in man, are themselves immunogenic, and are unable to recruit human effector functions, such as cytotoxicity. The development of human monoclonal antibodies would solve these problems, but they are difficult to produce. Human B cell lines tend to lose antibody production after a short time. Also, many therapeutically necessary target antigens are not recognized by the human immune system, being ignored as self-antigens.

One solution has been to 'humanize' murine monoclonal antibodies genetically, transplanting their antigen-binding sites onto human antibody frameworks[14]. There are several antibodies which have been 'grafted' in this way and whose therapeutic potential will soon be tested in humans. Included amongst these are antibodies to the lymphocyte antigens, CD4 and CD25, which could be used to suppress unwanted immune responses; antibodies against viruses, such as respiratory syncytial virus (RSV) and herpes simplex, and an antibody to epidermal growth factor receptor which has anticancer and possibly antipolyp potential.

A newer technology for rapidly producing human antibodies is emerging. This was made possible by several developments: firstly, the demonstration that the heavy and light chain variable domains (V_HV_L) on the antibody expressed in bacteria could join correctly to form a functional antibody fragment[15]. Secondly, the polymerase chain reaction (PCR) was found to be effective in cloning antibody gene libraries from pools of human B lymphocytes[16]. This permits easy access to the entire current antibody gene repertoire of a human. The third development was that of phage antibodies[17]. These genetically engineered bacteriophage particles contain antibody genes and display the corresponding antibody fragment on their surface. The relevant phage can be detected using antigen to bind to this surface antibody. It can then be used to infect bacteria which become phage 'factories' producing up to 10^{13} phage particles per litre of culture supernatant. The antibody genes can then be rescued and used to produce soluble antibody fragments or even complete antibodies.

In the past year, phage antibody libraries have been constructed using antibody genes derived from immunized mice or HIV-infected humans and have provided antibodies reactive with the immunizing antigens. Recently, a human phage antibody library has been constructed from the antibody genes of two healthy non-immunized blood donors and has already yielded antibodies to several antigens, raising the possibility of automated production of human antibodies. During construction of this library, the V_H and V_L genes were recombined randomly, thus creating new artificial antibodies not represented in the population of human B cells from which the genes were derived. These may be more likely to recognize human cell components, as B cells with this property are generally deleted or suppressed by the intact immune system. Many cancer 'antigens' and most targets for antibody-mediated immunosuppression (lymphocyte surface markers and circulating cytokines) fall into the category of self. This phage library may therefore be a richer source of therapeutically useful antibodies than any previously available. Antibodies to human immunoglobulin and to human tumour necrosis factor (TNF) have already been derived in this way. Thus, phage antibody libraries are a potentially limitless source of readily available human antibodies against many desirable molecular targets. Amongst these must be cytokines involved in the induction of the allergic response, such as GM-CSF as well as tumour antigens. The library could also prove a source of antibody to specific bacteria which is not available to certain individuals because of a B cell repertoire defect.

There are thus many possibilities for immunological help in ENT disorders, including immunological, infective and malignant, over the next few years. It is to be hoped that at least some of these will be realized.

REFERENCES

1. Harding SM. Human pharmacology of fluticasone. Allergologie. 1989;12:77,Abs. 04 04.
2. Austin CE, Foreman JC, Scadding GK. [D-Arg^0,Hyp^3,Thi^5,D- Tic^7,Oic^8]-bradykinin is an effective bradykinin antagonist in the human nasal airway. British Pharmacological Society Meeting Abstract, Rome, 1993.
3. Walls AF. Liposomes for allergy immunotherapy? Clin Exp Allergy. 1992;22:3–6.
4. Stanworth DR, Jones VM, Lewin IV, Nayyar S. Allergy treatment wit a peptide vaccine. Lancet. 1990;336:1279–81.
5. O'Hehir RE, Lamb JR. Strategies for modulating IgE synthesis. Clin Exp Allergy. 1992;22: 7–10.
6. Cookson W, Sharp PA, Faux JA, Hopkin J. Linkage between immunoglobulin E responses underlying asthma and rhinitis and chromosome 11q. Lancet. 1989;1:1292–5.
7. Cole PJ. Host–microbe relationships in chronic respiratory disease. In: Reeves D, Geddes AM, eds. Recent advances in infection. Edinburgh: Churchill Livingstone; 1989:141–51.
8. Riordan JR, Rommens JM, Kerem B-S, Alon N, Rozmahel R, Grzelczak Z et al. Identification of the cystic fibrosis gene: cloning and characteristics of complementary DNA. Science. 1989;245:1066–73.
9. Steuer MK, Matthias R, Schulze C, Brusw T. Intralesional therapy with natural interferon B in refractory squamous epithelial cancer of the ENT area. Laryngorhinootologie. 1992;71:618–25.
10. Clayman GL, Young G, Taylor DL, Savage HE, Lavedan P, Schantz SP. Detection of regulatory factors of lymphokine activated killer cell activity in head and neck cancer patients treated with interleukin-2 and interferon alpha. Ann Otol-Rhinol-Laryngol. 1992;101:909–15.
11. Gore ME, Riches P, Mallennan K et al. Phase I study of intra-arterial interleukin-2 in squamous cell carcinoma of the head and neck. Br J Cancer. 1992;66:405–7.
12. Mann EA, Spiro JD, Chen LL, Kreutzer DL. Cytokine expression by head and neck squamous cell carcinomas. Am J Surg. 1992;164:567–73.
13. Kohler G, Milstein G. Continuous culture of fused cells secreting antibody of predefined specificity. Nature. 1975;256:495–7.
14. Jones PT, Dear PH, Foote J, Neuberger MJ, Winter G. Replacing the complementary-determining regions in a human antibody with those from a mouse. Nature. 19986;321:522–5.
15. Skerra A, Pluckthün A. Assembly of a functional immunoglobulin Fc fragment in Escherichia coli. Science. 1988;240:1038–41.
16. Orlandi R, Gusson DH, Jones PT, Winter G. Cloning immunoglobulin variable domains expression by the polymerase chain reaction. Proc Natl Acad Sci USA. 1989;86:3833–7.
17. McCafferty J, Griffiths AD, Winter G, Chiswell DJ. Phage antibodies: filamentous phage displaying antibody variable domains. Nature. 1990;348:552–4.

Immunology and Medicine Series

1. A.M. McGregor (ed.). *Immunology of Endocrine Diseases.* 1986 ISBN: 0-85200-963-1
2. L. Ivanyi (ed.). *Immunological Aspects of Oral Diseases.* 1986 ISBN: 0-85200-961-5
3. M.A.H. French (ed.). *Immunoglobulins in Health and Disease.* 1986 ISBN: 0-85200-962-3
4. K. Whaley (ed.). *Complement in Health and Disease.* 1987 ISBN: 0-85200-954-2
5. G.R.D. Catto (ed.). *Clinical Transplantation: Current Practice and Future Prospects.* 1987 ISBN: 0-85200-960-7
6. V.S. Byers and R.W. Baldwin (ed.). *Immunology of Malignant Diseases.* 1987 ISBN: 0-85200-964-X
7. S.T. Holgate (ed.). *Mast Cells, Mediators and Disease.* 1988 ISBN: 0-85200-968-2
8. D.J.M. Wright (ed.). *Immunology of Sexually Transmitted Diseases.* 1988 ISBN: 0-74620-087-0
9. A.D.B. Webster (ed.). *Immunodeficiency and Disease.* 1988 ISBN: 0-85200-688-8
10. C. Stern (ed.). *Immunology of Pregnancy and its Disorders.* 1989 ISBN: 0-7462-0065-X
11. M.S. Klempner, B. Styrt and J. Ho (ed.). *Phagocytes and Disease.* 1989 ISBN: 0-85200-842-2
12. A.J. Zuckerman (ed.). *Recent Developments in Prophylactic Immunization.* 1989 ISBN: 0-7923-8910-7
13. S. Lightman (ed.). *Immunology of Eye Disease.* 1989 ISBN: 0-7923-8908-5
14. T.J. Hamblin (ed.). *Immunotherapy of Disease.* 1990 ISBN: 0-7462-0045-5
15. D.B. Jones and D.H. Wright (eds.). *Lymphoproliferative Diseases.* 1990 ISBN: 0-85200-965-8
16. C.D. Pusey (ed.). *Immunology of Renal Diseases.* 1991 ISBN: 0-7923-8964-6
17. A.G. Bird (ed.). *Immunology of HIV Infection.* 1991 ISBN: 0-7923-8962-X
18. J.T. Whicher and S.W. Evans (eds.). *Biochemistry of Inflammation.* 1992 ISBN: 0-7923-8985-9
19. T.T. MacDonald (ed.). *Immunology of Gastrointestinal Diseases.* 1992 ISBN: 0-7923-8961-1
20. K. Whaley, M. Loos and J.M. Weiler (eds.). *Complement in Health and Disease, 2nd Edn.* 1993 ISBN: 0-7923-8823-2
21. H.C. Thomas and J. Waters (eds.). *Immunology of Liver Disease.* 1994 ISBN: 0-7923-8975-1
22. G.S. Panayi (ed.). *Immunology of Connective Tissue Diseases.* 1994 ISBN: 0-7923-8988-3
23. G. Scadding (ed.). *Immunology of ENT Disorders.* 1994 ISBN: 0-7923-8914-X
24. R. Hohlfeld (ed.). *Immunology of Neuromuscular Disease.* 1994 ISBN: 0-7923-8844-5
25. J.G.P. Sissons, L.K. Borysiewicz and J. Cohen (eds.). *Immunology of Infection.* 1994 ISBN: 0-7923-8968-9

Index

ACTH, synthetic 100
adenoidectomy 55
adenoma of middle ear 77
AIDS, fungal infections associated 61
allergic response in nose 100
allergic rhinitis 93–114, 117–21
  clinical effects 106–7
    augmentation of response 107
    chronic problems 107
  diagnosis 107–8
    nasal challenge 108
    nasal sinuses 108
    skin prick testing 108
  environmental factors 96–7
  eosinophil involvement 102–3
  food-induced 118–21
    acute 118–19
    crossreacting antibodies 118–19
    delayed reaction 120–1
    diagnostic tests 119
    histamine 118
    histamine-releasing factors 118
  immunotherapy 217–19
    liposomes for 218–19
  late-phase responses 105
  mechanisms 93–5
  prospects 217–19
  T cell involvement 101–2
  treatment 108–13
    allergic avoidance 109
    during pregnancy 113
    immunotherapy 112
    pharmacotherapy 112
    surgery 113
allergy 154–5
alopecia areata 63
anaphylotoxins 14–15, 100
angiofibroma (juvenile nasopharyngeal angiofibroma) 83
angiotensin converting enzymes 145
antibodies
  designer 221–3
  diversity generation 24
    heavy chain constant region genes 26
    heavy chain variable region genes 26
    light chain genes 25
  functions 22 (table), 24
  murine 222
  phage 222
    libraries 222–3
antibody–antigen interactions 26–7
antigen-specific lymphocyte transformation test 181
antihistamines, non-sedating 112
antineutrophil cytoplasmic antibodies (ANCA) 79, 125–7, 129
aphthous ulceration 39–40
apoptosis (programmed cell death) 9
arachidonic acid metabolites 159
aspergilloma 65–7
aspergillosis 58 (table), 64
  acute invasive 66–9
    tropical 68–9
  chronic necrotizing 66
  paranasal sinuses 65–9
    hypersensitivity aspergillosis 66
    invasive aspergillosis 66–9
  pulmonary 59, 66
Aspergillus spp. 35, 41, 42, 60
  spores 60
Aspergillus niger 57
aspirin sensitivity 113–14, 154
asthma
  nasal polyps associated 154
  steroid-resistant 102
atopy 96
  genes 219
azelastine 112

bacterial culture from nose/paranasal sinuses 156 (table)
basophils 6, 100

degranulation 100
B cell 16, 17–18, 46
homing 47
IgE production 98
immature 47
null cells 18–19
Behçet disease 191–2
benign paragangliomatous tumour 90
betamethasone nose drops 109–10
blastomycosis 58
bone marrow suppressive drugs 35
bradykinin 105
bronchoalveolar lavage 138–9
Bruton's disease 53
Burkitt's lymphoma 42

C3b 10
C5a 100
calcitrol 139
cancer patients, acute invasive aspergillosis in 68
candidiasis 34, 41, 57, 58 (table)
chronic mucocutaneous 63
oesophageal 63
orophalangeal 36, 62–3
predisposing factors 62 (table)
severe resistant 36
superficial 58 (table)
carcinoid tumours 77, 89
catalase 59
cationic proteins 60
CD23 98–9
cerebral tissue 'tumours' 80
chemotaxins 6
childhood allergic diseases, environmental factors 97 (table)
cholesteatoma 108–9, 210 (fig.)
chordoma 83–4
chromomycosis 58 (table)
chronic ENT infections 219–20
Churg–Strauss syndrome 130 (table)
coccidioidomycosis 58
codeine 100
Cogan's syndrome 191
collagenase 10
complement 11–16
alternating pathway 11–12
factor B 11
factor D 11
properdin 11
components (C1–C9) 11–15
C3, C3bi deficiency 14
defence against infection 15
immune response induction 15
in inflammation 14–15
phagocytosis action 15
proteolytic fragments 12
serine proteases 12
conidiobolomycosis 57, 58 (table)
connective tissue diseases 188–92
corticosteroids 109, 110
cryptococcal meningitis 42
cryptococciosis 58
Cryptococcus 34, 35
Cryptococcus neoformans 60
cryptosporidiosis 34
cyclosporin 102, 218
cystic fibrosis 152, 153
cytokines 52, 105–6, 159–60, 218, 219, 223
cytomegalovirus 34
cytotoxic proteinase 11

Dandy's syndrome (idiopathic bilateral labrynthine failure) 181
delayed endolymphatic hydrops 186–8
Dermatophagoides pteronyssinus 93
dermatophytoses 57, 58 (table), 63–4
designer antibodies 221–3
diabetes mellitus 66
in rabbit 60
diseases with autoimmune markers 182
double-blind placebo-controlled food challenge 119
dynein 3
dysglobulinaemia 53

elastase 11
embryonal rhabdomyosarcoma 83
encephalocele 80
endothelial leukocyte adhesive molecule 6
enzyme-linked immunoabsorbent assay (ELISA) 182
eosinophil 6, 102–3, 105
eosinophil chemotactic factor 105
epithelium, nasal 2–4
ciliated cells 2–4
non-ciliated cells 4
epithelium, respiratory 2
Epstein–Barr virus 36
Escherichia coli 35

Fab antibody fragments 50
factor VIII-related antigen 76
Fc antibody fragments 50
fatty acids, medium chain 59
formyl-methionyl-leucyl-phenylalanine 6
functional dysgammaglobulinaemia 34
fungal infections 57–69
deep invasive 57
host defence 59 (table), 59–61
innate 59–61
immune defence 61
antibody 61
cell mediated immunity 61
leukocyte attraction 60
pathogenesis 58–9
subcutaneous 57

superficial 57

gingivo-stomatitis 40
glioma 80
β-glucan 9
granuloma cell tumour ('myoblastoma') 89
granulocyte 5–6
gustatory rhinitis 120

Haemophilus influenzae 41
hairy oral leukoplakia 36–8
heat shock proteins 6
herpes virus infection of larynx 86
herpes virus type-6 34
histaminases 159
histamine 103, 104, 158–9
sensitivity 107
histoplasmosis 34, 35, 41, 42, 58 (table)
HMB-45 marker 80
Hodgkin's disease 55
Hodgkin's tumour 42
human immunodeficiency virus-1 31–42
clinical consequences 34–6
changing patterns 35–6
infections 34–6
due to non-HIV related immunosuppression 35
tumours 34
cryptococcal meningitis 42
eczema 10
epistaxis 41
gingivo-stomatitis 40
hairy cell leukoplakia 36–8
immunopathogenesis 32–4
laryngeal nerve paralysis 42
nasal tumours 41
nasopharyngeal fungal infection associated 42
nasopharyngeal lymphadenopathy 41
nasopharyngeal tumours 42
oropharyngeal candidiasis associated 36
otitis media 42
paediatric disease 34
sinusitis 40
opportunistic infections 41
structure 31–2
viral replication 31–2
human immunodeficiency virus-2 31
human leukocyte antigens 192–3
human papilloma virus 86
5-, 12- and 15-hydroxyeicosatetraenoic acid (HETE) 159
hypergammaglobulinaemia 41
hypersensitivity diseases 63–4

idiopathic bilateral labyrinthine failure (Dandy's syndrome) 181
immotile cilial syndrome (Kartegener's syndrome) 154
immune complexes 6
immune deficiency 26–7, 52–3
immune system cells 5–9
immunity 1
non-specific 2–16
specific 16–26
immunochemical staining techniques 75–6
alkaline phosphatase-anti-alkaline phosphatase 76
avidin biotin method 75–6
peroxidase antiperoxidase method 75
immunocytochemistry 73–90
immunoglobulins 19–20
antibody 22–3
heavy chain 19–20
IgA 21–22
deficiency 52–3
MALT lymphocyte secretion 45–51
polymeric 49
secretory 49
IgA_1 49, 50
IgA_2 49, 50
IgD 23
cells producing 51–2
IgE 24, 95–6, 100
allergen-specific 158
binding factors 97
cell-bound 158
clone 88
in nasal polyp oedema fluid 156, 158
production control 97–8
receptor 10
IgG 13, 20, 51, 52
IgG_1 13
IgG_3 13
IgG_4 13
light chain 19–20
structure 19–20
immunological methods in diagnostic histopathology 74–5
immunological response to tumours enhancement 221 (fig.)
immunotherapy 112
immunological changes during 112 (table)
incus homograft 210–11
infection, cause of increased susceptibility 27 (table)
infectious mononucleosis 84
inner ear 169–94
anatomy 169–72
autoimmune disease 176–84
clinical features 180–1
genetics 192–4
investigations 181–2
pathophysiology 176–80
types I–IV 178–80
treatment 182–4

immunology 172–6
experimental studies 173–6
physiology 169–72
α-interferon 52
γ-interferon 61, 97, 98
interleukin-4 97–8
intermediate filament proteins 76

jugulotympanic paraganglioma 77–8
juvenile nasopharyngeal angiofibroma (angiofibroma) 83

kallidin 105
Kaposi's sarcoma 37 (fig.), 38–9, 41
auricular 42
nasopharyngeal 42
ulcerative 39–40
Kartagener's syndrome (immotile cilial syndrome) 154
kinines 104–5
Klebsiella spp. 35
Kveim test 145

lactoferrin 16
Langerhans cells 46–7, 48 (fig.)
laryngeal infections 86
laryngeal nerve paralysis 42
laryngeal squamous carcinoma 86–8
late-phase responders 105
Legionella pneumophilus 41
Leishmania 35
leukaemia, acute invasive aspergillosis in 68
leukocyte-function-associated molecules 7
leukotrienes
B_4 105
C_4 104
D_4 104
lipopolysaccharides 6
liposomes 218–19
low salicylate diet 114 (table)
lymphocyte 16–19
activation 19
B cell *see* B cell
MALT *see* MALT lymphocytes
T cell *see* T cell
tonsillar 46–7
lymphocyte inhibition test 181
lymphoid system 45–6
primary organs 45–6
secondary organs 45 (table), 46
lymphoma 41
malignant *see* malignant lymphoma
ulcerated 39–40
lysozymes 10, 16, 76

macrophages 139
malignant diseases of upper respiratory tract 221
malignant lymphoma 84–6
Hodgkin 85
non-Hodgkin 85 (table)
malignant melanoma 80
malignant schwannoma (neurogenous sarcoma) 80, 81 (fig.)
MALT lymphocytes 46
IgA secretion 47–51
mannan-binding protein deficiency 202, 220
mast cell 98, 99–102, 157
degranulation 100
mast cell-derived mediators 103–5
melanoma 76
melanotic neuroectodermal tumour of infancy (melanotic progonoma) 82
mellitin 100
membrane antigens 7d6
Meniere's disease 184–6
meningioma 78
microbicidal mechanisms 10–11
oxygen-dependent 11
oxygen-independent 10
middle ear 199–212
allografts 210–12
autologous temporalis fascia 211
tympano-ossicular 211
anatomy 199–200
immune competence 202
physiology 199–200
midline granuloma 79
monoclonal antibodies 74–5
monocytes, mannosyl-fucosyl receptors 9
mononuclear phagocytes 9–10
morphine 100
mucocoele 162
mucomycosis 42, 58 (table)
mucus abnormalities 220–1
mycetoma 58 (table)
Mycobacteria spp. 34, 41, 42
Mycobacterium avium intracellulare 40
'myoblastoma' (granular cell tumour) 89
mycoses
endemic systemic 57
opportunistic 57–8
myringitis, post-grafting 211–12

NARES syndrome 108
nasal allergy, local 157–9
nasal carcinoma 80
nasal papilloma 79
nasal polyps 151–66, 220
aetiology 162–3
allergy associated 154–5, 159
aspirin hypersensitivity associated 154
asthma associated 154
bacterial role 155–6
cystic fibrosis associated 153

histology 157
IgE levels 156, 158
immotile cilial syndrome associated 154
investigation 162
oedema 157
recurrence 164
respiratory disease associated 155 (table)
sinusitis 155–6
symptoms/signs 160–2
treatment 163–4
Young's syndrome associated 54
nasal ulcers, herpes simplex induced 41
nasopharyngeal carcinoma 82
natural killer cells 53 (fig.), 60
neurilemmoma 50
neuroectodermal tumours 89–90
neuroendocrine carcinoma 89
neurofibroma 80
plexiform 80
neurogenic tumours 80
neurogenous sarcoma (malignant schwannoma) 80, 81 (fig.)
neurone-specific enolase 76
neutral proteases 10
neutropenia 40
neutrophil 5–6
adhesion to endothelial cells 7
nexin 3
non-Hodgkin lymphoma 42
nude mice 61

OX T6+ cells 46
olfactory neuroblastoma 81–2
opsonization 9
otitis externa 64–5
otitis media, recurrent 220
otitis media with effusion 201–6
immune deficiency 201–2
immunology 203–6
management 206
mannan-binding protein deficiency 202
protein content of effusion 201
otomycosis 57
otosclerosis 206–8

paracetamol 114
Paracoccidioides brasiliensis 4
paraganglioma 90
paranasal sinus carcinoma 80
perilymph 171–2
pernicious anaemia 63d
phagocytosis 10
coiling 10
pityriasis versicolor 58
paracoccidioidomycosis (South American blastomycosis) 57, 58 (table)
plasminogen activator 10
platelet activating factor 6
plexiform neurofibroma 60
Pneumocystis carinii 34, 41
pneumonia 35
polyarteritis nodosa 190
polyendocrinopathy syndrome 63
polymerase chain reaction 22
polymorphonuclear leukocytes 60
primary system vasculitis 130 (table)
programmed cell death (apoptosis) 9
properdin 11
prostaglandins 158
D_2 158
D_4 154
pseudoallergy 100
Pseudoalleschere boydii 41

RAST test 64, 119, 120 (fig.)
relapsing polychrondritis 192
reverse transcriptase enzyme 32
rhinocerebral mucomycosis 69
rhinoscleroma (scleroma) 79
rhinosinusitis, chronic/recurrent 105
rhinoviruses 106
Rhizopus 60
Rynacrom (sodium cromoglycate) 110

S-100 protein 76, 80, 84, 89
saccharine test 4 (fig.)
Salmonella spp. 34
sarcoidosis 135–47
aetiology 137–9
age 136
bronchoalveolar lavage 138–9
clinical features 141 (table), 141–3
histology 141
immunohistology 139
immunology 137–9
incidence 136
investigations 144–6
biopsy 145–6
gallium scanning 145
Kveim test 145
radiology 146
serum angiotensin converting enzyme 145
pathogenesis 139–40
sex 136
site 136–7
treatment 146–7
schistosomes 93
schwannoma 76
scleroma (rhinoscleroma) 79
sensorineural hearing loss 180
serine proteases 12
sinusitis 220
sodium cromoglycate (Rynacrom) 110
South American blastomycosis (paracoccidioidomycosis) 57, 58 (table)
spindle cell carcinoma 88–9
sporotrichosis 58 (table)

squamous cell carcinoma 42
Staphylococcus aureus 41
stem cells 5, 9
Stevens–Johnson syndrome 40
Streptococcus pneumoniae 41
sympathetic cochleolabyrinthitis 180
sympathetic ophthalmia 180
syphilis 179
systemic lupus erythematosus 188–90

T cell 16, 18, 52
  allergic response involvement 101–2
  clones 98
  cytotoxic 52
  helper 98, 99 (fig.)
  radiosensitive 52
  receptor 17
  suppressor 52
  tonsillar 47
temporal arteritis 191
thrombocytopenia, autoimmune/drug-induced 41
tissue antigens 76
tonsillectomy 54–5
  immunological effects 55
tonsils 45–55
  antigen contact 46
  antigen fate 47
  germinal centre 47, 49 (fig.)
  immune function 52
  immunoglobulin secretion 47–52
  immunohistology 46–52
  inflammation 53–4
  M (microspore) cells 46
n-tosyl-L-arginine methyl esterase 103–4
toxoplasmosis 34
transferrin, unsaturated 59
trichophytin skin tests 63–4
tumour necrosis factor 6
  antibody 223

uveoparotid fever 143

Wegener's disease (Wegener's granulomatosis) 79, 123–31, 190–1
  aetiology 124–5
  age 123
  anti-neutrophil cytoplasmic antibodies in 125–7, 129
  clinical features 127–9
  differential diagnosis 130 (table)
  histology 127
  investigations 129
  natural history 131
  radiology 129–30
  sex 123
  site 123–4
  treatment 130–1
Western blot techniques 182

Young's syndrome 154

The Library,
Institute of Laryngology & Otology,
330/332 Gray's Inn Road,
London, W.C.1.

The Library,
Institute of Laryngology & Otology,
330/332 Gray's Inn Road,
London, W.C.1.